AYURVEDIC HEALING

2nd Revised and Enlarged Edition

By Dr. David Frawley

LOTUS
PRESS

Library of Congress Cataloging-in-Publication Data
Frawley, Dr. David
Ayurvedic Healing, 2nd Revised and Enlarged Edition
ISBN: 978-0-9149-5597-9
I. Subject   I. Title
Library of Congress Control Number 00-134620

Cover, page design and layout: Kerry Jobusch, KPComm

Published by:
Lotus Press
P.O. Box 325
Twin Lakes, Wisconsin 53181
Web: www.lotuspress.com
E-mail: lotuspress@lotuspress.com
(800) 824-6396

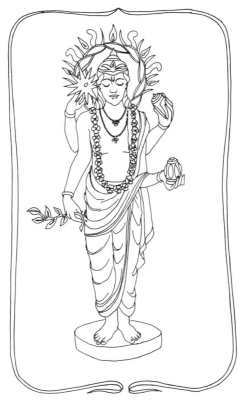

SRI DHANVANTARI NAMAH

Within all of us is the archetype of the Divine healer. This
Divine healer is the true healer in all beings, not any
particular individual or special personality. To heal ourselves we must set this Divine healer in motion within ourselves.

Dhanvantari, an incarnation of the God Vishnu, the immanent Divine consciousness, represents this Divine healer in the
tradition of Ayurveda. His statue is found at most Ayurvedic
schools and clinics. It is a reminder that however much we may
know or how skillful we become, everything still depends on
grace. This book is dedicated to the Divine healer within you.

TABLE OF CONTENTS

TABLE OF CONTENTS

FOREWORD

I started reading the manuscript of *Ayurvedic Healing* with a simple curiosity to see how a Western teacher and practitioner of Ayurveda interprets it. I ended my reading with profound admiration of his deep insight and clear grasp of the fundamental principles of this ancient Indian Science of Life.

It was a fascinating experience for me to observe how a western mind enters with perfect ease into the realms of intuitive knowledge of the East. This book is a splendid attempt to build a bridge of understanding between the eastern and western minds and their often opposite views of life. The author has succeeded in giving a reorientation of our ancient wisdom of India to suit the needs of the modern world. He has rightly pointed out that *"Ayurveda today is part of a new movement towards a global medicine that includes the best developments from all lands."* The author's effort in this and his other books will certainly help in creating a proper climate for such a synthesis.

Dr. Frawley enjoys some unique advantages as an Ayurvedic spokesman. He is primarily a Vedic scholar. Ayurveda is part of the Vedas, the oldest record of supreme knowledge and experience of mankind, the essence of which is man's harmony with nature and the individual's oneness with the universe. Ayurveda is to be viewed in such a wider perspective. Dr. Frawley has developed that vision. He is well acquainted with Sanskrit, the language of the original texts of Ayurveda. This has enabled him to reveal the deeper meanings of the terms and concepts mentioned in the texts. Literal translation of the Sanskrit terms into English almost destroys the sense of what was originally meant. Dr. Frawley is faithful to the spirit of the teachings in his translation and adaptation of them.

In addition he is a student of Yoga, the practical science of mind. He has acquired expertise in Vedic Astrology. He has studied and taught Chinese medicine. Naturally, with such a rare combination he is the most qualified person to introduce Ayurveda to the western world in light of its contemporary problems and life-style. His attempt symbolizes the world view of health.

The information given in this book covers almost all significant features of the Ayurvedic system and also of yoga. This includes constitutions of individuals, diet, health care, herbal therapies, specialized methods of relief, cure and revitalization such as oil massage, Pancha Karma, mantra, meditation, gems and, above all, the spiritual aspects of life. The main emphasis is naturally on diet and herbs with many home remedies.

Many Ayurvedic herbs have been acknowledged by modern researchers for their specific properties. It may be relevant here to quote the latest scientific study on the rejuvenation (Rasayana) concept of Ayurveda by a group of modern pharmacologists in India. They chose five plants for their experimental study. These were ashwagandha (Withania somnifera), shatavari (Asparagus racemosus), haritaki (Terminalia chebula), pippali (Piper longum) and guduchi (Tinosporia cordifolia). The study concluded that,

> Based on this experimental evidence we propose that the Rasayanas (rejuvenative substances) of Ayurveda harmonize the functions of the body by modulating the neuroendocrine-immune function. This strengthens the individual's general resistance by stimulating the immune function, a concept similar to 'prohost therapy'. The role of stress and emotion on immunological dysfunction is very well known, so is the role of stress in pathogenesis of many diseases. Therefore, it seems feasible that increased immuno-competence improves the quality of tissues so that they sustain effects of external and internal stress better.

Ayurveda Revisited
DR. SHARADINI A. DAHANUKAR AND DR. URMILA M. THATTE

Perhaps Rasayana therapy and yoga may prove to be the most effective integrated treatment for the health problems in which immune system and emotional problems are involved. Dr.

Frawley blazes a new trail in this direction by coordinating such intuitional and scientific wisdoms in his approach.

Lastly, Dr. Frawley has explained the spiritual aspect of life, a vital issue in the ultimate analysis of health and disease. Hindu spirituality believes in individualistic religion and pleads for freedom and spontaneity. This frame of mind transforms human emotions into Divine bliss and restores one's integrity of being, as the YOGA SUTRAS state (I.3.), "then the Seer returns to his own nature."

Ayurveda insists on spiritual and ethical discipline for mental health and normal development of personality. Dr. R.D. Lele, eminent physician and pioneer in Nuclear medicine in India has appreciated this aspect of Ayurveda in his book *Ayurveda and Modern Medicine.* He states, "The wisdom of Ayurveda lies in incorporating a code of conduct in the Science of Life as a means to ensuring mental health and happiness." Dr. Frawley has dealt with this aspect in all its details.

In conclusion, I must express my happiness as an Indian in welcoming Dr. Frawley to the community of distinguished commentators of Ayurveda and yoga. He deserves a place of honor in his own right.

DR. B. L. VASHTA
FEBRUARY 1989
BOMBAY, INDIA

Dr. B. L. Vastha (1919-1998) completed his educational course and obtained the qualification of Ayurvedic Visharad (proficiency in Ayurveda) in 1945. He was a professor of Ayurveda for some years, has written many books and is a regular columnist on health in leading Indian magazines. An eminent scholar of Ayurveda, Yoga and Naturopathy, he was also a consultant to major Ayurvedic companies in India.

PREFACE

*A*yurvedic Healing is oriented towards the practical treatment of disease. It is intended to serve as a handbook of Ayurvedic therapy, mainly on an herbal level. But it also explains relevant dietary, life-style and yogic methods to enhance herbal therapy, including the use of oils, aromas, colors, gems and mantras. In this way it outlines a complete and integral Ayurvedic approach to health and wellness.

On the first level of treatment, *Ayurvedic Healing* outlines general constitutional and life-style measures for health enhancement and disease prevention and gives home remedies for common diseases. We can treat many of our diseases ourselves or at least aid in their treatment. A few simple therapies as part of our daily regimen can work wonders for countering many health problems. Only when our life-style is out of harmony do severe diseases arise and professional health care becomes necessary.

On the second level of treatment, *Ayurvedic Healing* provides specialized medical knowledge and outlines specific remedies, including various herbal recommendations. However, accounts of diseases and their treatments are given here only in essence. Additional knowledge and experienced practice may be necessary to deal with severe conditions, acute symptoms or long standing complaints.

I have included relevant Western and Chinese remedies for reference purposes. They are not meant to set forth these systems in detail but to allow a point of connection with Ayurveda. Chinese and Ayurvedic systems have much in common and can be used to complement one another. Ayurveda as a global medicine encourages such dialogue and synthesis. As the United States, like Tibet in ancient times, is being influenced by both of these prime Asian healing systems, we may also eventually arrive at a similar synthesis of their approaches.

Please note that there is no final Ayurvedic way of treating a disease, which varies according to person, symptoms and environmental conditions. Ayurveda provides energetic guidelines for treatment but these must be applied flexibly on an individual basis. I have sometimes presented diseases in a slightly different way than in classical Ayurvedic texts. This has been done according to the need to revise Ayurveda according to our living situation today. Other Ayurvedic practitioners may view diseases from different angles. This reveals the expansiveness of the Ayurvedic vision that is as vast as life itself, not some inconsistency within it. Ayurveda provides guidelines for treatment but the ultimate factor is our own individual response and what actually works for us.

I would like to thank Dr. B.L. Vashta for going over the first edition. His help was invaluable in both the information and the inspiration behind the book and my Vedic work in general. Dr. Subhash Ranade was also helpful in the first edition and we have continued to work together on various Ayurvedic projects and books.

Since the first printing of this book over ten years ago (1989), Ayurveda has grown rapidly. Many new books are now available on the subject, several Ayurvedic schools have formed, and many more Ayurvedic herbs and health care products are available. Articles on Ayurveda are now common in yoga and health publications everywhere. Ayurveda is quickly emerging as a profession in the West and may soon enter the field of licensed health care throughout the world. *Ayurvedic Healing* is also meant as a textbook for students and an easy reference guide for Ayurvedic practitioners.

The present edition has been updated, reformatted and rewritten in light of such developments. I hope that these enhance the value of the book for its readers. I am especially thankful to Lotus Press for taking up not only this new edition but publishing so many of my books.

May this book contribute to the welfare of all beings!
May it stimulate the creative intelligence of all who come into contact with it!
Namaste! Reverence to the Divine Spirit within you!

DR. DAVID FRAWLEY (PANDIT VAMADEVA SHASTRI)
SANTA FE, NEW MEXICO
JANUARY 2000

INTRODUCTION

We are in the midst of a global paradigm shift in health care. At the center of this change is Ayurvedic medicine, a healing system which promotes health using natural, nontoxic substances and which recognizes the important role of the mind and emotions. A paradigm is a model used to explain how and why events happen the way they do, and as mankind's comprehension of the universe evolves, new paradigms emerge. The best example of paradigm shifts is in the field of modern physics. The classical Newtonian explanation of the world which for two hundred years was accepted as reality has now been replaced by quantum mechanics, superstrings, and field theory. In the old paradigm, every event had a definite cause and every action had an equal and opposite reaction. In the new paradigm, we describe events as possibilities instead of certainties and we recognize now the interconnectedness of all phenomena. The new explanation of the universe is, in a word, more holistic than the old reductionist view of explaining events in terms of separate, unrelated components.

In the same way, the medical paradigm shift which we are experiencing today represents a movement toward holism. The old medical paradigm viewed the human being as a machine, with separate systems, organs, and tissues; it separated mind and body into distinct categories. The new paradigm acknowledges the mutual interdependence of the physical body, mind, emotions, and the environment in creating health and disease. Neither is there separation in the emerging face of medicine between physician and patient. The new paradigm has removed the absolute authority from the doctor and has re-fashioned a model of shared responsibility between patient and physician—much in the same way that an electron forming a bond is shared between two nuclei.

Ayurvedic medicine, whose origins are shrouded in the midst of time, is a system for maintaining health and curing disease through adherence to natural rhythms and cycles. It employs a variety of natural means to bring harmony to the physiology including diet, herbs, spices, minerals, exercise, meditation, yoga, mental hygiene, sounds, smells, and mechano-procedures to eliminate toxic substances from the body. Most scholars believe that it appeared about 3500 years ago, but some insist on a much earlier date. Its wisdom grew and flourished in what is today India until the first millennium A.D. when a procession of mogul invasions from the north decimated much of what Ayurvedic physicians had come to understand about the nature of health and disease. A substantial portion of Ayurvedic wisdom was never recovered and will be lost forever, unless it is rediscovered by current and future vaidyas. Even today, references in existing publications are made to other intriguing texts which no longer exist and subjects which used to be taught in Ayurvedic medical colleges such as marma chikitsa (acupressure), suchi chikitsa (needling), medical astrology, and many other subjects remain as only fragmentary pieces of incomplete concepts or have disappeared from the curriculum entirely.

My involvement in Ayurvedic medicine dates back to my undergraduate days as a philosophy student at Brandeis University in the early 1970's. I had developed a strong interest in Vedic meditation and joined a School consisting of a diverse group of individuals who were devoted to exploring the Upanishads, Bhagavad Gita, and other ancient Vedic literature. My study and experience with that group provided me with the knowledge base and deep motivation to pursue a career using the inherent power of consciousness to bring health and happiness to people. The only problem was I didn't exactly know what kind of career that would be and I didn't see any listings in the New York Times classified section for "Consciousness Technician". At that time I had no interest in becoming a physician. Little did I know that forces were in play which would soon shape my life forever.

After graduating from college, I was told about a very inexpensive way to get to India and made arrangements with Benaras Hindu University in Varanasi, India to enroll as a graduate student in Sanskrit and Vedic Studies. Shortly after arriving in Varanasi I met an elderly woman at a reception for new students and began an innocent conversation. She began to describe for me an ancient system of healing which could cure serious medical conditions by changing their lifestyle, fine-tuning their diet, using natural herbal medicines, and recruiting the inherent healing capacity of the mind. It was that last part that caught my attention, and I proceeded to follow her around the reception pressing her for more information. Finally, she offered me the phone number of her nephew who could explain more. Her nephew turned out to be the Dean of one of the then 104 Ayurvedic medical colleges. When I met him it was like meeting my destiny, and before long I managed to become enrolled in classes as a student of Ayurvedic medicine. After completing my basic Ayurvedic training, I eventually earned my fellowship and finally a Ph.D. in Ayurveda. Subsequently, I returned to the United States and attended medical school and earned a conventional M.D. degree with advanced training in general internal medicine.

Today, in my medical practice at The National Institute Of Ayurvedic Medicine (NIAM), I generally do not use toxic pharmaceutical drugs, irritating allopathic medicines, vaccines, or serums. As a fully trained physician and vaidya who has been engaged in the practice of classical Ayurvedic medicine for the past eighteen years, I have come to the following conclusion: There is truly only one healing force in the universe and that is Nature herself. Neither the synthetic medicines of the modern allopath nor the botanical medicines of the herbalist can effect healing. Only the inherent and universal forces of Nature can do that and it is the physician's role to facilitate and promote this process with the aid of natural, non-harmful physical, mental, and spiritual therapies.

When I read the first edition of Dr. David Frawley's *Ayurvedic Healing* in 1989 I was gratified to find in one volume a comprehensive description of the principles of Ayurvedic diagnosis and treatments in clear and concise language. The current 2nd Revised Edition reflects some of the more important findings in the burgeoning field of Ayurvedic medicine. For example, mention is made of the use of the l-dopa-containing plant Mucuna pruriens (Kapikacchu) as well as the well-documented cholesterol-reducing effects of Commiphora mukul (Guggulu). Also the added sections on classical and modern Ayurvedic preparations will no doubt be of great interest to students.

This book offers both the physician and layperson practical guidance through the vast subject of Ayurveda. Reading through it again reminded me of the deep emotional response I had when I first began translating the Charaka Samhita and hearing its wisdom in its original voice for the first time. This book is not merely a source of information. Dr. Frawley, in the tradition of all who truly comprehend the message of Ayurveda, is a teacher, a motivator, a scholar, and a voice for self-empowerment. I am deeply honored to have Dr. David Frawley not only as a colleague, but as a truly valued friend. In concluding, let me lead you into the text that follows on an optimistic and patently realistic note as you turn the page. Almost all disease is curable. We each just have to discover our own unique path to balance and surrender to the Supreme.

Om Shanti

SCOTT GERSON, M.D.
EXECUTIVE DIRECTOR, BASIC AND CLINICAL RESEARCH
MEDICAL DIRECTOR, CLINICAL SERVICES
THE NATIONAL INSTITUTE OF AYURVEDIC MEDICINE

Part I
RIGHT LIVING THROUGH AYURVEDA

Ayurveda is the science that indicates the appropriate and inappropriate, happy or sorrowful conditions of living, what is auspicious or inauspicious for longevity, as well as the measure of life itself.

CHARAKA SAMHITA I. 41

Vata, Pitta and Kapha, the group of the three doshas, in their natural and disturbed states, give life to the body and also destroy it.

ASHTANGA HRIDAYA I.6

I:1
THE THREE DOSHAS
The Dynamics of the Life–Force

*A*yurveda, the science of life, is the natural healing system of India, its traditional medicine going back to ancient times. The same great Vedic seers and sages that produced India's original systems of yoga and meditation established Ayurveda as well.

Ayurveda originated as part of *Vedic Science*, an integral spiritual science that provides a comprehensive understanding of the entire universe of matter, mind and consciousness. Vedic Science includes yoga, meditation, mantra and astrology, and sets forth Ayurveda as its special branch for healing both body and mind. On this broad and profound background, Ayurveda includes herbal medicine, dietetics, bodywork, surgery, psychology and spirituality.

Ayurveda is the healing gift to us from the ancient enlightened Vedic culture. According to astronomical records in ancient Vedic texts, the Vedic system, including Ayurveda, was in practice before 4000 BC, when the vernal equinox occurred in the stars of Gemini and the now dry Sarasvati river was the greatest river in India. Ayurveda reflects healing wisdom of this ancient Sarasvati culture that was one of the great cradles of world civilization.

Ayurveda has gone through several stages of development in its long history. It spread east along with Indian culture into Indonesia and Indochina, and to the west to the Greeks, who developed a similar form of natural medicine. Buddhists added many new insights to Ayurveda and took it along with their religion to many different lands. Ayurveda became the basis of the healing traditions of Tibet, Sri Lanka, and Burma and also influenced Chinese medicine. Many great Buddhist sages, like Nagarjuna, perhaps the most important figure in the Buddhist tradition after the Buddha, were Ayurvedic doctors and authors. Ayurveda therefore is a rich tradition, adaptable to many different times, cultures and climates.

Today Ayurveda, in yet another stage of development, is reaching out to the western world and addressing modern conditions. Ayurveda is part of a new movement towards a global medicine that includes the best in the medicines of all lands. A new natural planetary medicine is emerging, largely through an examination of traditional medicines of native peoples throughout the world.

Ayurveda is probably the best place of synthesis for such a global medicine. It contains perhaps the broadest number of healing modalities. It retains much of the language of alchemy, which was a global medical and spiritual tradition in ancient times. The medicine of India has much in common with older Chinese and European traditions, and can serve as a point of integration between them. The medicine necessary to heal the planet and usher in a new age of world unity is already contained in this, perhaps the oldest of all healing systems.

THE THREE GREAT COSMIC FORCES

According to the ancient Vedic seers, there are three basic forces in existence. First is a principle of energy that gives movement, velocity, direction, animation and motivation. Life is nothing but a play of forces, continually changing and interacting. As modern science confirms, matter is energy and what seems solid is a static appearance of innumerable, subtle moving currents.

This energy of life is called *Prana*, meaning the primal breath or life-force. All energy follows a movement of inhalation and exhalation like the breath, expanding and contracting in a perpetual ebb and flow. All material energy is a development of the power of life itself. Energy is life and even inanimate energy holds a secret life-force. The ancient seers perceived the energy of the universe as the manifestation of Prana, ever seeking greater awareness, freedom and creative unfoldment.

Hidden in all energy is the working of a conscious will. Energy is will in action in the outer world. Behind will is sentience or consciousness as the power of determination. Prana is also the Purusha; energy is also the primal spirit. Life itself is being, the consciousness principle. There is an inner working of intelligence behind the movement of energy in the world. This natural or organic intelligence is conscious and sure in its plan and method; not by choice or intention but intuitively and spontaneously as a movement of pure beauty and harmony. Its glory is manifest in all nature, from the flowers to the stars.

The second of the triad of primal forces is a principle of light or radiance. Energy is light, *Jyoti*. Energy, as it moves, undergoes transformation, and gives off light and heat. Energy is an electrical force, which like lightning has its own luminosity. There is a natural warmth to all life and a natural light behind all energy. Behind all life is a principle of perception, a transparency that manifests as intelligence and consciousness. In all chemical reactions is concealed the power of light as the ability of consciousness to transform itself. Within the first spark is latent the light of the highest awareness. This principle of light goes along with life and guides its function.

The third of these forces is a principle of cohesion that allows for consistency and the development of form. Behind all manifestation is a common unity. There is an interlinking of forces into a single rhythm. There is an affinity of forces that links them together in one great harmony. This cohesiveness is not only a chemical property; it also reveals a conscious intent. It manifests the power of love, *Prema*. Love is the real force that holds all things together. Love unfolds the manifestation and ensures its continuity, sustaining all creatures in their life and awareness.

These three principles are one—life is light, which is also love. The energetic principle (life) possesses a radiance (light), which in turn has a bonding power (love). We must ever seek greater life, light and love because this is the nature of the universe itself.

In the *Vedas*, the great god Indra, the dragon slayer and wielder of the vajra (thunderbolt), symbolizes the power of life that can overcome all obstacles. The spirit of light is Agni, the god of fire, the divinity of vision and of sacrifice who upholds all

8

transformations. The spirit of love is Soma, the nectar of immortality that gives nourishment and delight to all. Hidden in cryptic Vedic mantras is the primal code of cosmic law, the key to the universal force on all its levels. Through these Vedic mantras we can learn to balance and control the forces of life. This not only creates health but also gives the basis for rejuvenation of the mind and the transformation of consciousness.

These three forces of life, light and love relate to the three great elements of air, fire and water. According to ancient mythology, in the beginning Heaven and Earth were one. There was no space between them for creatures to live. Then, by the will of the Creator, the gods came into being and separated Heaven and Earth, drawing apart the two firmaments. In the space between Heaven and Earth, the gods set in motion the life-force to give room for creatures to grow. This life-force became the atmosphere in which the elements of air, fire and water as wind, sun and rain provide for the development of life.

THE THREE DOSHAS

Ayurveda recognizes three primary life-forces in the body, or three biological humors called *Vata, Pitta* and *Kapha*, which correspond to the elements of air, fire and water. As the active or mobile elements, they determine the life processes of growth and decay.

The Ayurvedic term for humor is *dosha*, meaning that which darkens, spoils or causes things to decay. When out of balance, the doshas are the causative forces behind the disease process.

VATA is the biological air humor, also translated as wind. It means 'that which moves things'. Vata dosha is the motivating force behind the other two doshas, which are 'lame', incapable of movement without it. It governs sensory and mental balance and orientation, and promotes mental adaptability and comprehension.

PITTA is the biological fire humor, also translated as bile. Its meaning is 'that which digests things'. Pitta dosha is respon-

9

sible for all chemical and metabolic transformations in the body. It also governs our mental digestion, our capacity to perceive reality and understand things as they are.

KAPHA is the biological water humor, also translated as phlegm. It means 'that which holds things together.' Kapha dosha provides substance and gives support, and makes up the bulk of our bodily tissues. It also provides our emotional support in life, and relates to positive emotional traits like love, compassion, modesty, patience and forgiveness.

Each dosha exists in a second element that serves as the medium for its manifestation, acting as its container.

VATA, air, is contained in ether. It resides in the empty spaces in the body and fills up the subtle channels.

PITTA, fire, exists in the body as water or oil. It exists mainly in an acid form, as fire cannot exist directly in the body without destroying it.

KAPHA, water, exists in the medium of earth, which contains it. Our physical composition is mainly water contained within the boundaries of our skin and mucus membranes (earth).

QUALITIES OF THE DOSHAS

Each dosha has its primary qualities according to which we recognize them. An excess or deficiency of these qualities indicates an excess or deficiency of the particular dosha. This, in turn, brings about various pathological changes. According to Vagbhatta, one of the great Ayurvedic commentators:

Vata is dry, light, cold, rough, subtle and agitated in qualities.
Pitta is a little oily, is sharp, hot, light, unpleasant in odor, mobile and liquid.
Kapha is wet, cold, heavy, dull, sticky, soft and firm.
ASHTANGA HRIDAYA I. 11-12

Each dosha has one major quality of its own and shares another quality with one of the other two doshas. However, in terms of shared qualities there is a difference. Vata as air is lighter than Pitta as fire. Vata as air is colder than Kapha as water. Kapha as water is moister than Pitta, which has an oily quality (blood and acids).

PRIME ATTRIBUTES OF THE DOSHAS

VATA	Dry	Cold	Light
PITTA	Hot	Light	Moist
KAPHA	Heavy	Cold	Moist

ACTIONS OF THE DOSHAS

Their actions, on both the body and the mind, are described as follows:

> The root of the doshas, tissues and waste materials of the body is Vata. In its natural state it sustains effort, exhalation, inhalation, movement and the discharge of impulses, the equilibrium of the tissues, and the coordination of the senses.
>
> Pitta governs digestion, heat, visual perception, hunger, thirst, luster, complexion, understanding, intelligence, courage and softness of the body.
>
> Kapha gives stability, lubrication, holding together of the joints and such qualities as patience.
>
> ASHTANGA HRIDAYA XI. 1-3

VATA is the most important or primary of the three biological humors. It governs the other two and is responsible for all physical processes in general. For this reason, disturbances in Vata have more severe implications than the other two doshas, affecting the mind as well as the entire physical body. The quality of our life, through our care of the life-force, is the primary factor in both health and disease.

PITTA governs all aspects and levels of light and warmth in the body and mind. KAPHA is the material substratum and

11

support of the other two doshas and also gives stability to our emotional nature.

AGGRAVATED STATES OF THE DOSHAS

When aggravated, the doshas give rise to various symptoms and various diseases.

Vata in excess causes emaciation, debility, liking of warmth, tremors, distention and constipation, as well as insomnia, sensory disorientation, incoherent speech, dizziness, confusion and depression.

Pitta in excess causes yellow color of stool, urine, eyes and skin, as well as hunger, thirst, burning sensation and difficulty sleeping.

Kapha causes depression of the digestive fire, nausea, lethargy, heaviness, white color, chills, looseness of the limbs, cough, difficult breathing and excessive sleeping.

ASHTANGA HRIDAYA XI. 6-8

HIGH VATA (high air) results in the prana and the mind losing their connection with the body, causing decay and loss of coordination. There is hyperactivity at the expense of the vital fluids and the physical body begins to waste away.

HIGH PITTA (high fire) results in the accumulation of internal heat or fever, with inflammation and infections. We literally begin to burn ourselves up.

HIGH KAPHA (high water) results in the accumulation of weight and gravity in the body, which inhibits normal function and causes hypoactivity through excess tissue accumulation.

SITES OF THE DOSHAS

Each dosha has its respective site in the body.

Vata (air) is located in the colon, thighs, hips, ears, bones and organ of touch. Its primary site is the colon.

Pitta (fire) is located in the small intestine, stomach, sweat,

12

sebaceous glands, blood, lymph and the organ of vision. Its primary site is the small intestine.

Kapha (water) is located in the chest, throat, head, pancreas, sides, stomach, lymph, fat, nose and tongue. Its primary site is the stomach.

ASHTANGA HRIDAYA XII. 1-3

The doshas accumulate at these primary sites in the digestive system, giving rise to the disease process. Treating them at these locations by their respective methods, we can cut the disease process off at the root.

VATA (air) is produced from below, as gas from the colon.
PITTA (fire) is produced in the middle as bile and acids from the liver and small intestine.
KAPHA (water) is produced above as phlegm in the lungs and stomach.

The Five Forms of Vata

The five forms of Vata are 1. *Prana*, 2. *Udana*, 3. *Vyana*, 4. *Samana*, and 5. *Apana*. These words are formed by adding various suffixes to the root 'an', which means to breathe or to energize. They are also called *Vayus* or airs.

1. PRANA (pra-ana) means the forward or primary air or nervous force. Pervading the head and centered in the brain, it moves downward to the chest and throat, governing inhalation and swallowing, as well as sneezing, spitting and belching. It governs the senses, mind, heart and consciousness. It is our portion of the cosmic life energy and directs all the other Vatas in the body. It determines our inspiration or positive spirit in life and connects us with our inner Self. The term 'Prana' is also used in a broader sense to indicate Vata in general, as all Vatas derive from it.

2. UDANA (ud-ana) means the upward moving air or nervous force. Located in the chest and centered in the throat, it governs exhalation and speech. It is also responsible for memory, strength, will and effort.

13

Udana determines our aspiration in life. At death it rises up from the body and directs us towards various subtle worlds according to the power of our will and the karma that move through it. When fully developed it gives us the power to transcend the outer world, as well as various psychic powers. The practice of Yoga is involved primarily with developing Udana.

3. VYANA (vi-ana) means the diffusive or pervasive air. It is centered in the heart and distributed throughout the entire body. It governs the circulatory system and, through it, the movement of the joints and muscles and the discharge of impulses and secretions.

4. SAMANA (sama-ana) means the equalizing air. It is centered in the small intestine and is the nervous force behind the digestive system. Samana not only digests our food but also maintains balance and equilibrium in all the bodily systems.

5. APANA (apa-ana) means the downward moving air or the air that moves away. It is centered in the colon and governs all downward moving impulses of elimination, urination, menstruation, parturition and sexual activity.

As Udana, the ascending air, carries our life-force upwards and brings about the evolution or liberation of consciousness, Apana, the descending air, carries it down and brings about the devolution or limitation of consciousness. Apana supports and controls all the other forms of Vata, and derangements of it are the basis of most Vata disorders. As a downward moving force, when aggravated it causes decay and disintegration. Therefore, the treatment of Apana is the first consideration in the treatment of Vata.

The Five Forms of Pitta

The five forms of Pitta are 1. *Sadhaka*, 2. *Alochaka*, 3. *Bhrajaka*, 4. *Pachaka*, and 5. *Ranjaka*.

1. SADHAKA PITTA is the fire that determines what is truth or reality. It is located in the brain and the heart and allows us to accomplish the goals of the intellect, intelligence or ego. These

14

include worldly goals of pleasure, wealth and prestige and the spiritual goal of liberation. It governs our mental energy, mental digestion (the digestion of ideas or beliefs) and our power of discrimination. Its development is emphasized in Yoga, particularly the Yoga of Knowledge.

2. ALOCHAKA PITTA is the fire that governs visual perception. It is located in the eyes and is responsible for the reception and digestion of light from the external world. It aids in the acuity of the other senses as well.

3. BHRAJAKA PITTA is the fire that governs luster or complexion. It is located in the skin and maintains the complexion and color of skin. When aggravated, for example, it causes skin rashes or discolorations. It governs the digestion of warmth or heat, which we experience through the skin.

4. PACHAKA PITTA is the fire that digests things. It is located in the small intestine and governs the power of digestion. It is the basis and support of the other forms of Pitta, and is the first consideration in the treatment of Pitta, as our primary source of heat is the digestive fire.

5. RANJAKA PITTA is the fire that imparts color. It is located in the liver, spleen, stomach and small intestine, and gives color to the blood, bile and stool. It primarily resides in the blood and is involved in most liver disorders.

The Five Forms of Kapha

The five forms of Kapha are 1. *Tarpaka*, 2. *Bodhaka*, 3. *Avalambaka*, 4. *Kledaka*, and 5. *Sleshaka*.

1. TARPAKA KAPHA is the form of water that gives contentment. It is located in the brain, as the cerebro-spinal fluid, and in the heart. It governs emotional calm, stability and happiness, as well as memory. The practice of Yoga also increases the mental form of Kapha as contentment and bliss (Ananda).

2. BODHAKA KAPHA is the form of water that gives perception. It is located in the mouth and tongue as the saliva that

allows us to taste our food. Like Kledaka, it is also part of the first stage of digestion. It also helps lubricate the other sensory openings in the head.

3. AVALAMBAKA KAPHA is the form of water that gives support. It is located in the heart and lungs. It is the storehouse of Kapha (phlegm) and upon it depend the actions of the other Kaphas in the body. It is not simply the phlegm produced by the lungs, as that is an excess of Kapha generally. It corresponds to the basic plasma of the body, its primary watery constituent, which is distributed by lung and heart action.

4. KLEDAKA KAPHA is the form of water that moistens. It is located in the stomach, as the secretions of the mucous lining. It is responsible for the liquefaction of food and for the first stage of digestion.

5. SLESHAKA KAPHA is the form of water that gives lubrication. It is located in the joints as the synovial fluid and is responsible for holding them together.

THE SEVEN TISSUES

According to Ayurveda the human body is composed of seven *Dhatus* or tissue layers. These form concentric circles from the gross to the subtle.

1.Rasa Dhatu	Plasma, also called skin
2.Rakta Dhatu	Blood, particularly the hemoglobin portion
3.Mamsa Dhatu	Muscle tissue
4.Meda Dhatu	Fat or adipose tissue
5.Asthi Dhatu	Bone tissue
6.Majja Dhatu	Marrow and nerve tissue
7.Shukra Dhatu	Reproductive tissue

Kapha is responsible for all the tissues generally as earth and water form the basic substance of the body. It is specifically responsible for five—plasma, muscle, fat, marrow and reproductive. Pitta creates the blood, which holds the body heat, and Vata creates bone, whose porosity holds air.

Diseases of the doshas are usually reflected in the tissues that they govern. Pitta diseases usually involve the blood. Vata diseases usually involve the bone. Kapha diseases usually reflect the other tissues, particularly the plasma. However, any of the doshas can enter into any of the tissues and cause various diseases. Diseases are classified not only according to the doshas but also according to which tissues the doshas have entered. For example, most forms of arthritis consist of Vata (dryness and wind) invading the bones (asthi dhatu) called Vata in the bones (asthi gata Vata).

BODILY SYSTEMS

The human body is composed of innumerable channels that supply the various tissues of the body. The Sanskrit word for such channels is *srotas*, with the plural being *srotamsi*. Health consists of the proper flow through these channels. Disease is improper flow, which may be excessive, deficient, blockage, or flow out of the proper channel altogether. The excess doshas move into the channels causing these various wrong flows. The channels are similar to the different physiological systems of Western medicine but also contain subtler energy fields such as the meridian system of Chinese medicine. A complex symptomology of channel system-disorders exists in Ayurveda. Diseases are classified according to the systems they involve. Examination of the channels by various diagnostic measures is one of the main tools for determining the nature and power of disease.

Three channels connect with the outside environment and bring nourishment into the body in the form of breath, food and water. Seven channels supply the seven tissues of the body.

Three additional channels connect to the outside world and allow for the elimination of substances from the body. The waste product of breath is sweat, that of food is feces, and that of water is urine. These three waste materials are called the three Malas and they can also be damaged or obstructed by excess accumulations of the doshas.

The mind exists as a special system. It connects to the nervous system (majjavaha srotas) and the reproductive system (shukra-vaha srotas). The movement of energy in all the channels depends upon the stimulus that arises from the mind.

THE CHANNEL SYSTEMS (SROTAMSI)

PRANAVAHA SROTAS	Channels that carry Prana, the breath or life-force, primarily the respiratory system and circulatory system	Originates in the heart and the g.i. tract, primarily the colon
ANNAVAHA SROTAS	Channels that carry food, the digestive system	Originates in the stomach and left side of the body
AMBHUVAHA SROTAS	Channels that carry water or regulate water metabolism	Originates in the palate and pancreas
RASAVAHA SROTAS	Channels that carry plasma (rasa), the lymphatic system	Originates in heart and blood vessels
RAKTAVAHA SROTAS	Channels that carry blood (rakta), circulatory system	Originates in the liver and spleen
MAMSAVAHA SROTAS	Channels that supply muscles (mamsa), the muscular system.	Originates in the ligaments and skin
MEDAVAHA SROTAS	Channels that supply fat or adipose tissue (medas), the adipose system	Originates in the kidneys and omentum
ASTHIVAHA SROTAS	Channels that supply the bones (asthi), the skeletal system	Originates in adipose tissue and the hips
MAJJAVAHA SROTAS	Channels that supply the marrow and nerve tissue (majja), mainly the nervous system	Originates in the bones and joints
SHUKRAVAHA SROTAS	Channels that supply the reproductive tissue (shukra), the reproductive system	Originates in the testes or the uterus
SVEDAVAHA SROTAS	Channels that carry sweat (sveda), the sebaceous system	Originates in adipose tissue and the hair follicles

I.1 The Three Doshas

PURISHAVAHA SROTAS	Channels that carry feces (purisha), the excretory system	Originates in the colon and rectum
MUTRAVAHA SROTAS	Channels that carry urine (mutra), the urinary system	Originates in the bladder and kidneys
MANOVAHA SROTAS	Channels that carry thought, the mental system	Originates in the heart

Two special systems exist within the female as subsystems of the reproductive system.

ARTAVAVAHA SROTAS	Channels that carry the menstrual fluid (artava)
STANYAVAHA SROTAS	Channels that carry the breast milk, or the lactation system, treated as the subsystem of the menstrual system

I.2
THE SIX TASTES
The Energetics of Healing Substances

Ayurvedic diagnosis of disease is based on the three biological humors; treatment is according to the six tastes.
These apply not only to herbs but also to foods and minerals. They are based on the actual taste of the substance when
taken in the mouth and reveal an intricate dynamic of herbal
properties. These tastes are called rasas in Sanskrit, meaning
flavors or essences. They indicate the main impact of foods on
our senses.

The six tastes are *sweet, salty, sour, pungent, bitter* and
astringent. Each taste is made up of two of the five elements. The
six tastes are also classified as heating or cooling in energy. By
such qualities the tastes possess various therapeutic properties and
increase or decrease the doshas.

THE SIX TASTES

Taste	Found In	Energy	Elements	Doshas
SWEET	Sugars and starches	Cold	Earth and water	PV- K+
SALTY	Table salt or seaweed	Hot	Water and fire	KP+ V-
SOUR	Fermented food or acid fruit	Hot	Earth and fire	PK+ V-
PUNGENT	Hot spices like cayenne or ginger	Hot	Fire and air	K- PV+
BITTER	Bitter herbs like or goldenseal or gentian	Cold	Air and ether	KP- V+
ASTRINGENT	Herbs containing tannins like alum or witch hazel	Cold	Earth and air	PK- V+

Hottest		to		Coldest	
Pungent	Sour	Salty	Sweet	Astringent	Bitter

The six tastes have other important properties as heavy (creating weight) or light (weight-reducing), as well as moistening and drying. These qualities exist to different degrees as well.

Heaviest		to		Lightest	
Sweet	Salty	Astringent	Sour	Pungent	Bitter

Wettest		to		Driest	
Sweet	Salty	Sour	Astringent	Bitter	Pungent

The Six Tastes and Three Doshas

Three tastes increase each of the doshas and three decrease them. These are general rules. Many combinations and variations exist.

VATA (air and ether) is most increased by bitter taste, which most resembles it, then by astringent and pungent, which also contain the air element. It is most decreased by salty taste, then sour and sweet, which dominate in earth and water elements.

PITTA (fire and water) is most increased by sour taste, then pungent and salty, which are all heating. It is most decreased by bitter taste, then astringent and sweet, which are all cooling.

KAPHA (water and earth) is most increased by sweet taste, then salty and sour, which all abound in earth and water. It is most decreased by pungent taste, then bitter and astringent, which dominate in the air element.

TASTES AND DOSHAS

Dosha	Decreases	Increases
VATA	Sweet, sour, salty	Bitter, astringent, pungent
PITTA	Bitter, astringent, sweet	Pungent, sour, salty
KAPHA	Pungent, bitter, astringent	Sweet, salty, sour

Actions of the Tastes

Each taste has its specific therapeutic actions.

SWEET TASTE is building and strengthening to all body tissues. It harmonizes the mind and promotes a sense of contentment. It is demulcent (soothing to the mucus membranes), expectorant and mildly laxative. It counters burning sensations.

SALTY TASTE is softening, laxative and sedative. In small amounts it stimulates digestion, in moderate amounts it is purgative, and in very large amounts it causes vomiting.

SOUR TASTE is stimulant, carminative (dispels gas), nourishing and thirst relieving. It increases all tissues but the reproductive tissue, which it decreases.

PUNGENT TASTE is stimulant, carminative, and diaphoretic (promotes sweating). It improves metabolism and promotes all organic functions. It promotes heat and digestion and counters cold sensations.

BITTER TASTE is alterative (blood purifying), cleansing and detoxifying. It reduces all bodily tissues and increases lightness in the mind.

ASTRINGENT TASTE stops bleeding and other excess discharges (such as excess sweating or diarrhea) and promotes healing of the skin and mucus membranes.

AMOUNTS OF THE SIX TASTES NEEDED

Everyone needs a certain amount of each of the six tastes. The relative proportion differs according to the constitution or dosha of the individual. Too much of any taste can become harmful to any constitutional type, as can too little.

SWEET taste is needed in significant amounts for all doshas, as food is predominately sweet in taste. More is required for Pitta types, moderate for Vata, less for Kapha. It is necessary for maintaining tissue growth and development in all three doshas.

SALTY taste is needed in small amounts for all doshas, as it is strong in low concentrations. More is needed for Vata, moderate amounts for Pitta, less for Kapha. It is necessary for maintaining mineral balance and holding water.

SOUR taste is required in moderation for each dosha. More is needed for Vata, moderate amounts for Kapha, less for Pitta. It is necessary for maintaining acidity and countering thirst.

PUNGENT taste is needed in moderation for each dosha; more for Kapha, moderate amounts for Vata, less for Pitta. It is necessary for maintaining metabolism, improving appetite and facilitating digestion.

BITTER taste is needed in small quantities for each dosha; more for (Pitta) fire, moderate amounts for Kapha, less for Vata. It is necessary for detoxification and weight reduction, but also is depleting.

ASTRINGENT taste is needed in moderate amounts for each dosha, as a secondary food taste; more for Pitta, moderate amounts for Kapha, less for Vata. It is necessary for maintaining firmness of tissues and preventing excess discharges.

NUTRITIVE AND MEDICINAL VALUES OF THE TASTES

In terms of nutrition, sweet taste is most important generally for everyone because it possesses the highest nutritive value of all the tastes. Sour taste is moderately nutritive but can deplete the reproductive secretions that do not function well in an acid environment. Astringent taste has some nutritive properties, particularly for minerals; most green vegetables are regarded as astringent. Salty taste provides minerals and helps hold water but is not very nutritive in itself. Pungent taste has slight nutritive properties in various spicy vegetables, like onions, but is generally depleting. Bitter taste is the least nutritive, or tasty, and is a sign that vegetables are too old to eat.

In terms of medicinal properties, bitter and astringent tastes are the most commonly used. They treat severe fevers, infections and traumatic injuries that are the most immediate threat to life. Pungent is also very useful for stimulating our defensive reactions and breaking stagnation. These three tastes are the most common in plants, have the most immediate action, and are best for destroying pathogens. Sour, salty and sweet tastes have less medicinal value, and are more for long-term tonification.

AGGRAVATION OF DOSHAS BY THE SIX TASTES
Excess of the Tastes

Each taste in excess causes certain damage, first to the doshas that it aggravates then even to the doshas it alleviates (if in too large amounts). That is because our need for the different tastes is always within certain limits. We need more or less depending upon our constitution but too much or too little can cause trouble for anyone. We all need all of the six tastes but in different amounts and proportions.

For example, too much salt will initially aggravate Kapha by holding more water in the tissues. An excess, however, can even aggravate Vata, which it alleviates in normal amounts. This causes thirst, wrinkling of the skin and falling out of the hair.

Each taste differs in its power to aggravate the doshas. Bitter, pungent and salty tastes can have strong effects even in small amounts. Sour and astringent tastes require moderate amounts for their effects to manifest. Sweet taste requires the largest amount for its effects to come through.

The pure forms of each taste are more likely to aggravate the doshas. The complex forms are less likely to aggravate, as they require assimilation. They do not have so one-sided an action, nor are they as likely to disturb the immune system.

The pure forms of the six tastes are sugar (not only white sugar but any pure sugar), salt, hot spices, alcohol, pure astringents, and pure bitters. The first two are those most commonly taken in our culture. They are most responsible for the aggravation of the doshas, even those they usually alleviate.

25

PURE AND COMPLEX FORMS OF THE SIX TASTES

1. SWEET	Refined Sugar	Complex carbohydrates
2. SALTY	Table salt	Seaweed
3. PUNGENT	Hot peppers (cayenne)	Mild spices (cardamom, fennel)
4. SOUR	Alcohol	Sour food (yogurt, sour fruit)
5. BITTER	Pure bitters(goldenseal)	Mild bitters (aloe gel)
6. ASTRINGENT	Pure astringents (strong tannins)	Mild astringents (alfalfa, red raspberry)

Pure forms of the six tastes are more likely to aggravate the doshas when taken regularly, as in food or with food. Yet they also can possess strong medicinal properties for temporary conditions. Pure forms of the six tastes should be used with care or used therapeutically.

TASTES AND ORGANS
Each taste relates to certain organs and in excess damages.
- Sweet taste damages the spleen and pancreas
- Salty taste damages the kidneys
- Pungent taste damages and dries the lungs
- Sour taste damages the liver
- Bitter taste damages the heart
- Astringent taste damages the colon

However, too much of any taste, as we have seen, can damage the body as a whole. Sweet taste in excess builds up mucus and toxins; salty taste causes looseness; sour creates acidity; pungent causes burning and inflammation; bitter increases cold; and astringent causes contractions and blockages.

TASTES AND EMOTIONS
The six tastes are also the "flavors" of our various emotions. These can affect us in the same way as diet and herbs, and can increase the therapeutic or disease-causing effects of the tastes that correspond to them.

TASTES AND EMOTIONS

Hot Emotions	Anger, hatred, envy
Cold Emotions	Fear, grief, sorrow
Sweet—love	Salty—greed
Sour—envy	Pungent—hatred
Bitter—grief	Astringent—fear

Emotions have the same effect as food or herbs of the same energetic quality. Love nourishes us like the sweet taste but causes attachment. Bitter taste depletes us like grief. Astringent taste makes us contract like fear. Psychological factors, generally speaking, will outweigh physical factors. Anger can damage the liver as much as alcoholism. So herbs and diet are not enough if the taste of the mind has not changed.

Deficiency of the Tastes

A lack of each taste can also aggravate doshas, first those they alleviate, then if the lack is greater even those they aggravate. For example, too little sugar will first aggravate Vata and Pitta. But if the deficiency is to the point of malnutrition, it can even weaken a person with a Kapha constitution.

Usually in our culture bitter taste is used too little, then pungent and astringent. The lack of bitter taste in our diet causes us to accumulate toxins. The lack of spices keeps our digestive fire low. Hence, most of us can use more of these tastes. We usually have sweet and salty in excess, even if we are Vata types.

RELATIONSHIPS BETWEEN THE TASTES

These six tastes can be combined for various therapeutic actions. For example, pungent and bitter combine well for their drying and cleansing action (like the Western herbal combination of cayenne and goldenseal). Pungent, sour and salty combine well for their mutual action of stimulating digestion. Generally, tastes will further the action which they share in common, while reducing those they do not.

Some tastes balance or complement each other. For example, pungent taste aids in the digestion of sweet taste, as in the use of spices with sugars. Sweet taste helps alleviate the burning sensation of pungent taste, as in taking sugar with cloves. Pungent taste promotes sweating, while astringent stops it. Bitter taste counters the craving for sweet.

Six Tastes Pills

In India various herbal formulas are made combining all six tastes. Such pills are given, particularly to children, to insure that adequate amounts of all six tastes are received daily. These pills help educate our sense of taste and harmonize its function. A simple Ayurvedic version of the six tastes pill is made with:

SIX TASTES PILL NO. 1
Shatavari (sweet), amalaki (sour), rock salt, ginger (pungent), barberry (bitter), haritaki (astringent) in equal parts.
Dosage is 1/2 – 1 gram before meals or about 1/4 teaspoon.

We can modify this formula according to the three doshas. Vata types can take twice the amount proportionally of the sweet, sour and salty herbs, concentrating on the tastes that reduce it. Kapha can take twice the amount of the pungent, bitter and astringent herbs. Pitta can take twice the amount of the sweet, bitter and astringent. A good Western version can be made with:

SIX TASTES PILL NO. 2
Licorice (sweet), hawthorne berries (sour), sea salt, ginger (pungent), barberry (bitter) and red raspberry (astringent) in equal parts.
Dosage is 1/2 – 1 gram before meals or about 1/4 teaspoon.

These six taste pills are useful generally for strengthening digestion and improving absorption, for chronic digestive system disorders and as an intestinal corrective. They are particularly good for those with chronic low appetite and anorexia.

I.3
CONSTITUTIONAL EXAMINATION:
How to Determine Your Unique Mind–Body Type

Each one of us possesses all three doshas in our physical makeup. Kapha makes up our flesh and our secretions, the water in our body. Pitta gives us our warmth and capacity to transform substances in the body, our fire. Vata governs our energies and activities, giving us our air. We each replicate the great cosmic forces and through them our own physiology is part of the cosmic dance. However, the proportion of the doshas varies according to the individual. One dosha will usually predominate and place its mark upon us in terms of our appearance and disposition.

From the Ayurvedic perspective, the first step in treatment is to ascertain the natural constitution of the individual according to the predominant dosha as Vata, Pitta, or Kapha. The predominant dosha, in turn, reflects the main energies and qualities within the individual and their tendencies to either health or disease.

This constitutional approach is the essence of Ayurveda. It gives Ayurveda broad powers for disease prevention, health maintenance and longevity enhancement, as well as for the treatment of disease. Through it, we can prescribe a life plan for each individual to optimize our human and creative potential. It also allows us to apply Ayurveda along non-medical lines as a form of health education and life-style counseling.

Some individuals are strongly predominant in one dosha or another. These we might call *pure Vata* (pure air), *pure Pitta* (pure fire) and *pure Kapha* (pure water) types. Mixed types also exist, when two or more doshas stand in relatively equal proportion. Three different dual types exist as *Vata-Pitta* (air-fire), *Vata-Kapha* (air-water) and *Pitta-Kapha* (fire-water). An even type or *VPK* type is also found, making seven major types in all.

It should be noted that mixed types do not necessarily indicate better or worse health. They do serve, however, to complicate treatment. Efforts to balance one dosha may aggravate another. For dual types, therefore, it is often better to try to raise the third dosha, the one that is too low. Vata-Pitta (air-fire) types should try to increase Kapha (water). Pitta-Kapha (fire-water) types should try to increase Vata (air). Vata-Kapha (air-water) types should aim at developing Pitta . In this way it will be easier to understand which qualities need to be balanced.

Often we give numbers to denote the proportion of the three doshas in the body. Vata 4, Pitta 2, Kapha 1, would show a high-Vata, low-Kapha person. However, there is no fixed way of using numbers to denote the doshas and different practitioners may give them different values.

Different degrees of aggravation of the doshas exist as well. There is much difference between high Vata as insomnia and high Vata as paralysis, for example. And the doshas can become unbalanced in different ways, relative to their different attributes. High Vata, excess air, can manifest as dryness, causing rigidity or reduced motion. It can also manifest one of its other qualities as excess mobility, causing tremors, appearing almost opposite in attributes. The doshas provide us a simple background for understanding conditions, yet a more specific analysis is often necessary regarding the particular qualities out of balance.

In addition, outer circumstances can aggravate the doshas not predominant in an individual nature. For example, we live in a very Vata (high air) culture with constant travel, stimulation and communication. Vata disorders are more common here than in other cultures, even in individuals of other doshas. Such variations should not be lost sight of when we examine particular constitutions.

The dosha that you check most will usually indicate your predominant dosha. Generally speaking, we know ourselves well enough to determine our Ayurvedic constitution. Determining those of friends is more difficult. Consulting an Ayurvedic practitioner is helpful, but even here a difference of opinion sometimes exists. Different people may be more sensitive to one or another dosha in your nature depending upon various factors.

The natural constitution is most easily revealed by the fixed attributes of the physical body like frame, weight and complexion. Life-long habits and proclivities, and life-long disease tendency are also important. Though constitution tends to remain the same throughout the life, exceptional factors like a long-term illness can change it.

AYURVEDIC CONSTUTIONAL TEST
BODILY STRUCTURE AND APPEARANCE

	Vata	Pitta	Kapha
FRAME	Tall or short, thin; poorly developed physique	Medium; moderately developed physique	Stout, stocky, short, big; well developed physique
WEIGHT	Low, hard to hold weight, prominent veins and bones	Moderate, good muscles	Heavy, tends towards obesity
COMPLEXION	Dull, brown, darkish	Red, ruddy, flushed, glowing	White, pale
SKIN TEXTURE AND TEMPERATURE	Thin, dry, cold, rough, cracked, prominent veins	Warm, moist, pink, with moles, freckles, acne	Thick, white, moist, cold, soft, smooth
HAIR	Scanty, coarse, dry, brown, slightly wavy	Moderate, fine, soft, early gray or bald	Abundant, oily, thick, very wavy, lustrous
HEAD	Small, thin, long, unsteady	Moderate	Large, stocky, steady
FOREHEAD	Small, wrinkled	Moderate, with folds	Large, broad
FACE	Thin, small, long, wrinkled, dusky, dull	Moderate, ruddy, sharp contours	Large, round, fat, white or pale, soft contours
NECK	Thin, long	Medium	Large, thick
EYEBROWS	Small, thin, unsteady	Moderate, fine	Thick, bushy, many hairs
EYELASHES	Small, dry, firm	Small, thin, fine	Large, thick, oily, firm
EYES	Small, dry, thin, brown, dull, unsteady	Medium, thin, red (inflamed easily), green, piercing	Wide, prominent, thick, oily, white, attractive
NOSE	Thin, small, long, dry, crooked	Medium	Thick, big, firm, oily

31

	Vata	**Pitta**	**Kapha**
LIPS	Thin, small, darish, dry, unsteady	Medium, soft, red	Thick, large, oily, smooth, firm
TEETH AND GUMS	Thin, dry, small, rough, crooked, receding gums	Medium, soft, pink, gums bleed easily	Large, thick, soft, pink, oily
SHOULDERS	Thin, small, flat, hunched	Medium	Broad, thick, firm, oily
CHEST	Thin, small, narrow, poorly developed	Medium	Broad, large, well or overly developed
ARMS	Thin, overly small or long, poorly developed	Medium	Large, thick, round, well developed
HANDS	Small, thin, dry, cold, rough, fissured, unsteady	Medium, warm, pink	Large, thick, oily, cool, firm
THIGHS	Thin, narrow	Medium	Well-developed, round, fat
LEGS	Thin, excessively long or short, prominent knees	Medium	Large, stocky
CALVES	Small, hard, tight	Loose, soft	Shapely, firm
FEET	Small, thin, long, dry, rough, fissured, unsteady	Medium, soft, pink	Large, thick, hard, firm
JOINTS	Small, thin, dry, unsteady, cracking	Medium, soft, loose	Large, thick, well built
NAILS	Small, thin, dry, rough, fissured, cracked, darkish	Medium, soft, pink	Large, thick, smooth, white, firm, oily

WASTE MATERIALS/METABOLISM

URINE	Scanty, difficult, colorless	Profuse, yellow, red, burning	Moderate, whitish, milky
FECES	Scanty, dry, hard, difficult or painful, gas, constipation	Abundant, loose, yellowish, diarrhea, with burning sensation	Moderate, solid, sometimes pale in color, mucus in stool

I.3 Constitutional Examination

	Vata	**Pitta**	**Kapha**
SWEAT/ BODY ODOR	Scanty, no smell	Profuse, hot, strong smell	Moderate, cold, pleasant smell
APPETITE	Variable, erratic	Strong, sharp	Constant, low
TASTE PREFERENCES	Prefers sweet, sour or salty food, cooked with oil and spiced	Prefers sweet, bitter or astringent food, raw, lightly cooked without spices	Prefers pungent, bitter or astringent food, cooked with spices but not oil
CIRCULATION	Poor, variable, erratic	Good, warm	Good, warm Slow, steady

GENERAL CHARACTERISTICS

ACTIVITY	Quick, fast, unsteady, erratic, hyperactive	Medium, motivated, purposeful, goal seeking	Slow, steady, stately
STRENGTH/ ENDURANCE	Low, poor endurance, starts and stops quickly	Medium, intolerant of heat	Strong, good endurance, but slow in starting
SEXUAL NATURE	Variable, erratic, deviant, strong desire but low energy, few children	Moderate, passionate, quarrelsome, dominating	Low but constant sexual desire, good sexual energy, devoted, many children
SENSITIVITY	Fear of cold, wind, sensitive to dryness	Fear of heat, dislike of sun, fire	Fear of cold, damp, likes wind and sun
RESISTANCE TO DISEASE	Poor, variable, weak immune system	Medium, prone to infection	Good, prone to congestive disorders
DISEASE TENDENCY	Nervous system diseases, pain, arthritis, mental disorder	Fevers, infections, inflammatory diseases	Respiratory system diseases, mucus, edema
REACTION TO MEDICATIONS	Quick, low dosage needed, unexpected side effects or nervous reactions	Medium, average dosage	Slow, high dosage required, effects slow to manifest
PULSE	Thready, rapid, superficial, irregular, weak/ like a snake	Wiry, bounding, moderate/ like a frog	Deep, slow, steady, deep, rolling, slippery/ like a swan

33

MENTAL FACTORS AND EXPRESSION

	Vata	Pitta	Kapha
VOICE	Low, weak, hoarse	High pitch, sharp Moderate, good	Pleasant, deep, good tone
SPEECH	Quick, inconsistent, erratic, talkative	Moderate, argumen-tative, convincing	Slow, definite, not talkative
MENTAL NATURE	Quick, adaptable, indecisive	Intelligent, penetrating, critical	Slow, steady, dull
MEMORY	Poor, notices things easily but easily forgets	Sharp, clear	Slow to take notice but will not forget
FINANCES	Earns and spends quickly, erratically	Spends on specific goals, causes or projects	Holds on to what one earns, particularly property
EMOTIONAL TENDENCIES	Fearful, anxious, nervous	Angry, irritable, contentious	Calm, content, attached, sentimental
NEUROTIC TENDENCIES	Hysteria, trembling, anxiety attacks	Extreme temper, rage, tantrums	Depression, unresponsiveness, sorrow
FAITH	Erratic, changeable, rebel	Determined, fanatic, leader	Constant, loyal, conservative
SLEEP	Light, tends towards insomnia	Moderate, may wake up but will fall asleep again	Heavy, difficulty in waking up
DREAMS	Flying, moving, restless, nightmares	Colorful, passionate, conflict	Romantic, sentimental, watery, few dreams
HABITS	Likes speed, travelling, parks, plays, jokes, stories, trivia, artistic activities, dancing	Likes competitive sports, debates, politics, hunting, research	Likes water, sailing, flowers, cosmetics, business ventures, cooking

Total (50)   V_____   P_____   K_____

MENTAL NATURE

Vata (Airy) Mentality

Vata types have emotional tendencies towards fear and anxiety. They are mentally changeable, excitable, and indecisive and have good but erratic mental powers. They are good at both grasping and forgetting. They are quick at both attachment and detachment, fast at getting emotional and expressing emotions, as well as forgetting them. Their minds and senses are sensitive, but unsteady. They will not have much courage and tend towards cowardice. Generally they will be of a solitary nature and not have a lot of friends. However, they are good at forming friendships with people outside their social sphere. They do not make good leaders, but they will not be good followers either. They will not be very materialistic and are not much concerned with accumulating possessions or money. They spend money quickly and easily.

Pitta (Fiery) Mentality

Pitta types are prone to fiery emotions like irritability and anger. They are logical, critical, perceptive and intelligent. They are quick to get emotional and have no trouble expressing anger. They are articulate, convincing and self-righteous. They usually possess strong wills, are dignified and make good leaders. While very helpful and kind to friends and followers, they are cruel and unforgiving to opponents. They are bold, adventurous, daring and reckless. They are inventive, ingenious and possess good mechanical skills. Their memories are sharp and not sentimental. They are more concerned with the accumulation of power than with material resources but will gather material resources to gain their ends.

Kapha (Watery) Mentality

Kaphas incline to watery emotions, like love and desire, romance and sentimentality. They are kind, considerate and loyal, but also slow to respond, conservative, shy and obedient. They tend to have many friends and to be very close to their fam ily, community, culture, religion and country, but they can be closed-minded outside their sphere of habitual activity. They travel less and are happier at home. They easily get attached and find it hard to be detached. While they can display affections easily, they are slow to express emotions, particularly anger. Mentally, they are steady with good forethought but need time to consider things properly.

PHYSICAL AND PSYCHOLOGICAL TYPES

As mental nature is subtler than physical nature, more variations are possible. As it is more changeable than physical nature, it can more easily take on temporary disturbances different than the physical constitution. Mental disturbances, therefore, are more likely to be different from the physical constitution than are physical diseases. The mind is also very easily disturbed by the disease process and not always in a way that is of the same quality as the disease. Generally, all diseases make us afraid. They bring up the basic fear of death, tending to aggravate Vata or create anxiety in the mind.

MENTAL NATURE AND ASTROLOGY

Differences between the physical and mental nature are often revealed through astrology, which gives us a more accurate and detailed picture of the mind than simple Ayurvedic examination. The birth chart itself is a picture of the energies of the mind or astral body. The physical body can also be read from it by isolating certain factors within it. Hence, in treating the mind it is good to consult astrology. It affords a unique overview of the life, personality and the purposes of the soul in the incarnation.

MENTAL AND SPIRITUAL DISPOSITION

In the Vedic system, mental nature is judged according to the gunas, the three prime attributes of nature (Prakriti) as sattva, rajas and tamas. These indicate the mental traits respectively of clarity, distraction and dullness. The doshas have a secondary importance in this regard. These three qualities reflect the level of development of the soul. They are not simply intellectual proclivities or emotional types. They show the sensitivity of the mind, its capacity to perceive truth and to act accordingly.

The mind itself is called sattva, clarity, as sattva is the basic clear quality of the mind that allows for perception to occur. Sattva means what possesses the same nature as truth or reality (sat). The mind is naturally clear and pure but becomes darkened by negative thoughts and emotions. When pure it produces enlightenment and self-realization. Sattva is the divine or godly nature. It brings about internalization of the mind, the movement of the consciousness inward and the unification of the head and the heart.

Rajas, which means stain or smoke, is distraction or turbulence in the mind that causes us to look outward and lose ourselves in the external world. It is the mind agitated by desire. Rajas is disturbed thoughts and imaginings. It includes willfulness, anger, manipulativeness and ego. It involves the seeking of power, stimulation and entertainment. In excess it creates a wrathful (asuric) nature.

Tamas, which means heaviness and lethargy, is dullness, darkness and inability to perceive. It is the mind clouded by ignorance and fear. Tamas creates sloth, sleep and inattention. It involves lack of mental activity and insensitivity, and domination of the mind by external or subconscious forces. Tamas creates a servile or animal nature.

Usually rajas and tamas go together. Tamas creates the darkening of awareness, which allows rajas to project various false imaginations or ego ideas. Rajas, similarly, in excess, depletes our energy through over-activity and makes us tamasic, dull and lethargic.

Rajas and tamas are necessary forces in nature. Rajas creates energy, vitality and emotion and relates to prana. Tamas creates stability and allows fixed forms to take shape, thus it underlies our physical body. But these two qualities are out of place in the mind and in the perceptual process. For objective awareness to occur, the mind must be calm. It must be free of distraction or inertia. It must be like a mirror in order for us to see, like a lake free of ripples to reflect the moon. We should give rajas and tamas their proper place in the lower aspects of our nature as body and prana but should free the mind from their compulsions.

DISEASE TENDENCY OF THE THREE MENTAL TYPES

In Ayurveda, the main cause of disease is said to be 'failure of intelligence', *prajnaparadha*. This is not simply lack of intellectual knowledge or verbal acuity, but a failure of natural wisdom. It is a lack of understanding of the natural harmony of life—living out of harmony with nature, the universe and the Divine. This failure of our natural intelligence to operate is caused by external conditioning factors, like fear and desire. It inhibits creative living and traps us in convention or habit. It manifests as lack of faith in life and in the Divine, and becoming careless or irresponsible about health.

Mental disorders specifically are usually caused by failure of intelligence, or inadequate sattva. This comes from poor education (lack of moral or ethical values in upbringing), causing harm to others, excess stimulation and entertainment, dishonesty, or untruthfulness. Such physical factors as wrong diet, eating too much sugar or meat, and excess sleep contribute to it.

Sattva is improved by spiritual cultivation, yogic practices, mantra, meditation, spending time in nature, a pro-sattva diet, and a life regimen in harmony with ones constitution. Ayurveda encourages us to try to develop sattva whatever we may do.

Guna Types and Disease Potential

SATTVIC TYPES have the greatest freedom from disease. Their nature is harmonious and adaptable. They strive towards balance and have peace of mind that cuts the psychological root of disease. They are considerate of others and take care of themselves and their bodies. They see all life as a learning experience and try to see the good in all things, including disease.

RAJASIC TYPES have good, or even excess, energy but can burn themselves out through excessive activity. Their disease symptoms are frequently acute and recovery is possible with the right remedial measures. They are impatient and inconsistent in dealing with disease and do not always take the time or responsibility to get well. They often blame others for their condition, which postpones healing.

TAMASIC TYPES are prone to chronic diseases and low vitality. Their energy and emotions tend to be stagnant or blocked. Their diseases are deep seated, obstinate and difficult to treat. They do not seek proper treatment and usually have poor hygiene. They will accept their disease as fate and will not take advantage of the methods that may cure them. They are often caught in bad habits, addictions and attachments that they are unable to question.

THE THREE MENTAL TYPES AND THE THREE DOSHAS

An important method of balancing the three doshas is to move from their tamasic and rajasic sides to their sattvic (spiritual) side. It is usually not possible to transcend ones predominant dosha, but one can move to its higher level of functioning. For example, a Kapha type can move from greed, a tamasic emotion, to devotion, a sattvic emotion; this transforms a negative emotional disease tendency to a power of health and enlightenment.

All of us contain various degrees of these three mental qualities, just as we all have the three doshas. Without sattva we could not perceive anything at all. Without rajas we could not move. Without tamas we would have no stability or consistency. The right balance of all qualities is also sattva, which means balance.

There have been a number of attempts to correspond the three doshas to the three prime gunas. Actually any of the three doshas can correspond to any of the three gunas. We have presented the larger picture in the next table.

We should examine our mental constitution according to the proportions of sattva, rajas and tamas that we find in ourselves.

This will give us a better idea how to improve our minds and balance our disease tendency through yoga and the cultivation of character.

When we combine the three qualities and the three doshas the following picture of mental development in human beings emerges. Each dosha is divided according to the three qualities. We see that no dosha is necessarily better than another in terms of mental nature. Their temperaments vary, but higher and lower spiritual levels exist within each type.

Ultimately, seven different guna types can be ascertained for each dosha (like the seven different doshic types). These are pure sattva, pure rajas, pure tamas, sattva-rajas, sattva-tamas, rajas-tamas and all three in equal proportion. Totally pure sattva (shuddha sattva) gives enlightenment.

All of us should examine these mental traits and see which most fit our nature. We should reduce qualities that are negative, such as disease-causing habits, by the appropriate remedial measures. These include meditation, prayer, mantra, puja or various other forms of self-examination, or surrender to the Divine. Our culture as a whole today is very rajasic. Therefore, some rajasic traits may be more due to circumstances than indicative of our own disposition.

Vate (Airy) Mental **Nature**

Sattvic (Harmonious)	Energetic, adaptable, flexible, quick in comprehension, good in communication, strong sense of human unity, strong healing energy, true enthusiasm, positive spirit, able to initiate things, good capacity for positive change and movement
Rajasic (Disturbed)	Indecisive, unreliable, hyperactive, agitated, restless, disturbed, nervous, anxious, overly talkative, superficial, noisy, disruptive, false enthusiasm
Tamasic (Darkened)	Fearful, servile, dishonest, secretive, depressed, self-destructive, drug addict, prone to sexual perversions, mentally disturbed, suicidal

Pitta (Fiery) Mental Nature

Sattvic (Harmonious)	Intelligent, clear, perceptive, enlightened, discriminating, good will, independent, warm, friendly, courageous, good guide and leader
Rajasic (Disturbed)	Willful, impulsive, ambitious, aggressive, controlling, critical, dominating, manipulating, angry, wrathful, reckless, proud, vain
Tamasic (Darkened)	Hateful, vile, vindictive, destructive, psychopath, criminal, drug dealer, underworld figure

Kapha (Fiery) Mental Nature

Sattvic (Harmonious)	Calm, peaceful, content, stable, consistent, loyal, loving, compassionate, forgiving, patient, devoted, receptive, nurturing, supportive, strong faith
Rajasic (Disturbed)	Controlling, attached, greedy, materialistic, sentimental, needing security, seeking comfort and luxury
Tamasic (Darkened)	Dull, gross, lethargic, apathetic, slothful, coarse, slow comprehension, insensitive, a thief

I.4
Examination of Disease
The Patterns of Imbalance

D iseases reflect the predominant dosha that produces them. We can understand the nature of a disease, like that of physical constitution, according to the doshic attributes that it presents. We can treat it with the remedies appropriate for the dosha involved.

Some diseases are characteristically of one dosha or another. The majority of diseases are of a Vata nature, as Vata tends towards decay. Ayurvedic books list more Vata disorders than Pitta and Kapha together with eighty Vata disorders, forty Pitta disorders, and twenty Kapha. Kapha diseases are characterized primarily by phlegm. Pitta diseases are indicated by fever or burning sensation. Vata diseases show up as pain or debility.

- Kapha (water or phlegm) diseases include most respiratory disorders, colds, fluís, asthma, bronchitis, swollen glands, edema, and benign tumors. The main attributes of Kapha disorders are dampness, excessive tissue growth, and cold.
- Pitta (fire or bile) diseases include most febrile and infectious diseases, liver disorders, ulcers, acidity, boils, skin rashes. The main attributes of Pitta disorders are heat, redness, and oiliness.
- Vata (air or wind) diseases include most nervous system disorders, insomnia, tremors, epilepsy, paralysis, and arthritis. The main attributes of Vata disorders are dryness, cold, impaired or abnormal movement, and wasting away of tissues.

In general, all diseases can be divided into Vata, Pitta or Kapha types according to the dosha most commonly involved with them. Yet the same disease may be caused by different doshas. Most common colds are of a Kapha nature with phlegm and congestion as the main symptoms. Others may be Pitta in quality with a higher fever and severe sore throat. Though any one disease may be of many types, the treatment for all diseases follows the same main lines and principles, that of the aggravated dosha.

THE DOSHAS AS THE SITES OF DISEASE

Most diseases can occur from an imbalance of any of the three doshas. For example, arthritis may come about from high Vata, high Pitta or high Kapha. Yet each disease is usually characterized more by one dosha than another, like arthritis which is mainly a Vata disorder because Vata relates to the bones.

To understand this point better we should realize that the doshas can damage each other. The doshas, as the underlying forces of the body, are not only the factors that cause disease but also the sites where disease occurs. They relate to the tissues, organs and systems that they rule; so, diseases involving the nervous system show Vata as the site of the disorder. Diseases of this system ruled by Vata will more commonly be Vata. Yet they may be of a Pitta or Kapha nature, as these other doshas when high can damage Vata.

Usually, a dosha will aggravate the factors it rules. It will be the site as well as the causative factor in the disease process. Thus high Kapha (phlegm) damages the lungs, a Kapha organ. But an excess dosha may take the disease site of another dosha. This often indicates a more severe condition, in which the dosha has already damaged its own sites. For example, high Kapha, after damaging the lungs, may then damage the nervous system, as in asthmatic wheezing or epilepsy due to phlegm blocking the channels, thus affecting Vata. The doshas affect each other and, in severe diseases like cancer, all three doshas may be out of balance, making treatment very complicated.

According to Ayurveda it is not necessary to know the names or forms of diseases. It is more important to know the attributes of the doshas and their states of imbalance behind different diseases. From this standpoint treatment is simpler and more holistic. Once the aggravated dosha is ascertained, along with its site of manifestation, an integral regimen for reducing it can be implemented. It is the underlying energy of the disease which has to be countered, not merely its face that has to be identified. Ayurveda sees all diseases according to the three doshas. For it no really new diseases can be found, only variations in the same basic disease-causing factors.

Excess of the Doshas

According to Ayurvedic source books the classical symptoms of the aggravated or elevated doshas are as follows:

Vata's actions when aggravated are collapse, spasms, piercing pain, numbness, depression, breaking, striking and biting pain, constipation, cracking of the joints, contraction, retention of waste materials in the body, excitability, thirst, trembling, roughness of skin, porosity of tissues, dehydration, agitated movement, stiffness, astringent taste in the mouth and dark or reddish brown discoloration.
—We see in these the drying and disruptive powers of the wind.

Pitta's actions when aggravated are burning sensation, redness, feeling hot, boils, sweating, pus formation, bleeding, necrosis, exhaustion, fainting, inebriation, pungent and sour taste in the mouth and all discolorations but white and brown.
—We see in these the burning and fermenting action of fire.

Kapha when aggravated creates phlegm, hardness of tissues, itching, cold sensation on the skin, heaviness, congestion, obesity, edema, indigestion, excessive sleeping, white color, and sweet and salty tastes in the mouth which take time to notice.
—These reflect the heaviness and stagnation of water.

Ashtanga Hridaya XII. 49-54

Deficiency of the Doshas

Disease is primarily caused by the doshas that are too high or aggravated. Low doshas are not thought to possess the strength to cause disease, but they do have their symptoms. Vata when low

45

resembles high Kapha. Pitta when low resembles both high Vata and high Kapha. Kapha when low resembles high Vata. The symptoms of the doshas when low or deficient are as follows:

Vata when low causes lassitude of the limbs, deficiency of speech and enthusiasm, and confusion of perception, as well as increase in phlegm and the production of toxins (ama).

Pitta when insufficient causes weakness of the digestive fire, cold, and lack of lustre.

Kapha when low results in a feeling of emptiness in the stomach, palpitations, and loosening of the joints.

Ashtanga Hridaya XI. 14-16

SYMPTOMS OF AGGRAVATED DOSHAS

The following list gives, in a comprehensive way, the disease symptoms common to each of the three doshas. These can be added to the factors of constitutional examination for greater clarity. Examination of pulse, tongue and abdomen, as well as questioning the patient, are important.

	Vata	Pitta	Kapha
COLOR as in complexion, discharges, discolorations	Black, brown, blue black, blue, pink, decrease or absence of normal color	Red, purple, yellow, green, black, smoky	White, pale
PAIN	Most severe; throbbing, biting, churning, beating, tearing, variable,migratory, intermittent	Medium; burning, steaming	Least; heavy, dull, constant
FEVER	Moderate temperature; variable or irregular fever, thirst, anxiety, restlessness	Highest temperature; burning sensation, thirst, sweating, irritability, delirium	Low-grade fever; dullness, heaviness, constant elevated temperature

I.4 Examination of Disease

	Vata	Pitta	Kapha
DISCHARGES	Gas, sound (discharge of gas, cracking of joints, etc	Bleeding, pus, bile	Mucus, salivation
MOUTH	Astringent taste, dry.)	Bitter or pungent taste, increased salivation	Sweet or salty taste, profuse salivation, mucoid discharges
THROAT	Dry, rough, pain and constriction of esophagus	Sore throat, inflammation, burning sensation	Swelling, dilation, edema
STOMACH	Decreased secretions, irregular appetite, frequent eructation (belching, hiccup), sense of constriction	Excessive appetite, sour or pungent eructation, burning sensation, ulcers, cancer	Slow digestion, sweet or mucoid eructation
LIVER AND GALL BLADDER	Dry, rough, scanty secretions, irregular activity	Soft, excessive bile production, gall stones, inflammation, abscesses, increased activity	Enlarged, heavy, firm, scanty bile, decreased activity
INTESTINES	Dry, peristalsis disorders, distention, gas, constipation	Profuse secretions, quick peristalsis, inflammation, ulceration, abscesses, tumors, cancer, bleeding, perforation	Mucus coating, slow peristalsis, obstruction, distention, edema, tumors
FECES	Constipation, painful and difficult bowel movements, dry, small in quantity	Diarrhea, watery stools, quick or uncontrollable evacuation, burning sensation, increased frequency, moderate amount	Solid, decreased frequency, large amount, containing mucus, with itching

	Vata	**Pitta**	**Kapha**
URINE	Scanty, difficult to discharge, increased frequency or absence of urination,colorless	Profuse, with burning sensation, increased frequency, yellow, turbid, brown or red incolor	Profuse, decreased frequency, mucoid, white or pale
SWEAT	Scanty, irregular	Profuse, hot	Moderate, constant
MIND AND SENSES	Delusion, fear, apathy, sorrow, loss of consciousness, insomnia, desire for hot and dislike of cold things	Weakness of senses, intoxication, restlessness, violent emotions, delirium, loss of sleep, dizziness, fainting, desire for cold things	Slow perception, lack of desire, lethargy, stupor, excessive sleeping, desire for hot things
ONSET OF DISEASE	Rapid, variable, irregular	Medium, with fever	Slow, constant
TIME OF DAY WHEN AGGRAVATED	Dawn, dusk	Noon, midnight	Mid-morning, mid-evening
SEASON WHEN AGGRAVATED	Fall, early winter	Summer, late spring	Late winter, early spring
EXOGENOUS AGGRAVATING FACTORS	Wind, cold, dryness	Heat, sun, fire, humidity	Dampness, cold

THE DISEASE PROCESS

OJAS, THE ESSENTIAL ENERGY OF THE IMMUNE SYSTEM

Ojas is the essential energy of the body. It literally means 'vigor'. It is the subtle essence of the reproductive system and of all the vital secretions. It is the special Ayurvedic concept of a source fluid underlying all our physical capacities. Ojas is not a physical substance. It is the sap of our life energy and exists on a subtle level in the heart chakra. When it is sufficient, there is health. When it is deficient, there is disease. Disease strikes at the locations where it is weak. In modern terms, we could say it is something like the essential energy of the immune system. Ojas is defined as:

> The ultimate essence of the reproductive fluids and the heat of the tissues. Located in the heart, it pervades the entire body, giving stability and support. It is moist, of the nature of nectar (Soma), transparent, slightly red and yellow in color. When it is destroyed one dies; when it is sustained, one lives.
>
> Ojas is decreased by such factors as anger, hunger, worry, sorrow and overwork. Then one experiences fear and lack of strength. One constantly worries, with disturbed senses. Lacking color, weak in mind, one becomes wasted. Such qualities as patience and faith disappear.

Other factors that decrease Ojas include excessive sexual activity and the use of drugs or stimulants, as well as stress, anxiety, devitalized food, unnatural environment and life-style.

Ojas is replenished by special foods like milk and ghee (clarified butter), and by special tonic herbs like ashwagandha, shatavari and guduchi. Meditation practices, mantras such as Om, and sexual moderation are also helpful, as Ojas is essentially sattvic (pure) in nature.

When low, Ojas causes chronic, degenerative diseases, as well as mysterious and hard to treat infectious and nervous disorders. The modern disease AIDS has all the symptoms of a disease of low Ojas. Less severe chronic low-energy conditions are also related to low Ojas; chronic low-grade infections like Epstein-Barr virus or chronic hepatitis. Ojas decreases with age, and the diseases of old age reflect low Ojas, just as low Ojas causes premature aging.

THE SIX STAGES OF DISEASE

According to Ayurveda, the disease process can be summarized in a simple way. The doshas undergo increase by aggravating factors (diet, climate, seasons, life-style, emotions, etc.). This causes weakening of the digestive fire, which in turn allows an undigested food mass (called Ama in Sanskrit) to arise. This, with the increased dosha, blocks the channels and becomes deposited in any weakened site in the body, from which the disease then manifests.

Ayurveda recognizes six stages in the disease process according to the development and movement of the aggravated doshas. These are called:

1. Accumulation (sancaya)
2. Aggravation (prakopa)
3. Overflow (prasara)
4. Relocation (sthana samsraya)
5. Manifestation (vyakti)
6. Diversification (bheda)

The first two refer to the increase of the doshas in their respective sites. The other four show their spread to different parts of the body.

1. Accumulation

The doshas begin to increase in their respective locales. Causes include wrong diet, seasonal maladjustments, wrong life style, psychological disturbance, and all the usual factors that increase a particular dosha.

- Vata (air) accumulates in the colon causing distention, gas, constipation, insomnia, fear, fatigue, dryness and seeking of warmth.
- Pitta (fire) accumulates in the small intestine producing burning sensation, fever, hyperacidity, bitter taste in the mouth,

yellow coloring of urine and stool, desire for cold things, and anger.
• Kapha (water) accumulates in the stomach resulting in lassitude, heaviness, pallor, bloating, indigestion and desire for light food.

2. Aggravation

The doshas continue to increase in their respective sites, bringing about an increase in the symptoms manifested there and, by the pressure of this accumulation, reflected symptoms elsewhere.

• Vata causes light-headedness, increased constipation, abdominal pain or spasms, further accumulation of gas with rumbling in the bowels, along with upper abdominal distention.
• Pitta causes increased acidity, acid regurgitation, burning pain in the abdomen, excessive thirst, loss of strength, difficulty sleeping.
• Kapha causes loss of appetite, indigestion, nausea and increased salivation, heaviness in the head and heart, and excess sleeping.

3. Overflow

The doshas have now filled up their respective sites and begin to overflow into the rest of the body. They enter into the plasma and blood, spreading out of the G.I. tract. The doshas are no longer localized and can now penetrate into the organs and tissues of the body.

They move in different directions causing various disorders and dysfunctions. The nature and location of these complications depends upon the direction the doshas move. They can move in any direction, up, down, to one side or the other, but will go the way it is easiest for them to travel. They come into close contact with the tissues and waste materials of the body and become mixed with either of them. There will be a worsening of symptoms at their respective sites.

- Vata causes dry skin, pain or stiffness of the joints, lower back pain, convulsions, spasm, headache, dry cough, intermittent fever, as well as continued abdominal pain with constipation and painful bowel movements and general fatigue.
- Pitta causes inflammatory skin diseases, conjunctivitis, gingivitis, dizziness, headache, high fever, bilious vomiting, as well as diarrhea with burning sensation.
- Kapha causes cough, asthma, swollen glands, low-grade fever, vomiting, swelling of the joints, and mucus in the stools

4. Relocation

The doshas now relocate themselves in other sites in the body where they begin to cause specific diseases. Generally the doshas move to the tissues that they are most connected to:

- Accumulated Vata moves to the bones
- Accumulated Pitta moves to the blood
- Accumulate Kapha moves to the lymphatic system

However, the doshas can move to any sites in the body that are weak. For example, in arthritis, the doshas deposit themselves in the joints and accumulate there. Or, if a person has eaten too many sweets the doshas move to the pancreas and cause diabetes. Disease symptoms become fixed at the relocation phase, whereas in the overflow state they move around.

5. Manifestation

The doshas manifest specific symptom complexes at these particular sites. We can now identify the disease as asthma, diabe-

tes, arthritis, or whatever it may happen to be. The disease onset
is now major and treatment becomes difficult.

6. Diversification

At these particular sites the doshas manifest their special char-
acteristics. The disease can be identified according to its doshic
attributes.

For example, a Vata type arthritis will evidence severe pain,
cold, stiffness, dry skin, and constipation. A Pitta type arthritis
will show fever, burning sensation, red swelling of the joints and
loose stool. A Kapha type will demonstrate swelling, edema,
phlegm and congestion.

The general rule in treatment is that it is always easier to treat
the doshas while they are still located in their original sites. The
stages of accumulation and aggravation, therefore, are relatively
easy to cure. The stage of overflow is the transitional stage.

At the relocation phase only the preliminary symptoms of the
disease are in evidence and vitality is still strong, so treatment is
still simple. The last two stages present a fully developed disease.
It has matured and will take time and effort to rectify.

THE THREE DISEASE PATHWAYS

Three pathways for diseases are differentiated: *outer, inner,*
and *central.*

1. THE INNER DISEASE PATHWAY (antar marga) consists of the
   digestive tract defined mainly in the three sections of the
   stomach, small intestine and large intestine. This pathway is
   called inner because the digestive tract forms a channel
   through the inside of the body. Diseases here are easy to
   treat since it is possible to expel them from the body directly through the digestive tract, which is the main route for
   eliminating toxins. They include mainly diseases of the
   digestive tract.

2, THE OUTER DISEASE PATHWAY (bahya marga) consists of the plasma (skin) and blood, the two outer or superficial tissues. Diseases here are more difficult to treat because they have already entered into the tissues, but they still have not yet entered deeply enough to cause really serious diseases. They include skin diseases and toxic blood conditions.

3. THE CENTRAL DISEASE PATHWAY (madhyama marga) consists of the deeper tissues of muscle, fat, bone, nerve, and reproductive tissue. It is called the central disease pathway because it occurs between the outer pathway, the skin, and the inner pathway, the g.i. tract. The most sensitive points and organs of the body are affected, such as the head, heart, bladder and the joints of the bones. Diseases here are deep-seated and thus difficult to treat. Most severe, chronic and degenerative diseases, from arthritis to cancer, come from this area.

The outer and central disease pathways make up the seven tissues of the body. The first two, skin and blood, are the outer and the next five, muscle, fat, bone, marrow and reproductive fluid, the middle. Diseases are also classified by which tissue the dosha resides in, like Pitta in the muscle tissue (inflammation of the muscles) or Kapha in the bones (Kapha-type arthritis).

MOVEMENT OF THE DOSHAS THROUGH THE DISEASE PATHWAYS

The factors that make the doshas move from the digestive tract to the tissues are—"excessive exercise, too much hot or sharp food, wrong life-regimen and by being transported by Vata."

The doshas move from the inner tissues back to the digestive tract by—"purification of the openings of the channels", particularly by oleation and sweating therapies, as well as by the control of Vata (breath-control, pranayama) and by following a right life-regimen.

We see, therefore, that all diseases are produced by an accumulation of the doshas. Almost any disease can be caused by any of the three doshas. Yet while the general disease process is the same in all diseases, it varies according to stages, movement of the doshas, and the sites where they become deposited. Ayurveda thus affords us a simple, yet comprehensive understanding of the disease process that allows us to treat the disease at the right stage. By understanding this process and following the right regimen for our constitution, we prevent the doshas from accumulating and cut off the disease process at its very root.

SPIRITUAL ASPECTS OF HEALING

According to Ayurveda, all diseases have two primary causes. First, they arise from physical or biological causes—the imbalance of the biological humors, the elements and prime energies of the physical body. The treatment for this consists of physical or medical methods with a naturalistic basis including herbs, diet, body-work and yoga postures.

Second, diseases can arise from karmic causes—from the effects of wrong actions that we have done in this or previous lives, meaning from psychological or spiritual causes. These wrong actions include not only moral failings but also wrong occupation, problems in relationship or emotional difficulties. The treatment may require changes in life-style and attitudes. Such causes include not living up to our spiritual purpose or in life, not following our 'dharma'. Diseases can arise from wrong actions in previous lives, primarily those that harmed other beings.

Karmic diseases require some form of atonement or sacrifice, an 'inner rectification'. For this Ayurveda uses yoga and a system of divine or spiritual therapy (daiva chikitsa) which includes the use of gems, mantras, prayers, rituals and meditation. These are not medieval superstitions but reflect a profound understanding of the deeper levels of the mind and healing the soul.

According to Ayurveda, the human being consists of three bodies—the physical, astral and causal—or what could be called in western terms, body, mind and soul. Its diagnosis and treatment, though focused on the physical, considers the other two bodies as well. Many Ayurvedic methods work to correct disorders in the energy field behind the physical body, as well as the field of consciousness behind it. Most disease conditions involve both physical and spiritual factors, and require treatment on both levels.

The word 'God', for many of us in our culture, has negative connotations, largely because of its misrepresentation by fundamentalist religions. Yet a lack of faith in the Divine, which is something like a lack of faith in life or a positive will to live, is found behind many diseases. Disease is often a lack of love, including a lack of caring for oneself and one's physical body.

Therefore, the first step in healing is to open up to the Divine or cosmic will and accept the flow of grace. This requires understanding that ones life has a purpose in the development of the soul and in the spiritual evolution of humanity. It involves seeking the truth in whatever way is closest to our heart, following the spiritual path that is truest to our nature. Yet this must include respecting the right of others to follow their own paths that might be very different from ours. We might call this process 'first healing the soul,' remembering that the soul, in the yogic system, is our inner consciousness.

Western medicine has tried to remove religion from medicine. This has been an important and necessary step in the evolution of the mind. Organized religion's dogma, authoritarianism and repressive nature have no place in the realms of knowledge, which require freedom and objectivity in order to develop properly. Yet while something has been gained by ridding medicine of the outer forms of religion, something has been lost by removing the inner aspects.

The essence of healing is integration. Faith, love, devotion, the sense of the unity and sacred nature of humanity and all life are missing in modern medicine. These qualities do not create any dogma, nor do they impose any idea, will or discipline on another. They give the space and the freedom to grow and to see. They create the grace and flow of the cosmic life-force necessary for healing to occur. Without them we are broken and withered inside and our lives have little meaning. Without them the magic, wonder, beauty and purpose in life are taken away. Most of us today are sick because this spiritual meaning is not present in our lives. We are trapped in the tedium and stimulation of the outer world with practically nothing to nourish our hearts.

Ayurveda cannot accept medicine without religion. From its hallowed ancient perspective, that is like healing without love. This does not mean Ayurveda wishes to impose its religious background on anyone. Along with the regular tools and methods of natural healing, it provides yogic methods that can be adapted to various religious or spiritual orientations. As the Mother of healing Ayurveda transmits this grace of the Divine Mother.

If not a sign of spiritual crisis or change, disease is at the least, a spiritual opportunity. According to the *Upanishads*, disease is the highest form of asceticism (tapas), through which the truth of life can be revealed. Disease may be a sign of wrong action but it can also indicate that the soul is directing its energy inwardly away from the body. Either way it requires a spiritual reexamination, particularly if the disease is severe. Therefore, self-examination is the first step and fundamental basis for understanding and resolving any disease.

All life is learning and a development of self-knowledge. We must view disease in this light in order to understand it. We must, therefore, not just treat disease, but use disease as a tool for understanding ourselves. Once this communion with our inner consciousness is gained, we will find an inner harmony and joy that can overcome all external difficulties.

I.5
AYURVEDIC LIFE–REGIMENS
Balancing the Doshas

According to Ayurveda, though diseases are of many kinds and pathogens are of many varieties, they are mainly produced by disharmonies of the three doshas of Vata, Pitta and Kapha. Ayurvedic treatment aims at balancing the doshas to neutralize the disease process. It is not, as with western medicine, so concerned with the classification of disease or with the identification of pathogens. In merely treating external pathogens only the symptoms, not the underlying causes, are dealt with. In balancing the doshas the root of the disease process is cut off. The fundamental treatment for the doshas is not clinical but comes from our own right living methods. In this way Ayurveda always brings us back to self-healing.

Ayurvedic curative aids are not necessarily complex, nor do they always have to be administered by another person. They involve diet, herbs, life-style, yoga and meditation that we can implement for ourselves. The more complex remedies (extensive or strong herbal prescriptions or chemical drugs) and the more specialized methods (such as surgery) become necessary only when the disease process has been allowed to continue unchecked for a long time.

The basic rule is—*whatever we can do for ourselves to improve our own health is more effective in the long run than what another person can do for us*. Only when we have failed in our own efforts does the health care professional or clinical facility become necessary. Even then their value is temporary, to bring us back to the point of properly caring for ourselves. Often small things we do for ourselves, such as giving up wrong foods, do more than taking many medicines or consulting many doctors.

There is no substitute for our own right living. It cannot be bought at any price and another person cannot provide it for us. As long as we are not living in harmony with our constitution we cannot expect to be really healed by any method. The beauty of Ayurveda is that it gives each one of us the knowledge and the means to live in balance. It provides the right regimen for our particular type covering all aspects of our nature, physical, psychological and spiritual. But Ayurveda can only succeed with our own time and effort, devotion and dedication.

One of the failings of modern culture is that it deprives us of the time that we need to take care of ourselves. We are caught in a process of expending energy but not of renewing it. However, if we really value our well-being we will take the time. The responsibility is ours, and there is no one else to blame if we do not make the effort.

AYURVEDIC LIFE-REGIMENS

Ayurvedic treatment is founded on following the appropriate life-regimen according to our unique constitution. I do not like the word 'routine' because it implies a rigid discipline followed mechanically, a rut or a groove to fall into. 'Discipline' is also a misleading term because it implies trying to impose some external pattern upon our resistant nature. It is more a matter of discovering, through sensitivity to life, the natural movement of our own being. It is 'yoga', a coordinating and harnessing of our resources for their maximum energetic effect.

We must establish the right rhythm in our lives. This maintains a certain harmony and consistency, but remains flexible and responds to the challenges of the moment. The rhythm of right action creates a momentum that gives power to our lives and improves all of our faculties.

We must live creatively in order to be truly healthy and happy. Creativity is not chaotic. It establishes an order, but one that gives freedom, because through it our energies are no longer dispersed through wrong or untimely usage. This order of creativity is the order of intelligence that gives each thing its right place. It mirrors the profound beauty and order of nature that is never rigid but yet never chaotic.

Ayurvedic regimens keep us in harmony with the cosmic life-force. They are the rhythms of creative living, as natural as the breath. They require an effort to establish in the beginning to counter the inertia created by our life out of balance, but they soon develop a self-sustaining and expanding force of their own that will guide us to yet greater unfoldment.

These regimens help us establish a daily, monthly and yearly program for optimal health. All serious students of Ayurveda should implement such a program in their own lives. They should write it down and keep track of how well they follow it. Conditions before implementing the program should be carefully noted, along with the results of following it on an ongoing basis. Then we can really begin to practice self-healing as a way of life. If we do these regimens consistently there is no limit to how much we can improve our own state of being over time.

TAKING CONTROL OF OUR OWN KARMA

What we do every day makes for who we are. Our actions determine the content of our consciousness as well as the energy level of our physical body. An occasional visit to a healer, no matter how famous or expensive, cannot substitute for our own action or substantially alter its effects. The healing methods that we ourselves put into practice are of the greatest importance, not what someone else does for us. The latter are palliative; only the former can be curative because they alone indicate a change of our own nature.

What we do every day determines not only who we are in this life but also who we will become in the next life. According to the *Upanishads*, "As is a man's will, so is his action, as is his action, so he becomes." (BRIHADARANYAKA UPANISHAD V.4.5) We must first have the right will and the true resolve to live in harmony. This is called *kratu* in Sanskrit, meaning intelligence in action. Through it we take control of our own karma and cease to be victims of our unconscious actions.

What we do every day is our real religion because it shows what we truly value in life. From it derives the deeper tendencies that we take into our next life. Our wrong habits are not only bad

61

for the health problems they cause us in this life, they also create a predisposition to such problems in future lives. We may be able to escape their immediate effects, but they will come to us eventually.

AYURVEDIC REGIMENS AND THE TREATMENT OF DISEASE

Ayurveda simply and succinctly explains diseases and their treatment according to the three doshas. Kapha constitution individuals tend to Kapha type or congestive diseases. Pitta constitutions usually have Pitta or inflammatory diseases. Vata people similarly have a predominance of Vata or nervous diseases. Ayurvedic life regimens, therefore, afford us a methodology for preventing, as well as curing, disease.

However, it is possible to temporarily come down with a disease caused by a dosha other than that predominant in one's constitution, so the nature of the disease itself should be carefully examined. Diseases of a dosha different than one's constitution, as a rule, are easier to treat.

A disease can be identified through its underlying doshic imbalance according to the symptoms and syndromes it presents. Therefore through recognizing the underlying doshic imbalance we can treat a condition even if we do not know technically what it is. For example, if an individual has cough, congestion, profuse white phlegm, excessive salivation and other such high Kapha signs, we can implement an anti-Kapha therapy even if we do not know the condition is bronchitis or another lung disease.

Any natural form of healing takes time, as well as our own efforts. It may take a month of a natural herbal remedy, particularly for a long-standing disorder, to provide a noticeable effect. It may take several months of following a constitutional regimen to create major health changes. Nor can we expect the mild remedies of natural healing, such as herbs or bodywork, to succeed if our own life is out of balance, if our diet, work and stress of life-style are antagonistic to them. We cannot expect to get better through natural healing methods if our life is out of harmony with nature.

Mild natural remedies work on a subtle internal level by correcting and improving the life-force. This is like growing flowers. The natural healer provides the seed but the water, sunshine and love must come from us because the seed is planted in the soil of who we are. If that soil is not prepared properly, the seed may not be able to flourish, even if it is good.

So, dear friends, if you are serious about natural healing, you must have faith. You must have patience. And you must put YOURSELF to work. No one else can heal you any more than anyone else can live life for you. Be respectful of your own life and give reverence to the Divine spirit within you. Be the master of your own destiny.

LIFE-REGIMENS AND OTHER TYPES OF TREATMENT

Ayurvedic life-regimens are simple, non-invasive, non-traumatic and generally do not interfere with other forms of treatment. They can often be taken along with allopathic medicine. They can enhance almost any therapy, physical or psychological.

Self-care methods aim mainly at pacifying (shamana) the doshas. For severe cases, Ayurveda supplements them with stronger elimination methods (shodhana) like Pancha Karma.

DANGER OF EXCESS TREATMENT

Physical disease often results from an over-fixation upon the physical body and the material world. If we put too much energy into our physical condition we may aggravate the disease process. We must give the body its proper care, but need not let it dominate over the other aspects of our nature. We should make the required healing efforts with faith and patience, while devoting the greater part of our energy for the real spiritual and creative issues of our lives.

Many of us today suffer from excess treatment. We have taken too many medications and seen too many different doctors or healers. Our bodies are disturbed by too strong efforts to make them well. Therefore, in healing ourselves we should proceed with gentleness, patience and simplicity. By taking too many remedies we may not make things better, even if our condition is not good, we can make things worse. Moreover, we must give therapies adequate time to work and not switch them too quickly. Nor should we combine many different kinds of treatments at once, particularly those of a strong or forceful nature, which may conflict with one another.

AYURVEDIC LIFE–REGIMENS

Sattvic Living

All human beings should follow a sattvic or pure life-style that gives peace and clarity of mind. The remedial measures in Ayurveda are generally of a sattvic (harmonious) nature.

Physical purity includes pure diet, with raw or freshly cooked vegetarian food, pure air and water, proper exercise of a calming nature, as well as physical cleanliness.

Purity of mind includes truthfulness, honesty, humility, equanimity, non-violence, friendliness and compassion to all beings. Emotional impurities like anger, hatred, pride, lust and fear are given up; gossip and worry are to be set aside. These are the main bad mental habits that destroy the natural clarity and equipoise of mind.

Purity of life-style includes right livelihood (an occupation that does not bring harm to others), pleasant speech, harmonious or pleasant environment, and avoidance of distraction, noise and all violent or degrading forms of entertainment.

Sattvic life-style includes devotion to the Divine or to truth, compassion, service to humanity, study of spiritual teachings, reverence for spiritual teachers, and the practice of yoga and meditation.

Purity itself, however, should not become a fault through self-righteousness, hypersensitivity or fanaticism. Good humor and moderation should always be maintained. Natural harmony and adaptability are what is necessary, not the imposition of an artificial standard.

DIET AND HERBS

Diet is the most important long-term physical remedial measure. Its effects take time to manifest, often one to six months, but are enduring. As a remedial measure it is constant, though requiring modification for season, age or specific diseases. Our physical body is composed of food; we cannot expect its condition to change without changing our diet.

Herbs are like subtle foods. They can be taken in small or large doses. Large doses (more than one ounce of herbs per day) should usually not be taken without special study or professional guidance. In small doses herbs are like strong food supplements; and they can and should be taken on a regular basis by almost everyone. They are part of our necessary food articles and provide subtle nutrition. Right nutrition is not only taking our daily bread but also taking our daily herbs.

OILS AND MASSAGE

Massage and external application of oils are necessary for most of us on a regular basis. This may be no more than applying a common oil, such as sesame, to the feet or head twice a week. Therapeutic touch communicates to our body and breaks stagnation along its surface. Oil massage nourishes the heart and calms the mind. It gives elasticity to the muscles and ligaments and strengthens the bones.

Essential oils and fragrances are also an important part of life. They open the mind and heart and purify the air and aura. Incense works along the same lines. It aids in purification and helps create an atmosphere receptive to the Divine powers.

COLORS AND GEMS

The right use of colors has a harmonizing effect on the mind and emotions through the senses. Our impressions feed the mind and affect the doshas.

Gems help balance the aura and harmonize the cosmic influences projected upon us through the stars. They are not merely for ornamentation but offer an additional method of attunement with the subtle energies of life. It is helpful to wear or use gem-stones that help balance one's physical and mental nature. This is shown through astrology and Ayurveda.

LIFE-STYLE

Life-style is probably the most important factor in physical and mental health. Right life-style does not mean suppressing our nature, but bringing out its deeper powers. In Ayurveda, this includes not suppressing our natural urges like eating, sleeping, sex, elimination, urination, sneezing, weeping, coughing, or yawning.

Life-style considerations for everyone involve such physical factors as right amount of rest, sufficient exercise, right exposure to sun, heat or cold, and a pleasant and natural environment. The mental factors and ethical attitudes of right life-style are the principles of sattvic living. Such factors as right relationship and right attitudes are included here, as well as right livelihood.

YOGA AND MEDITATION

Yoga and meditation relate to the spiritual aspect of life. According to Ayurveda the soul is the source of life and health. We must live according to the purpose of our soul in order to have peace and well-being. Disease generally indicates that we have lost contact with our soul and its creative force.

Each of us should perform some daily yoga and meditation. This may include yoga postures, breathing exercises, mantra and visualization, as well as meditation practices aimed at silencing the mind. Without this our life has no real center around which the other practices of right living can be organized.

It should be noted that although Ayurveda includes different remedial measures as part of the system of Vedic science, all are not specific to it. Gem therapy is more appropriately part of Vedic astrology. Yoga therapy is a branch of treatment in itself, including a more specific use of asanas, pranayama and mantra. It is important to consult practitioners of these other systems for a more detailed guidance on these subjects.

Spiritual methods vary more according to differences of culture and individual temperament than do physical health measures. The mind is not as defined an entity as the physical body and requires greater flexibility in its treatment. These are general guidelines to be adapted with intelligence and consciousness.

In addition, the doshas do not comprehend all aspects of our nature, which are not simply physical or health based. It is not necessary to stereotype oneself according to one's dosha. All that is required is to prevent the problems that arise from not compensating for it. The doshas are guidelines for tuning into our unique nature, but the full attunement is ultimately an individual affair.

Classical Remedial Measures for the Doshas

Vata is treated by mild application of oils, mild sweating and purification methods; by sweet, sour, salty and warm food, and by oil massage; by staying indoors, by firm guidance, by anointing the eyes, by wine made from grain or sugar; by warm oil enemas, by moderate cleansing enemas, by comfortable living; by medicines that stimulate the digestive fire, by all kinds of oils, particularly by oil enemas with sesame oil or meat or animal fat broths.

Pitta is treated with the ingestion of ghee (clarified butter), by purgation with sweet and cold herbs; by sweet, bitter and astringent foods and herbs; by application of cool, delightful and fragrant essential oils; by the wearing of precious gems around the neck; by frequently anointing the head with camphor, sandalwood and vetivert oils; by relaxing in the moonlight, by beautiful songs, by a cool wind; by unrestrained enjoyment, by friends, by a devoted son; by a beautiful and attractive wife; by ponds with cool water, by houses with large gardens; especially by loving emotions; and by milk and ghee as laxatives.

Kapha is treated by strong emetic and purgation methods according to the rules; by food that is dry, little in quantity, sharp, hot and pungent, bitter and astringent in taste; by old wine, by sexual enjoyment, by staying up at night; by all kinds of exercise, by mental activity, by dry or strong massage; by smoking of herbs and, generally, by taking pleasure in physical hardship.

ASHTANGA HRIDAYA XIII. 1-12

The Ayurvedic methods traditionally used to balance the doshas are complex. They are not our modern "take this pill and come back in a week," but consider all aspects of life. It is important not only what we do but how we do it. We may take the right remedies, but if we take them with the wrong attitude they cannot be expected to work.

Vata people tend to do things hastily, irregularly or erratically. Pitta people tend to be fanatical or forceful and may apply things in a rigid or authoritarian manner. Kapha types are slow or conservative in what they do. All that we implement to balance our constitution should be based on an attitude that also compensates for it. It is not simply what we do but the manner and attitude in which we do it.

SYNOPSIS OF TREATMENT

Below is an outline of the main therapies for each dosha. These therapies are described specifically in other chapters.

ANTI-VATA THERAPY
Comprehensive Therapy for Reducing Excess Air

All anti-Vata (anti-air) therapies are nurturing, warming, moistening, calming and grounding. They should be done with patience, peace, consistency and regularity.

DIET

A nutritive, strengthening diet is indicated with predominately sweet, sour and salty tastes. Food should be warm, heavy and moist with frequent and regular meals. Spices should be used in cooking to regulate digestion. Cold water or ice should be avoided, as well as stimulating beverages such as coffee, though a small amount of wine or alcohol can be taken with meals.

HERBS

- Digestion—spices and salts: asafoetida, rock salt, garlic, ginger, cumin, fennel, coriander, cardamom, cinnamon, and ajwan.
- Elimination—bulk and tonic laxatives like psyllium and flaxseed, mild laxatives like Triphala, and oily purgatives like castor oil.
- Energy—special anti-Vata tonics: garlic, ashwagandha, bala, shatavari, black musali, white musali, kapikacchu, and amalaki. Other useful herbs include ginseng, dang gui, lycium berries, marshmallow, comfrey root, Solomon's seal, and saw palmetto.
- Mind—anti-Vata nervine herbs: calamus, ashwagandha, haritaki, jatamamsi, valerian, nutmeg, asafoetida, and basil. Other useful herbs include zizyphus seeds, biota seeds, and camomile.

OILS AND MASSAGE

Oil therapy is specific for Vata with warm, heavy oils like sesame and almond applied on a regular basis. The best sites are the feet, the top of the head, the back and the lower abdomen. Massage for Vata should be warm, moist, mild, nurturing, relaxing and not inducing pain or discomfort.

The best essential oils for Vata are warming, calming and clearing like sandalwood, camphor, wintergreen, cinnamon, and musk. These are also good for use as incense.

COLORS AND GEMS

Most colors are good for Vata (which tends towards depression), especially bright colors like yellow, orange and white and a small amount of red. Vata, however, is sensitive and lighter or more pastel shades are preferable to bright or metallic tones. Dark colors, grays, browns and blacks, should be avoided. Green and blue can be used in moderation or with warmer   colors.

The right gemstones are stabilizing and grounding for Vata. Special gems for the nervous system are best—emerald, jade, and peridot set in gold or yellow sapphire, topaz and citrine and other golden colored stones set in gold. Ruby or garnet can be helpful and improve circulation and energy.

YOGA

Calming and grounding asanas are indicated such as sitting and lying postures, as well as backbends and inverted poses done gently. Calm deep breathing practices are helpful, such as alternate nostril pranayama or Soham pranayama. Calming and fear-dispelling mantras like RAM, SHAM, HUM, HRIM, SHRIM are specific.

MEDITATION

Raja yoga is indicated for Vata types, which is an integral yoga combining knowledge, devotion and psychophysical techniques. The right attitude for meditation involves giving up worry, fear and anxiety, negativity and lack of faith.

LIFE-STYLE

Make sure to always get adequate sleep and do not stay up late at night. Practice moderate sunbathing and mild exercise. Avoid wind and cold, overwork or physical hardship. Avoid excess talking, thinking, or traveling. Practice moderation in sex and reduce excess stimulation including television, movies and radio. Develop peace and take care of your body with diligence.

PURIFICATION PRACTICES/PANCHA KARMA

Enema therapy is indicated as the main anti-Vata treatment in severe conditions. Nourishing herbs like licorice, ashwagandha and shatavari or oils like sesame are used for tonifying enemas. Vata dispelling herbs like calamus, ginger, fennel and rock salt work well for cleansing enemas.

Nasal therapy is also indicated with the taking of Vata clearing herbs like calamus, ginger and basil in the form of snuffs, decoctions, medicated oils or ghees.

ANTI-PITTA THERAPY

Comprehensive Therapy for Reducing Excess Fire

All anti-Pitta (anti-fire) therapies should be cooling and calming, moderately cleansing and nurturing. They should be implemented with an attitude of peace, restraint and moderation.

DIET

A balanced strengthening and reducing diet is indicated with mainly sweet, bitter and astringent tastes, along with adequate intake of raw food and juices. Food should be cool, heavy and a little dry, even in taste, without excessive spices. Water should be taken cool. Coffee and alcohol should be avoided but tea can be taken.

HERBS

- Digestion—digestive bitters like aloe, gentian, and barberry for medicinal purposes. Cooling or mild spices like turmeric, fennel, coriander, cumin, and mint are best for flavoring food.
- Elimination—bitter laxatives like aloe, cascara sagrada, rhubarb root and senna in acute conditions. Mild laxatives such as milk, ghee or rose, or bulk laxatives like psyllium husk powder are good in milder conditions.

- Energy—calming and cooling tonics: shatavari, bala, amalaki, saffron, aloe gel, licorice, and guduchi. Other useful herbs include comfrey root, Solomon's seal, marshmallow, dandelion root, burdock root, fo-ti, and rehmannia.
- Mind—cooling and calming herbs: gotu kola, bhringaraj, sandalwood, rose, and lotus seeds. Other useful herbs include skullcap, passion flower, betony, chrysanthemum, and hibiscus.

OILS AND MASSAGE

Use cooling oils such as coconut, sunflower or ghee for massage. For medicated oils, brahmi (gotu kola) or bhringaraj (eclipta), are best. They can be applied to the top of the head, forehead and heart.

Fragrances and flower essences are specific, such as sandalwood, vetivert, henna, rose, lotus, jasmine, gardenia, honeysuckle, and iris. They can also be used in the form of incense.

COLORS AND GEMS

The cooling colors white, blue and green are best, but generally any overly strong or very bright colors should be avoided, particularly red. Grays and browns are all right but dark black is not good.

Cooling gems are indicated such as moonstone, clear quartz crystal, emerald, jade, peridot, blue sapphire, and amethyst set in silver or white gold.

YOGA

Cooling and calming asanas are indicated such as most sitting or lying postures, and shoulderstand. Cooling pranayamas like shitali and lunar pranayama are best, as well as cooling and calming mantras like OM, SHAM, SOM, SHUM, and SHRIM.

MEDITATION

Yoga of knowledge or self-inquiry is generally appropriate, such as Vedanta, Zen, or Vipassana, along with giving up of anger, hostility, argument and an overly critical nature.

LIFE-STYLE

Too much sun and exposure to heat or heaters should be avoided. One should resort to cooling breezes, cool water, moonlight, gardens, flowers, and lakes. One should practice sweetness of speech, forgiveness and contentment.

PURIFICATION PRACTICES/PANCHA KARMA

Purgation is indicated with strong laxatives like rhubarb root, senna and aloe. For self-care, milder laxatives can be used—aloe gel, Triphala or psyllium husk powder.

ANTI-KAPHA THERAPY
Comprehensive Therapy for Reducing Excess Water

All anti-Kapha (anti-water) therapies are reducing, lightening, stimulating, drying and clearing. They should be applied with force and determination, as well as detachment.

DIET

A reducing diet emphasizes pungent, bitter and astringent tastes. Food should be warm, light and dry, prepared with hot spices. Occasional fasting or skipping a meal is good. Avoid eating early in the morning or late at night. Cold or ice water should be avoided as well. Herbal teas are good and regular tea can be taken as well.

HERBS

- Digestion—hot spices are indicated: cayenne, black pepper, dry ginger, pippali, mustard, cloves, cinnamon, garlic for improving metabolism. Bitters such as aloe, turmeric, barberry and gentian are useful for reducing the need for sugars and fats.
- Elimination—a combination of bitter laxatives like aloe, cascara sagrada, rhubarb root and senna along with spices like ginger, basil or cayenne.
- Energy—pungent or bitter tonics: garlic, pippali, cinnamon,

73

saffron, ginger, elecampane root, shilajit, guggul, myrrh and aloe gel.

- Mind—stimulants and mind-clearing herbs: calamus, gotu kola, basil, guggul and myrrh. Other useful herbs are sage, bayberry, skullcap and betony.

OILS AND MASSAGE

Dry or strong massage is good or massage with such light oils as mustard or flaxseed (linseed) oil. Rubbing alcohol or warm herbal oils prepared in alcohol, like wintergreen, camphor, eucalyptus, cinnamon, mustard and cayenne, are excellent.

Use stimulating and cleansing fragrances and incenses like musk, camphor, cloves, cinnamon, cedar, frankincense and myrrh.

COLORS AND GEMS

Use warm and bright colors like yellow, orange, gold and red. White should be avoided along with the white or pale shades of blue and green, and also pink. Brown, gray and black colors can be used in moderation.

Warm gems are indicated: ruby, garnet and cat's eye set in gold. Reducing gems such as blue sapphire, amethyst, and lapis, set in gold, can be good but should be combined with the warmer stones.

YOGA

Strong workouts are indicated with more active asanas, headstands if possible, and stretching of the chest. Solar pranayama, bhastrika (breath of fire) and other strong deep breathing exercises are good. Best are stimulating and clearing mantras like AIM, HRIM, HUM, and OM.

MEDITATION

The yogas of devotion (bhakti yoga) or service work (karma yoga) are generally best. Usually the divine is worshipped as a particular deity or incarnation, like Rama, Krishna, Christ,

Buddha or the Goddess. Renunciation of greed, desire, attachment and sentimentality is indicated for clearing the mind.

LIFE-STYLE

Strong and aerobic exercise should be done with walking, running and outdoor activity. Sunbathing is good with exposure to warm and dry breezes, and avoidance of cold and damp environments. One should follow a disciplined life, working hard, not sleeping early at night, and avoiding sleep during the day. Keep the mind stimulated with new thoughts, projects and information. Travel and pilgrimage are excellent.

PURIFICATION PRACTICES/PANCHA KARMA

Therapeutic vomiting is indicated with such expectorant herbs as calamus, lobelia, licorice, and salt in high dosages. For self-care, expectorant herbs can be taken in lower dosages including bayberry, sage, elecampane and ginger.

Balancing the Doshas in the Modern World

The factors of imbalance implicit in our modern life-style must be considered when implementing these life-regimens. Various aspects of our culture aggravate different doshas. Our dietary emphasis on sugars, ice cream, ice water, soft drinks, carbohydrates, meats and foods fried in oil increases Kapha. Our competitive social and business practices, our emphasis on personal achievement and success, as well as such habits as smoking and drinking aggravate Pitta.

However, the great majority of our practices increase Vata. Eating of junk food or food that has been microwaved aggravates Vata because the prana in the food has been depleted. Vata is aggravated by such modern life-styles as frequent traveling, particularly by plane. This dissociates us from the ground, literally raising us high into the air. Any form of transportation that removes us from direct contact with the earth increases Vata, even riding in cars. High speed increases Vata. The faster we drive the more that our Vata, our nervous energy, becomes hyper. Fast forms of sports, excessive running or skiing, for example, also have this effect.

We must consider the physical problems such practices create over time, particularly for people who work in these fields. Simple therapies should be done to compensate for them, such as having a foot massage; applying sesame oil to the feet; doing inverted yoga postures; or just walking barefoot on the earth.

The mass media has an influence that strongly aggravates Vata. We are affected not only by its message, which is change and mobility, but also by the subtle radiations that it emits. The physical body has a vital or energy sheath, the basis of Vata (the life-force). This can be short-circuited by excess exposure to waves given off by televisions and computers. We have become habituated to perpetual stimulation. The emphasis on superficial information keeps our minds in a state of want (emptiness that increases Vata) and perpetual distraction. Sitting in front of a computer all day can have an over-stimulating effect; playing computer games even more so.

Rock music, or any other frequent exposure to loud sounds or a high noise level, disturbs the nervous system and aggravates Vata. Sound is the quality that corresponds to ether (part of Vata, composed of air and ether), so excess or disharmonious sound will increase Vata.

Most drugs derange Vata, including both medicinal and recreational types, largely through their over-stimulation or disruption of nerve function. Stimulant drugs (uppers), weight reduction pills and pain-relieving drugs as well as amphetamines and cocaine are strongly disruptive. Marijuana and tobacco, followed by coffee and caffeine-containing soft drinks affect Vata in a milder way. Mind-altering drugs such as LSD or ecstasy aggravate Vata in a potentially severe manner. Artificially induced, temporarily heightened sensitization of the nervous system leads to either long-term desensitization or hypersensitivity. Symptoms of such Vata derangement include insomnia, constipation, dry skin, weight loss, vertigo or light headedness, loss of memory, loss of sensory acuity or coordination, tremors, palpitations and anxiety.

A number of New Age practices are highly Vatogenic (air-increasing). Channeling, forceful meditational practices, excessive imagination, or anything that may disrupt the connection of our life-force with our physical body, can increase Vata.

Excess sexual indulgence aggravates Vata by removing from our body its strongest energy of water (the reproductive fluid) to keep it in check. Our life style of easy divorce, frequent sexual partners, and broken families takes its toll here. The family or home itself has a Kapha or watery nature that is disrupted by excessive change. Such disturbances derange the Vata or life-force of all of its members, particularly the children who are more impressionable (who have not yet established a life center of their own).

There is no moral judgement in these statements but merely a question of energetics. Other cultures have their own characteristic imbalances as well. To the degree that we are involved in such activities, we invite imbalance.

These factors that imbalance Vata (and sometimes Pitta) are primarily rajasic. They also reduce sattva, harmony of mind. Our primary social values are materialistic ñ money, pleasure, fame and power. Our primary social behavior is constant action, stimulation, entertainment, and seeking—moving from one thing to another. We must consider the spiritual implications of our life styles. Health and harmony of the physical life should be the basis of the development of consciousness. If it is not possible or desirable to change the nature of our activity, we can at least adopt the appropriate remedial measures to compensate for its side effects.

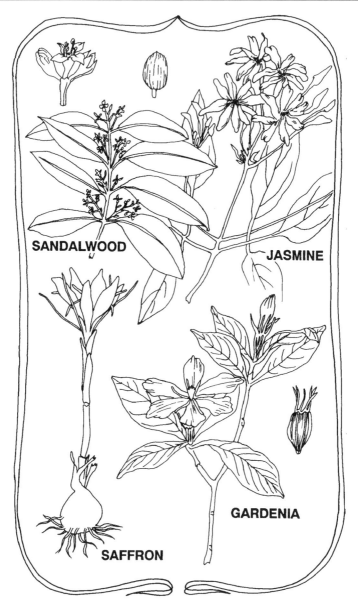

SANDALWOOD

JASMINE

SAFFRON

GARDENIA

I am food, I am the eater of food, and I eat the eater of food. I consume the entire universe. My light is like the Sun.

Taittiriya Upanishad II.9.6—PRIVATE

I.6
AYURVEDIC DIET
Personalizing Your Dietary Regimen

Dietary Therapy

Right diet is the main factor in the treatment of the physical body that is built up by food. Without changing our diet we cannot expect the body, which is its product, to change fundamentally whatever else we may attempt.Wrong diet is the main physical cause of disease. By correcting the diet, we eliminate the fundamental causes of disease. In its constitutional approach, Ayurveda emphasizes the correct diet for the individual as the basis for health.

Herbs and foods follow the same energetics and can be looked at according to the same principles. Both involve taste, energy, elements and doshas. Herbs provide subtle nutrition while foods provide more gross or substantial nourishment. Herbal therapy also requires the support of the proper diet to be effective. Diet can enhance, or counter, the effect of healing herbs. Generally, an inharmonious diet will either neutralize or greatly limit the effect of the right herbs and render them ultimately ineffective.

Diet can be an effective treatment in itself. Though dietary results are slower to manifest, over a period of time they are as certain as herbs. Dietary treatment is usually the safest therapy. It can be used by itself when herbal knowledge may not be adequate for a proper prescription. Diet is the essence of effective self-care.

Ayurveda is concerned primarily with the energetics of food as a means of balancing the doshas. It is not as concerned with the specific nutritional requirements, the actual mineral, vitamin and chemical content of food. From its view there is no standard diet for everyone, or any minimum daily requirements. Its concern is that the food we take in, and the manner in which we take it, is in harmony with our nature. Its primary classification of food is according to the doshas. This affords us a simple yet comprehensive understanding of what is good for us and why.

79

DIET AND THE MIND

In Vedantic philosophy the mind is considered to be the essence of food. The *Upanishads* state, "The food that is eaten is divided threefold. The gross part becomes excrement. The middle part becomes flesh. The subtle part becomes the mind." (Chandogya Upanishad VI.4.1.) According to the common adage, "We are what we eat." What we eat affects our emotions and can create a predisposition for both psychological and physical disorders. Just as wrong emotions can upset our digestion, so wrong digestion can upset our emotions.

We should consider also the spiritual qualities of the food we take in. Does it enhance our mental processes and peace of mind? Or is it disturbing? It is for this reason that meat, however nourishing, is not a good food. It has the energy of death and brings the forces of violence and decay, and the negative emotions of fear and hatred along with it.

The *Upanishads* also tell us, "The water that is drunk is divided threefold. The gross part becomes urine. The middle part becomes blood. The subtle part becomes the life-force." (Chandogya Upanishad VI.4.2.) What we drink nourishes our life-force. Drinking stale water, such as tap water or distilled water, and drinking alcohol, coffee or other stimulating beverages, will disturb our prana and derange our emotions and thoughts.

AYURVEDIC PRINCIPLES OF DIETETICS

While care should be taken about the nature of food, other factors of food intake should be considered as well. These include right preparation of food, right combination of foods, right amount of food, right frequency of meals and right times and places for eating. Right emotional or mental state is necessary; good food taken in a bad mood or ill dosha can cause disease. Also important is right attitude in the person preparing the food, which should be done with care and good feelings.

Seasons

The diet should be adjustable for climate and seasonal variations. An anti-Vata diet should be given emphasis in the fall. An anti-Pitta diet should be followed more in the summer and late spring. An anti-Kapha diet should be followed more in the winter and in early spring.

Individuals whose constitutions are equal in two of the doshas, what we call dual types, should vary their diet by season. Vata-Pitta types should follow an anti-Vata diet more in the fall and winter and anti-Pitta in the spring and summer. Vata-Kapha types should follow an anti-Vata diet in the summer and fall and anti-Kapha in the winter and spring. Pitta-Kapha types should follow an anti-Pitta diet in summer and fall and anti-Kapha in winter and spring.

Climate

- An anti-Vata diet is more appropriate to cold, dry, windy climates, like the high desert or high plains regions.
- An anti-Pitta diet is more suitable for hot climates including the southern United States and the lower desert of the southwest.
- An anti-Kapha diet is more appropriate in damp and cold regions like the Midwest, most of the east and northeast, and the Pacific northwest.

- Just like dual constitutions, dual climates also exist. The hot desert is a Pitta-Vata climate, while the southeast is largely a Pitta-Kapha climate.

Age and Sex

In old age an anti-Vata diet is more appropriate. In middle age an anti-Pitta diet is better. In childhood an anti-Kapha diet should be given special consideration. Men should consider a more anti-Pitta diet because male energy is more Pitta (fiery). Women should consider a more anti-Kapha diet because female energy is more

Kapha (water). Such general factors, however, should enhance, not replace, the basic diet for balancing one's dosha.

QUALITIES OF FOOD

Food is usually neutral, neither too hot nor too cold in energy. For this reason the heating or cooling effects of foods are mild. For heating or cooling to manifest, either large quantities or long-term consumption is necessary. Foods can be made hot by cooking and by the addition of spices; colder by taking them cold or raw. Anything very hot, like pepper, or very cold, like bitter herbs, cannot have much food value.

Foods are primarily heavy or light, though most tend to be heavy. It can be made lighter through the use of spices or by consuming less. Foods also are drying or moistening; most often they are moistening. They can be made drier by evaporation or dry-preparing them. They can be made moister by cooking or by the addition of liquids or oils.

DIETS FOR THE THREE DOSHAS

For the treatment of most diseases the diet prescribed will be opposite in nature to the dosha causing the disease. It will generally be the same diet as that for one's constitutional dosha; the diseases we get are usually caused by it. These diets should be applied considering the variations mentioned above and according to the proper dietetics. It is not only the types of foods we have to watch, but also our manner of eating.

Nor is it just a simple matter of avoiding the food that is bad for us. We must also improve our digestion through the use of spices, herbs and other regimens. Without these aids even the food that is good for us may not be digestible.

It should be noted that the quality of foods varies according to freshness, preparation and combination, as well as other factors already mentioned. The system presented here is only a general guideline. Some difference of opinion as to food quality may exist among different practitioners (even more so than about the quality of herbs).

Classification is also according to food categories. Each food type has its general degree of increasing or decreasing the dosha. When both the category and the specific food are high for increasing a dosha, the effect is greater. Foods not listed can generally be judged by category or by comparing them to related foods.

Foods are classified according to different degrees of increasing or reducing the doshas: * low degree, ** high degree.

Therefore, under the **YES** column:
- * **low degree for reducing the dosha**
- ** **high degree for reducing the dosha**

Under the NO column, a food marked:
- * **low degree for increasing the dosha**
- ** **high degree for increasing the dosha**

The best foods for each dosha are marked ** in the yes column. The worst foods are marked ** in the no column. A food that is * on the no column, for example, may be taken occasionally, or easily antidoted. On the other hand, a food marked ** on the no column should be generally avoided. Our predominant diet is what matters; we have some latitude within that field, except when we are very ill. Often the qualities of foods can be balanced by using the appropriate spices and condiments, particularly when their dosha aggravating affects are low.

ANTI-VATA DIET
Diet for Decreasing the Biological Air Humor

GENERAL CONSIDERATIONS

Vata types are most likely to suffer from emaciation, malnourishment or wasting away of tissues. Therefore dietary therapy, improving food quality and quantity, is one of the most important treatments for all Vata disorders. Vata types should generally try to eat more food and eat more frequently. They require a calming, grounding, nourishing diet. Food should be warm, heavy, moistening and strengthening.

The dominant tastes recommended for them are sweet, sour and salty. Pungent, bitter and astringent should be taken with discretion. Pungent taste, however, is excellent as a spice (rather than as food) for regulating appetite unless the individual has extreme enervation or hypersensitivity.

Vatas suffer from a variable digestive power. The heavy and nutritive foods that are good for them are not always digested properly. Care must be taken that the digestive fire is adequate for the food, or toxins may be produced from the improperly digested food mass.

DIETETICS

Meals should be small and frequent but regular. Food should be taken warm or cooked. Fast food, instant food and junk food should be avoided. Not too many different food types should be combined in the same meal. Mild spices and salt can be used.

Meals should not be taken when nervous, anxious or afraid, when excessively thoughtful or worried. Attention should be given to eating. Watching television, reading or other forms of nervous stimulation should be avoided during meals.

Vata types do better if they do not eat alone and if their food is cooked for them. So if you have a Vata friend, one of the best things you can do is to cook a meal for him or her. Vata individuals should learn to cook in order to help balance out their constitutions.

They also have the most irregular and erratic eating habits, and are most in need of a dietary regimen. They are likely to forget to eat, not want to cook, or when they do cook burn their food. On the other hand, when given a good meal they may overeat.

Vata people are more likely to suffer from food allergies; some foods that are normally good for them may have to be taken with care. Nightshades (potatoes, tomatoes, eggplant, peppers, and chilies) are the most typical in this regard. Yet often it is not the food that is the problem for Vata people, but their hypersensitivity, which can render anything indigestible. So rather than restricting the diet, it is usually better to take herbs and follow regimens to lower Vata.

FRUIT

Most fruit is fine for Vata as it is pleasant, harmonizing, clearing and increases body fluids. The main exception is dry fruit, which is particularly gas-forming (Vatogenic).

However, fruit is generally too light to really lower high Vata. It should be taken in moderation, seasonally, and not mixed much with other foods. Vata types should not become fruitarians (even if they live in Hawaii). Fruit contains a high percentage of the ether element. It can increase ungroundedness, lack of concentration, lack of will power and other high Vata traits if it becomes excessive in the diet.

YES	Apples (cooked)*, apricots*, bananas**, blueberries*, cherries*, dates (raw or soaked)**, figs (raw or soaked)**, grapes**, grapefruit**, lemons**, limes**, mango**, oranges**, papayas**, peaches*, pears*, persimmons*, pineapple**, plums*, pomegranate*, prunes (soaked or raw)**, raspberries*, strawberries*
NO	Dry fruit generally**, apples (uncooked)*, cranberries*, melons*,

VEGETABLES

Vata types cannot live primarily on a vegetable diet because it is too light for them, but they can tolerate most vegetables if they are cooked. Preparing them with oils and spices and eating them along with whole grains makes them better. Vatas should take raw vegetables and salads only moderately or in season with a fair amount of oil or dressing.

Cabbage family plants (cabbage, broccoli, cauliflower, Brussels sprouts, kale, and kohlrabi) cause gas. Mushrooms are diuretic and drying and can aggravate Vata. Raw onions are gas forming but cooked they are one of the best anti-Vata foods. Again, be careful of allergic reactions to nightshades.

Many vegetables in the no category, like potatoes, can often be made acceptable through application of spices, oils (sesame or ghee), cheese, sour cream, or salt.

YES	Avocado**, chilies**, beets*, carrots*, cilantro*, corn (fresh)*, green beans*, mustard greens*, okra*, onions (cooked)**, parsley*, peas (fresh)*, radish**, seaweed*, squash*, sweet potatoes**, turnips*, watercress*, yams**
NO	Alfalfa sprouts**, artichoke*, asparagus*, bell peppers*, broccoli**, Brussel sprouts**, cabbage**, cauliflower*, celery*, chard*

GRAINS

Most whole grains are good for Vata, as they are both nourishing and heavy. They can be digested by Vata types when other foods cannot. Following a long-term whole grain diet can alleviate many Vata diseases.

Grains that are drying (diuretic) like corn or rye can aggravate Vata. Yet even these are good in some Vata disorders that involve Ama or dampness (as the use of barley to treat arthritis).
Breads are more likely to aggravate Vata because yeast tends to cause gas. Their overall Vata-reducing property is less. Dried grains such as granola and most chips such as corn chips, tend to aggravate Vata.

YES	Basmati rice*, brown rice**, khus khus**, oats**, quinoa*, wheat**
NO	Granola and dried grains**, barley*, buckwheat*, corn*, millet*, rye*

BEANS

Most beans strongly aggravate Vata (cause gas). They are usually drying (diuretic) and promote constipation. Their quality is rajasic and so they can be over-stimulating. Tofu is one of the better beans for Vata but more sensitive Vata types may still find it hard to digest. Most Vata types will have to take some beans for protein, even those not the best for them. They should learn to cook the beans to antidote Vata, using spices like hing (asafoetida), cumin, ginger, and cayenne.

YES	Mung**, tofu*
NO	Aduki*, chick peas*, fava beans**, kidney beans*, lima beans*, peanuts*, pinto**, soy beans**, split peas*, urad dal*

NUTS AND SEEDS

Most nuts and seeds are good for Vata, particularly taken lightly roasted with salt. They are warm, heavy and moist and nourish the lungs, reproductive system and the nerves. But they are also hard to digest and cannot be taken in large quantities at a time. Dry roasted, they are more likely to cause difficulties in digestion (this also applies to peanuts).

YES	Almonds**, Brazil nuts**, cashews**, coconut*, filberts**, pecans**, pinenuts**, pistachio**, pumpkin seeds*, sesame seeds**, sunflower seeds*, walnuts**

DAIRY

Most dairy products are good for Vata because they are heavy, nourishing and moistening. But as dairy products tend to be cooling, heavy, or hard to digest, they should be taken with a proper consideration of the digestive fire. Most dairy products are better taken warm or with spices; milk should be taken by itself. Fermented dairy products are usually better for Vata as they are already predigested.

YES	Butter**, buttermilk*, cheese*, cottage cheese**, cream*, farmerís cheese (paneer)**, ghee**, goat milk*, kefir**, milk**, sour cream**, rice milk*, yogurt**
NO	Ice cream**, soy milk*

ANIMAL PRODUCTS

Meat and fish lower high Vata and are among the most effective foods in this respect. Vatas, more than the other types, can most honestly claim to benefit from meat in their diet, including red meat of all kinds. They sometimes find that it restores their health when nothing else seems to work (particularly if they have been raised on it). Yet even for these conditions, chicken and fish are usually enough. Eggs are also very good for reducing Vata.

While meat may be helpful short-term for some Vata conditions, in general it is not necessary. Meat is tamasic and has many side effects, including being difficult to digest, increasing Ama and dulling the mind. Because Vata types are the most sensitive they can pick up the negative energy of killing from the meat which disturbs their minds. Even in very high Vata conditions special tonic herbs can be used rather than meat and with greater effectiveness.

Oils

Most oils are good for Vata. Oil, being moist and warm, is the main substance indicated for lowering high Vata because it possesses the opposite properties. But oils can be hard to digest. They can be better applied externally because they can be absorbed more easily through the skin. Most of the vegetable oils tend to be light and are inferior to ghee and sesame oil for lowering Vata.

YES	Almond**, avocado*, butter**, coconut*, flaxseed*, ghee (clarified butter)**, mustard*, olive**, peanut*, sesame**
NO	Canola*, corn*, margarine**, safflower*, soy*

Sweeteners

Most sweeteners or sweet foods are good for Vatas. They need more sugar than other types for maintaining strength of the tissues and body fluids. Only natural sugars should be used; refined sugar is an artificial food that depletes the prana. However, pure sweets cause many difficulties in food combining. As Vata types most commonly suffer from gas, they must be particularly careful in how they combine sweets with other foods. Complex carbohydrates tend to be safer and more calming. Although sweet taste is good for Vata it is not an excuse for indulging in sugars, pastries and candies.

YES	Fruit sugar**, honey*, jaggery**, maple syrup**, molasses**, raw sugar**
NO	White sugar*

SPICES

Most spices are good for Vata, for regulating appetite and dispelling gas. They are particularly useful with heavy or sweet food to allow Vata types to digest them properly. Really hot spices, however, like pepper or mustard, can be overly drying or stimulating and aggravate some high Vata conditions. Yet, particularly in the winter, Vata individuals will find them helpful.

Vata types are most in need of salt, particularly for improving digestion, for which purpose rock salt is best. It should not be taken in excess as salt has the power to aggravate all three doshas. A good combination for Vatas is salted ginger along with the meals.

YES	Asafoetida**, basil**, bay leaves**, black pepper*, cardamom**, cayenne*, cloves**, coriander**, cumin**, cinnamon**, dill*, fennel**, fenugreek**, garlic**, ginger**, horseradish*, oregano**, mint*, mustard*, nutmeg**, paprika*, rock salt**, rosemary*, saffron**, sage**, sea salt*, soy sauce*, tamarind**, turmeric*

BEVERAGES

Vata types need to take adequate fluids. Water itself, however, is not nourishing enough. Dairy is preferable if problems digesting it do not exist. Herbal teas are excellent, particularly spicy teas like cinnamon and ginger taken with milk and a natural sweetener. Tonic herbs are also excellent. Sour fruit juices are good or water with lemon or lime.

Alcohol, particularly wine or Ayurvedic herbal wines such as draksha, is good in small quantities, 1-3 ounces, with or immediately before meals.

VITAMINS AND MINERALS

Vatas do well with oily vitamins like A, D and E. Sour vitamins like Vitamin C are also excellent. Minerals are good for them, particularly zinc and calcium, but they can be heavy and hard to digest and are best taken with spices.

ANTI-PITTA DIET
Diet for Lowering the Biological Fire Humor

GENERAL CONSIDERATIONS

Pitta types require a diet that is cool, slightly dry and a little heavy. They usually possess the best appetites and strongest digestions and can get away with excessive eating or with bad food combinations. The effects of wrong diet may manifest more through toxic blood and infectious diseases than through simple digestive upsets. The correlation between wrong diet and disease is not as easy to make in their case.

Tastes that decrease Pitta are sweet, bitter and astringent. It is increased by sour, salty and pungent. Sharp or strong tastes increase Pitta; mild or bland tastes decrease it. Hence, Pitta types should avoid tasty food.

DIETETICS

Pitta types should take food cool, raw, not heavily spiced and not cooked with a lot of oil. They should avoid fried and overly cooked food, and be careful not to clog the liver by a too rich diet.

Meals should not be taken when angry, irritable or upset. Pitta types should cultivate clarity rather than a critical nature in terms of what they eat. Food should be taken in an attitude of emotional calm and thankfulness. Three regular meals are usually sufficient. Eating late at night should be avoided.

FRUIT

Most fruit is good for Pitta as it is mainly cooling, calming, harmonizing and thirst relieving. Even sour fruit can be taken seasonally and bananas are OK occasionally, except in acute conditions like ulcers or urinary tract infections. Most fruit juices are good, particularly pomegranate, grape, pineapple and apple.

YES	Apples**, blueberry*, cranberry**, dates**, figs**, grapes**, limes*, mango*, melons**, oranges (sweet)*, pears**, persimmon**, pineapple**, plums*, pomegranate**, prunes**, raspberries*
NO	Apricots*, bananas*, cherries**, grapefruit**, lemons*, papaya*, peaches*, strawberries*

VEGETABLES

Most vegetables are good for Pitta, particularly if taken raw (though when in cases of debility or low energy, or during the winter, it is still better for Pitta types to take them cooked). They are also good steamed and taken with ghee but should not be fried, particularly deep fried. Nightshades, particularly tomatoes, but sometimes also peppers, eggplant and potatoes can aggravate Pitta by their acid content, as can chard and spinach.

YES	Alfalfa sprouts**, artichokes**, asparagus**, bell peppers*, bitter melon**, broccoli**, Brussels sprouts**, cauliflower**, cabbage**, celery**, cilantro**, corn (fresh)*, cucumber**, eggplant*, green beans**, kale**, lettuce**, mushrooms**, okra**, parsley*, peas (fresh)**, potatoes*, squash*, sunflower sprouts**
NO	Avocado*, beets*, carrots*, chard*, chilies**, onions (raw)**, onions (well cooked)*, radishes*, seaweeds*, spinach*, sweet potatoes*, tomatoes**, turnips*, watercress*, yams*

GRAINS

Most whole grains are good for Pitta, as they are strengthening and harmonizing but not overheating. Even those that increase Pitta do so only slightly; they should only be avoided as primary staple foods in the diet or in acute conditions. Most whole grain breads are also good, as is pasta.

YES	Barley**, basmati rice**, blue corn*, Brown rice (long grain)*, khus khus**, millet*, granola**, oats**, quinoa**, wheat**
NO	Brown rice (short grain)*, buckwheat*, corn*, rye*

BEANS

Pitta types, with their good digestive fires, are better able to digest beans than the other types. Even for them beans require spices like cumin so that they do not upset the digestion. Most beans are rather neutral for Pitta. When cooked in lard, as with many refried beans, they aggravate Pitta.

YES	Aduki**, chick peas*, kidney*, lima**, mung**, soy*, split peas*, tofu**
NO	Lentils**, peanuts*

NUTS AND SEEDS

Nuts are generally oily and warm and increase Pitta, all the more so if they are roasted and salted. However, they are less likely to increase Pitta than meat or fish, particularly when fresh; so they are preferable to these foods when strong nourishing food or protein sources are required.

YES	Coconut**, sunflower**
NO	Almonds**, Brazil nuts**, cashews**, filbert**, pecans**, pinenuts*, pumpkin seeds*, sesame*, walnuts**

OILS

Oils are Pitta (hot) in nature and should be generally avoided by Pitta types, except for those that are cooling. Animal oils are the hottest, then oil from nuts and seeds. Vegetable oils are the least warm in nature. Ghee and butter are best for Pitta as they possess a strong cooling nature.

YES	Butter**, coconut**, ghee**, sunflower*, soy*, Almond**,canola*
NO	corn*, flaxseed*, olive*, margarine*, mustard**, peanut**, safflower*, sesame**

I.6 Ayurvedic Diet

DAIRY

Pitta types are best able to digest dairy products, particularly milk. They do well with milk fasts for harmonization of body and mind. Sour dairy products, however, increase Pitta, as they possess enzymes that give them a warm energy. Pitta individuals can better digest ice cream than the other types.

YES	Cheese (unsalted)*, cottage cheese**, cream**, farmerís cheese (paneer)**, milk**, rice milk**, soy milk**
NO	Buttermilk*, cheese (salted)**, ice cream*, kefir**, sour cream**, yogurt**

ANIMAL PRODUCTS

Meat has a Pitta-increasing nature and provokes anger and aggression. Red meat is most severe in this respect. Pitta types like meat because it makes them feel strong and powerful but it often brings out their bad side. They usually do not need it and can get by as lacto-vegetarians. Should they take meat, white meat is preferable. Egg white is better for them than egg yolk. Most fish is not good for them because it is heating. This includes shellfish.

SWEETENERS

Pitta types can best handle sugar. They often need something sweet to cool and calm them down and harmonize their emotions, but for this same reason they can overindulge in sweets and suffer in the long run for it. Honey is cool in nature when fresh but becomes hot or Pitta increasing when it is over six months old.

YES	Fruit sugar**, honey (fresh)*, jaggary*, maple sugar**, raw sugar**
NO	Honey (old)*, molasses*, white sugar*

SPICES

Spicy food is one of the main causes of high Pitta. Nevertheless, Pitta types can take some spices, those that are neutral or cool in energy, particularly when eating heavy food. They should generally avoid salt but in the summer heat salt can be helpful for maintaining body fluids (along with sour juices). Pittas do well taking coriander in food, or cilantro (coriander leaf).

YES	Cardamom*, cilantro**, cloves*, coriander**, cumin*, dill*, fennel**, mint*, rosemary*, saffron**, turmeric*
NO	Asafoetida**, basil*, bay leaves*, black pepper**, cayenne**, cinnamon*, fenugreek*, garlic**, ginger*, horseradish**, oregano**, mustard**, nutmeg*, paprika**, rock salt*, sage*, sea salt*, soy sauce*, tamarind*

BEVERAGES

Pittas need adequate fluid intake. Cool spring water is good. Tea can be taken (black or green), but not coffee. Astringent herb teas are good such as alfalfa, raspberry leaf, hibiscus, dandelion and comfrey, but not too many spice teas except a little mint. Dairy is good, particularly milk. Pomegranate, pineapple or cranberry fruit juices are excellent, or vegetable juices such as celery and other green vegetable drinks. Avoid alcohol, beer and wine.

VITAMINS AND MINERALS

Pitta does well with B vitamins. Vitamin K is also good for stopping bleeding. They can use vitamin A for their eyes, which are often sensitive to light. Minerals like calcium and iron are important. Pitta types can usually digest raw vegetables well enough to extract most of what they need. They also can handle large mineral supplements without weakening the digestive fire, which tends to occur with the other doshas.

ANTI-KAPHA DIET
Diet for Decreasing the Biological Water Humor

GENERAL CONSIDERATIONS

Kapha types do best with a diet that is warm, light and dry. They should avoid food that is cold, heavy and oily. Accumulation of mucus in the system is a sign of taking too much Kapha-promoting foods.

Tastes that increase Kapha are sweet, salty and sour; those that decrease it are pungent, bitter and astringent. As most food is sweet in taste, Kapha types should take less food. Their main dietary therapy is in eating less and taking more herbs.

DIETETICS

Kapha individuals need to eat less in quantity and less frequency. They should have three meals a day with the main meal at noon, the other two light in nature. They also need to take less time in eating or in preparing food for themselves. They can direct the energy they give to eating towards preparing food for others (like their Vata friends).

It is better for them not to eat in the evening, particularly heavy foods. They should fast seasonally or one day a week. It is good for them to avoid breakfast. They should not sleep after eating. Generally, they should eat between 10 am and 6 pm, particularly rich, heavy or greasy food.

They should be careful not to use food as an emotional support for feeling loved or feeling secure, or as an attachment.

FRUIT

Fruit increases water in the system and may cause the formation of mucus. It is not generally prescribed for Kapha types, particularly when combined with other foods, particularly with milk or sugar. But fruit is light in nature and usually does not strongly increase Kapha, which is heavy. Some sour fruit, like lemon and grapefruit, can help reduce fat and dissolve mucus (not if taken with sugar, though honey is ok). Sweet fruit depresses the digestive fire. This is its main negative action in Kapha types.

YES	Dry fruit (generally)**, apple*, cranberry*, pomegranate*
NO	Bananas**, blueberry*, cherries**, dates**, figs**, grapes**, grapefruit*, lemon*, lime*, mango**, melons**, oranges**, papaya*, pears*, peaches*, persimmons**, pineapple**, plums**, pomegranate*, prunes*, raspberry*, strawberry*

VEGETABLES

Most vegetables are fine for Kapha, as they tend to be dry and light. Many vegetables, such as carrots and celery, are diuretic (reduce water). However, they should be taken warm, preferably steamed and with spices to counteract their generally cold nature, except in warm weather when they can be taken raw. Little oil should be used in their preparation and not much salt.

YES	Alfalfa sprouts**, artichokes*, asparagus**, beets*, bell peppers*, bitter melon*, broccoli**, Brussels sprouts**, cabbage**, carrots*, cauliflower*, celery**, chard**, chilies**, cilantro**, eggplant**, green beans**, kale**, lettuce**, mushrooms**, mustard greens**, parsley**, peas*, potatoes*, radish**, spinach**, sunflower sprouts**, turnips**, watercress**
NO	Avocado*, corn (fresh)*, cucumber**, okra*, seaweeds*, squash*, sweet potatoes**, tomatoes*, yams**

GRAINS

Many grains are not good for Kapha, as they are heavy and increase weight. Grains good for Kapha are nourishing with diuretic and expectorant (drying) properties. Kapha types do well on a diet of whole grains and steamed vegetables. Breads, however, tend to increase Kapha, as they are more sticky and mucus forming.

YES	Barley**, buckwheat*, corn**, dry or popped grains generally**, millet*, quinoa*, rye**
NO	Basmati rice*, brown rice*, khus khus**, oats**, wheat**, white rice**

BEANS

Most beans are good for Kapha, as they are drying and increase air. Tofu slightly increases Kapha, but it is still much better than dairy, meat or nuts and is one of the safer protein sources for Kapha.

YES	Aduki**, kidney*, lima**, lentils**, mung*, peanut*, soy**, split peas*, tofu*
NO	Chick peas*

NUTS AND SEEDS

Most nuts and seeds are not good for Kapha, as they are heavy and mucus forming. They tend to increase congestion. Again, as a protein source, they are preferable to dairy or meat and need not be avoided altogether.

YES	Pumpkin seeds*, sunflower seeds*
NO	Almond**, Brazil nuts**, cashew**, coconut**, filbert**, pecan**, pinenut**, sesame**, walnut**

OILS

Most oils are not good for Kapha, as they are moist and heavy (of the same nature as Kapha). They should be used in small amounts. Animal fats such as lard should be strictly avoided as they are much heavier than vegetable oils. Light oils, especially mustard, are best.

YES	Canola**, corn*, flaxseed**, mustard**, safflower**, soy*, sunflower**
NO	Almond**, avocado**, butter**, ghee*, margarine*, olive*, peanut*, sesame**

DAIRY

Kapha types should generally avoid dairy products, except for buttermilk or goat milk. Dairy products are especially mucus forming and promote congestion. For Kapha types dairy is often harder to digest than meat and may cause food allergies. Soymilk can be taken as a dairy substitute.

YES	Buttermilk*, goat milk**, soy milk**
NO	Cheese**, cottage cheese*, cow's milk**, cream**, ice cream**, kefir**, rice milk*, sour cream**, yogurt**

ANIMAL PRODUCTS

Kapha types generally do not need animal products, as they are less likely to suffer from tissue deficiency. Of meats, fowl, which is light in nature, is the least aggravating to Kapha. Chicken is better for Kapha than cheese but any form of meat will tend to increase Kapha in the long run. White or lean meat is better for them; fat should not be eaten. Eggs generally aggravate Kapha as well.

SWEETENERS

Sweet taste is the most highly aggravating for Kapha. Too much of it is perhaps their main dietary indiscretion and causes most of their diseases. The exception is honey, which has expectorant properties and a long-term drying effect.

YES	Honey (old)*
NO	Brown sugar**, fruit sugar**, honey (raw)**, jaggery*, molasses*, maple syrup**, white sugar**

SPICES

All spices are good for Kapha including the hot and peppery ones. Spicy taste is opposite in properties to Kapha, as it is hot and dry. They increase the metabolism to prevent fat and water from accumulating in the tissues. Salt, however, should be avoided, except in small amounts during the summer or when sweating a lot. Kaphas do well with peppery food (black pepper or cayenne).

YES	Asafoetida**, basil**, bay leaves**, black pepper**, cardamom**, cayenne**, cilantro*, cinnamon**, cloves**, coriander*, cumin*, dill*, fennel*, fenugreek**, garlic**, ginger**, horseradish**, mint*, mustard**, nutmeg**, oregano**, paprika**, parsley*, rosemary*, saffron*, sage**, soy sauce*, turmeric**
NO	Rock salt*, sea salt**, tamarind*

BEVERAGES

Kapha types need to drink less water and should avoid all ice and cold water. They can take regular tea, herbal teas, spice teas like ginger and cinnamon, and astringent teas like alfalfa, dandelion root or chicory root. Teas can be taken with honey but sugar and milk should not be used frequently. Coffee is all right taken occasionally.

VITAMINS AND MINERALS

Kapha types need less vitamins and minerals and more spices and enzymatic agents. Usually B vitamins are good for them but oily vitamins (A, D and E) should not be taken in excess. Heavy mineral supplements can also weaken digestive power further because of their heavy nature.

Sattvic or Yogic Diet for Improving the Mind

From the quality of Sattva is born knowledge, from Rajas comes greed, and from Tamas derives confusion, delusion and ignorance.
BHAGAVAD GITA XIV.17

Ayurveda, as a branch of yoga, is primarily a peaceful (sattvic) form of healing. Sattvic healing methods are natural, gentle, non-violent, non-traumatic, and non-invasive. They include such methods as herbs, diet, aromatherapy, bodywork, and yoga therapy.

Rajasic methods are forceful, rough, invasive, and traumatic. The healer's motivation is often the seeking of money or other personal goals. Surgery is the most typical rajasic therapy. Tamasic methods are heavy, dulling, insensitive, and inorganic. Drugs, though initially rajasic in their action, are tamasic in the long-term. Such harsher methods may be necessary in extreme or acute conditions but are quite limited as primary therapies for chronic diseases or for health maintenance.

The Sattvic diet was originally devised for the practice of yoga and the development of the mind. It is good for those who use their minds a lot because it improves mental quality and energy. It is important for treating mental disorders because it helps restore harmony and balance to the mind.

A Sattvic diet is good for convalescence from disease or after toxins have been removed. It aids in tonification and rebuilding of a higher quality tissue in the body, particularly for those who wish to improve their state of consciousness. It is often combined with rejuvenation (rasayana) therapies, particularly rejuvenation of the mind (Brahma rasayana).

A Sattvic diet consists of pure foods that are light in nature and mildly cooling in energy that do not disturb the mind. Foods rich in the life-force or prana are best. These include organic fresh fruit and vegetables. All foods produced by harming living beings are to be avoided, such as meat and fish. Foods prepared in toxic environments or with an excess of chemical fertilizers or sprays are also not acceptable.

A sattvic diet is generally healthful and balancing for all three doshas, with some modifications per type. However, as a sattvic diet is for improving the mind, it may not be nourishing enough for those who do physical labor. It sensitizes the mind but this may not be helpful for those who are already hypersensitive and easily disturbed by noise and stress. As such it may not be grounding enough for Vata (high air) conditions.

The classification of foods here follows the three Gunas or qualities of primal Nature. Sattva is pure, light, clear, calming, harmonizing, opens the mind and promotes wakefulness. Rajas is cloudy, agitated, turbulent, energizing and disturbs the emotions. Tamas is dark, heavy, dulling and promotes lethargy. It contracts and closes the mind.

Sattvic Diet and the Six Tastes

• Of the six tastes only sweet taste is considered generally sattvic. By this is meant naturally sweet taste as in fruit. It is pleasant, harmonizing and nourishing and reflects the energy of love.

- Pungent, sour and salty tastes are rajasic. They are stimulating and potentially irritating.
- Bitter and astringent tastes are tamasic. Their long-term affect is to cause rigidity.

Pungent taste irritates the nerves by its dispersing property. Sour and salty aggravate the emotions through heating the blood. Bitter and astringent have a constricting affect that can hold in toxins or weaken our energy. This classification of the six tastes is general and mainly in terms of food value. The effects of the tastes vary as to quantity and usage of the tastes.

Too much sweet food becomes tamasic or dulling. This is particularly true of old or artificially prepared sweets. Some bitter herbs, like gotu kola, are sattvic because bitter taste being composed of air and ether elements opens the mind. Some spices with sweet fragrances, like ginger or cardamom, are sattvic. Excessive eating is tamasic, while light eating is sattvic. A sattvic diet is bland and even in taste, not going to any extremes.

FRUIT

Fruit is sattvic (pure) in nature. It is sweet, light and promotes contentment. It has large amounts of the element ether, which controls and balances all the other elements. All fruit is generally good for a yogic diet or improving the mind. It harmonizes the stomach, relieves thirst, calms the heart and improves perception. It both cleanses and nourishes body fluids. It is preferable to take it fresh and in season.

Some yogis, however, avoid heavy, sweet fruit, such as bananas, as they are mucus forming and may clog the channels.

VEGETABLES

Most vegetables are good for a sattvic diet, though not as much as fruit. This is because vegetables contain a greater amount of bitter and astringent tastes than fruit.

Mushrooms are regarded as tamasic because they are allied with decay. However, Chinese Buddhists include many mushrooms as good for a diet promoting meditation, something that has proven true in my own experience. But the mushrooms must be collected fresh or properly dried. Otherwise they can easily cause indigestion.

Pungent vegetables—garlic, onions, radishes and chilies—are rajasic and tamasic and can stimulate the sexual nerves. Excess of cabbage family plants—cabbage, broccoli, Brussels sprouts and mustard, and cauliflower—are rajasic or gas forming. Potatoes and sweet potatoes can be a little heavy or mucus forming in excess. Otherwise fresh or steamed vegetables or vegetable juices are quite sattvic. Celery is particularly good for the brain.

GRAINS

Grains, like fruit, are sattvic in nature, especially rice (basmati or long grain brown rice). Wheat and oats are also good. Whole grains are preferable but breads are also sattvic, though to a lesser degree. Grains are usually the main staple food in a sattvic diet because they allow for an even release of energy over a long period of time that allows the mind to stay clear, grounded and focused.

BEANS

Beans are usually rajasic in nature, as they are irritating, gas forming and heavy. Exceptions are mung beans, aduki beans and tofu, which go well with Sattvic diets. Equal parts split mung beans and basmati rice (called kicharee) is the basic yogic staple diet and the main simple food for purification or for convalescence in Ayurveda.

NUTS AND SEEDS

Seeds and nuts are sattvic in nature. They should be taken fresh or lightly roasted, not heavily roasted and salted, which reduces their value. Almonds, pine nuts, pecans and walnuts are particularly good. As nuts are a little heavy, they should not be taken in large quantities. Nuts and seeds go rancid (become tamasic) easily.

DAIRY

Dairy products are naturally sattvic in nature. Pasteurized, however, they lose much of this quality. Milk is produced by the love of the cow for its calf. When the cow is separated from its calf this quality of love in the milk is easily lost. For this reason if we do use dairy products, and they can be very helpful for certain body types, we should strive to use raw, organic or humanely prepared items.

A milk fast, or buttermilk fast, is an important part of a yogic diet and helps revitalize the skin and plasma. Milk is a good food for convalescence, particularly from conditions of blood loss or wasting diseases. It can be used almost like an IV for hydrating the tissues. Yogurt is also good but is a little heavy and should not be taken in excess or it can clog the channels. Cheese is generally heavy and so not recommended on a regular basis, except for lighter cheese, cream cheese, farmer's cheese (paneer) and cottage cheese.

OILS

Most oils are heavy and not recommended in large amounts. Ghee or clarified butter is sattvic, promotes intelligence and perception and can be freely used. It can be added to grains or to cooked vegetables. Sesame oil is sattvic, as is coconut. Olive oil is also good but not with garlic (which makes it rajasic).

SWEETENERS

Sweet taste in moderation is sattvic, but refined sugars are tamasic. Yogic diet takes raw sugars in small amounts, including honey (preferably unheated) and raw sugar, particularly jaggary. It is said that sweet feeds Shakti (the power of awareness).

SPICES

Most spices are rajasic but a number of exceptions exist. Sattvic spices include ginger, cinnamon, cardamom, turmeric, basil, fennel and coriander. They help balance the effect of too much fruit, dairy or other dampness forming foods. Some yogis also use black pepper

103

or pippali to dry excess mucus and keep the channels open. Here rajas is used to counter tamas, thus producing sattva indirectly. Such strategic variations should be kept in mind.

Salt should avoided except in the summer or in hot climates. Then it is best combined with lime.

BEVERAGES

Pure spring water is good, as are sattvic herb teas like ginger, or milk. Coffee and other stimulants should be avoided. Green or black tea (in moderation), however, is fine and is thought to improve mental functioning.

DIETETICS

Meals should be simple and infrequent, usually three a day. The main meal is usually taken around noon, with no heavy food before 10 am or after sunset. Sattvic meals require preparation with love and awareness. These enhance the sattvic (spiritual) and life-supporting properties of any food.

HERBS

Most tonic herbs such as ashwagandha, shatavari, amalaki, ginseng, astragalus or comfrey root are sattvic and can be an important energy supplement to a Sattvic diet. Chyavan Prash, Brahma Rasayana and such Ayurvedic jellies are very sattvic.

Many herbs for the mind are useful in a sattvic diet. Gotu kola (brahmi) gives clarity, calm and coolness to the mind. Calamus is particularly good for clearing the channels, promoting perception and improving speech. Other good sattvic herbs for the mind are jatamamsi, shankha pushpi, lotus, and bhringaraj. Good Western and Chinese herbs for the mind that are sattvic in nature include skullcap, sage, zizyphus, and biota seeds.

Rajasic and Tamasic Diets

Rajasic and tamasic foods disturb or dull the mind and produce diseases. Rajasic foods aggravate Vata and Pitta. Tamasic foods increase Kapha and Ama (toxins). Rajasic foods cause hyper-activity, restlessness, irritability, and insomnia, increase toxins in the blood, cause bleeding and promote hypertension. Tamasic foods cause hypoactivity, lethargy, apathy, excess sleep, and accumulation of phlegm and waste materials.

Rajasic food includes most overly tasty food. It is excessively spicy, salty and sour—chilies, garlic, onions, wines, pickles, excess salt, mayonnaise, sour cream, and vinegar. Meat is also rajasic (irritating), particularly red meat, though it has tamasic properties as well. Food too hot in temperature is rajasic. Most fried food or roasted and salted food is rajasic. Rajasic food is usually taken with stimulating (rajasic) beverages like coffee or alcohol.

Tamasic food is stale, old, recooked, rancid, artificial, greasy or heavy. It includes all 'dead' food, all meat and fish, particularly pork and animal organ parts. Most canned food is tamasic as well. Poor quality dairy products are at least in part tamasic, particularly those produced by factory farms. Excessive intake of fats, oils, sugars and pastries is tamasic. White sugar and white flour have a long-term tamasic effect (though short-term white sugar is rajasic). Food that is too cold is also tamasic.

SATTVIC DIET AND DIETS FOR THE DOSHAS
SATTVIC VATA DIET/ SPIRITUAL ANTI-AIR DIET
Vata constitutions are prone to rajas or agitation. Their diet, therefore, includes food articles that are sattvic or tamasic in order to counter this. For a sattvic Vata diet, tamasic items should be eliminated including garlic and onions, meat and fish. Rajasic spices, which are sometimes used for Vata like cayenne, black pepper, mustard, and asafoetida should be used with discretion. Salt should not be used in excess.

SATTVIC PITTA DIET/ SPIRITUAL ANTI-FIRE DIET
Pitta types tend towards rajas, but not as much as Vata. They can easily follow a sattvic diet. The regular anti-Pitta diet is predominately sattvic. Pittas only need to remove a few rajasic items

from their diets. Such are mainly beans (other than mung, aduki and tofu) and meat, which should not be taken. Excess of sugar and overeating are also contrary to this approach.

Sattvic Kapha Diet/ Spiritual Anti-water Diet

Kapha people incline to tamas, as they easily develop heaviness, inertia, congestion and stagnation. Generally, many rajasic foods and spices are recommended for them to counter this. A sattvic Kapha diet is, therefore, more restrictive than the usual anti-kapha diet. It requires, in addition to the regular Kapha diet, reducing hot spices, avoiding beans (except mung, aduki and tofu), and avoiding meat. Sattvic spices should be freely used, particularly ginger, cinnamon and cardamom, and whole grains like corn or millet for strength.

I.7
AYURVEDIC THERAPIES
The Methods of Reintegration 1
TONIFICATION AND REJUVENATION

Tonification and Reduction

Ayurveda employs a whole range of therapies. Yet they can all be simply defined under two groups, *tonification* and *reduction*, also called supplementation and elimination. Reduction, *langhana*, means "to lighten"; Tonification, *brimhana*, means "to make heavy".

Reduction therapies decrease excesses in the body and are indicated for overweight, accumulation of toxins, and aggravated doshas. They aim at eliminating the factors that cause disease. Tonification methods nourish deficiencies in the body and are indicated for underweight, debility, or tissue weakness. They work at building up inadequate energy or lack of substance in the body that may bring disease about.

Reduction methods are indicated in the acute stage of disease, when the attack is strong, like sweating therapies for a common cold or bitter herbs for fevers. They are also employed to eliminate deep-seated toxins as part of disease prevention, internal cleansing programs, like using purgatives to cleanse the colon.

Tonification is indicated in chronic disease, in convalescence, for the debilitated or malnourished, or after reduction methods have been used. *The usual rule is first to reduce and then to tonify*. If we tonify first we may feed toxins or excess doshas in the body and make conditions worse. In this regard, most of us can benefit from some reduction methods, if only to purify our systems to make use of tonic herbs. However, there are conditions when an individual is too weak for reduction methods and tonification must be given first. The two methods may be combined to some degree, particularly for long-term therapies.

This twofold division of therapies is similar in Chinese Medicine. In Chinese Medicine, reduction is used for external pathogenic factors like heat, cold, wind, dampness or dryness. Therapeutic methods, such as promoting sweating, elimination or

107

urination, are employed to remove these factors and the diseases that they cause. Tonification is of yin, yang, chi or blood, the primary constituents of the body.

Reduction therapy is called *discontenting* (asantarpana) because it includes practices of discipline, hard living and giving things up. It makes us doubt ourselves and question who we are and what we are doing. It stimulates us to change and give up wrong habits.

Tonification is called *gladdening* (santarpana) therapy because it consists of methods to give us greater nourishment, care, relaxation, ease and enjoyment. Tonification therapy aims at making us feel better about ourselves. It encourages faith, love and positive attitudes.

INDICATIONS OF REDUCTION AND TONIFICATION

Reduction is indicated primarily for Kapha constitutions, while tonification is mainly for Vata. This is because the main attribute of Kapha is heaviness, while that of Vata lightness. Kaphas accumulate excesses in the form of excess weight, water or mucus. Vatas are prone to deficiencies in the form of underweight, dryness or debility. Pittas usually require a mixed therapy, with some degree of both reduction and tonification. Generally Pittas need to reduce heat and inflammation but rebuild tissue damaged by them.

The anti-Kapha life-regimen and diet is generally reducing. The anti-Vata life-regimen and diet is generally tonifying. Those of Pitta fall in between. The reduction methods for Kapha are strong like fasting or vomiting therapy. For Vata they are mild, enema therapy or a nutritive diet. For Pitta they are moderate like purgation.

Tonification methods for Vata, conversely, are strong, with powerful tonic herbs such as ashwagandha or ginseng. Tonification for Kapha is mild, with herbs for supplementation that are not too heavy, like elecampane or pippali. Tonification for Pitta is moderate with cooling tonics such as shatavari or aloe gel.

Tonification and Rejuvenation

Tonification therapy is indicated for the elderly, for pregnant women, for women who have just given birth, for children, for the debilitated, emaciated, convalescent, those suffering from anemia, malnutrition and nervous exhaustion. It is the primary therapy for Vata types and conditions.

The main season for tonification therapy is the fall, when the dryness and lightness of Vata prevails. Yet it can be initiated any time when significant debility exists. Most of us require a certain degree of tonification in the late fall to give us the weight and strength to endure the vicissitudes of winter. It is particularly useful in cold climates or when we will be doing outdoor work and exercise in the cold.

Tonification is contraindicated in Ama conditions (where an undigested food mass exists), for the obese, during colds or flus, congestive disorders, fevers or infectious diseases. It should be applied with care when allergies exist. As tonic foods and herbs are hard to digest, the state of the digestive fire must always be considered before administering them.

MEANS OF TONIFICATION

Tonification is described as nourishing the body with:

Meat, milk, raw sugar, ghee and honey, with oil enemas; by sleeping and resting freely; by oil massage; by baths and by comfortable life-style.
ASHTANGA HRIDAYA XIV. 9-10

The main method is dietary: rich, nutritive food, along with strong, tonic herbs, mild massage, rest and relaxation. It includes much oleation therapy with both external as well as internal use of oils.

Work, both physical and mental, should be reduced as much as possible. One should go to bed early and sleep as much as desired. Sexual activity should be reduced. According to the *Yoga Sutras*, the classical work on yoga, sexual abstinence is the best means of gaining energy. Breathing exercises such as Pranayama or Qi Gong also build energy in a primary way. Stimulation, including most of our mass media entertainment, should be reduced as it disperses the prana.

It is preferable to take a vacation in nature, like a mountain cabin, or at least stay in a comfortable and peaceful place for awhile. It may not be possible for us to do all of these; but tonification therapy can still be effective if we persist in several major tonification procedures over time.

Tonification is much simpler than elimination therapy. Many different methods and routes of elimination exist like purgation, vomiting or sweating while tonification involves one primary method, increased nutrition. Yet tonification is not just a matter of eating more. Ayurveda uses ways to increase nutrition through the skin, the nose and the colon as well as the mouth through different oil applications. These allow a broader tonification therapy and show the comprehensive nature of the Ayurvedic approach.

EXTERNAL APPLICATION OF OILS

In reduction or detoxification approaches, oils are applied externally to help liquefy toxins, so they can be eliminated more easily. In tonification therapy, oils are applied to nourish the body through the skin. The effects of such nutrients extend to the bones and the nerve tissue, a direct penetration.

Because external application of oils bypasses the digestive tract, many oils can be used that can be difficult to digest. Good oils for tonifying oil massage include sesame, almond, olive, coconut, and avocado, as well as various special medicated sesame oils. As mentioned previously, care must be taken because external oils tend to depress the digestive fire and the other fires of the body (like Bhrajaka Pitta that imparts luster to the skin).

INTERNAL USE OF OILS

Oils are the main substances for tonification internally as well. We should add such oils to our diet in the form of ghee, but-

110

ter, sesame oil or various animal fats and meat broths if we are not vegetarian. These oils go well with rice, beans or curries. Spices like turmeric, ginger and black pepper are necessary so that we digest these oils properly.

Tonifying Enemas

Oils can be taken through the rectum in the form of enemas. Vata types can take an enema of 1/2 cup of warm sesame oil mixed with 1/2 cup of warm water in the evening (and preferably hold it at least twenty minutes) as part of tonification therapy.

Tonic herbs can be taken through the rectum. Ashwagandha, shatavari or licorice can be made into decoctions and taken rectally. Milk decoctions or meat and bone soups can be used. These can be very helpful, particularly in debility conditions and serve something like an I.V. to hydrate the tissues.

Tonifying Nasal Medications/ Nasya

Tonic substances can be taken through the nose. Ghee, sesame oil or herbs to nourish the brain, such as gotu kola, calamus or licorice, work well this way. One can take a few drops of such Nasya mixtures into the nose daily. Note, if you do take herbal decoctions into the nose, make sure that there is a little salt and sesame oil along with the herbs so that they donít irritate the mucus membranes of the nose.

Foods for Tonification Therapy

A tonification diet is similar to an anti-Vata (anti-air) diet, but can be adjusted according to the doshas. This diet can be used as a strengthening diet for conditions of debility and for finding meat substitutes. It can be followed to increase vigor for doing harder work, even for those who are otherwise healthy.

Dairy Products

Dairy products are the best forms of animal food because they do not involve killing the animal. They are effective meat substitutes and important foods for debility and convalescence. Milk or buttermilk fasts are good for rebuilding energy, particularly after dehydration, tissue loss or poor digestion.

Milk is good for restoring vigor and vitality. It strengthens the lungs, stomach and reproductive system and increases Ojas. Ghee is the best food for restoring vitality, nourishing the nerves and improving Ojas. It also strengthens the digestive fire. Buttermilk, though not as building, is the easiest to take and improves absorption.

Good dairy products for tonification therapy include ghee, butter, cream, milk, buttermilk, yogurt, sour cream, cottage cheese, cream cheese, and cheese. Again, make sure to take these with the appropriate spices like ginger, cardamom or cayenne to render them more digestible and less likely to produce mucus.

OILS
Oils are the essence of tonification therapy and are important meat substitutes as well. Helpful oils include ghee, butter, sesame, almond, olive, and avocado. But most other oils are also good. However, avoid light oils like canola, corn or mustard.

NUTS AND SEEDS
Nuts and seeds strengthen the nerves and the reproductive system and improve vitality. They are excellent meat substitutes. Nut butters are also good. Good nuts for tonification therapy include almonds, pecans, walnuts, pinenuts, cashews, coconut, black sesame seeds, and lotus seeds.

GRAINS
Whole grains have good strengthening properties. They are mild and easy to digest in convalescence but are not as directly strengthening as dairy or nuts. Strongest are wheat, oats and brown rice. Whole grain breads can also be helpful. Wheat gluten itself is very good. Kicharee—equal parts basmati rice and split mung beans—is one of the best basic foods for tonification or reduction methods. It can be digested when nothing else can.

BEANS

Beans are good sources of protein and work as meat substitutes. As they increase Vata, however, they are better meat substitutes for Kapha and Pitta. A few are especially good foods for convalescence and improving vitality, such as black gram, chickpeas, mung, and tofu.

STRENGTHENING FRUITS AND VEGETABLES

Most fruits and vegetables are too light to be really strengthening. There are some exceptions: sugars in fruit improve vigor and rebuild tissues. Strengthening fruits include dates, raisins, figs and jujubes, and juices like pomegranate and black grape.

Some mushrooms are considered good meat substitutes and to be Chi or energy tonics in Chinese medicine and can be quite helpful, including ordinary mushrooms, shitaki, portabella mushrooms and chanterelles. Starchy vegetables can be tonifying like okra, potatoes, sweet potatoes, yams and Jerusalem artichokes. Onions, particularly cooked in ghee, are one of the most strengthening foods.

STRENGTHENING SPICES/CURRIES

Spices can have the very yang, warming, strengthening effect of meat when combined with oils like ghee. The combination of spices and oils in curries is the basis of Indian cooking, which normally does not use meat.

The best strengthening spices are garlic, ginger, cinnamon and pippali, which give vigor. Black pepper, cardamom, cloves, fennel, cumin, cayenne and asafoetida are also useful, particularly cooked in oils such as ghee and taken along with other tonic foods.

SUGAR AND SALT

Raw sugars give strength and build all tissues, but care should be taken with food combination. Ayurveda considers jaggary, crude raw sugar, to be the best because it is the richest in minerals and the easiest to digest. Other helpful sugars include raw honey, raw sugar, maple syrup, rock candy, molasses, malt sugar, lactose, and fructose. Adequate salt intake is part of the tonification diet, particularly rock salt.

Rejuvenation

Rejuvenation (Rasayana) is a special form of tonification therapy. It follows deep cleansing like Pancha Karma, and the elimination of excess doshas from the body, because real renewal is only possible once the factors of decay have been taken away. Though its methods are similar, it is different from general tonification therapy that can be given in any debilitated condition.

Rejuvenation diet is essentially the same as tonification diet. The herbal treatment is similar as well. The emphasis is on substances to increase Ojas (primary vitality) and improve sattva (mental clarity). For this reason some of the heavier substances for tonic therapy, such as meat, are not recommended for rejuvenation.

When rejuvenation of the mind (Brahma Rasayana) is the aim, sattvic and tonification diets must be combined. Special herbs for the mind like gotu kola, calamus and shankha pushpi are used. One should engage in asana, pranayama and meditation, preferably in a retreat situation for a period of at least two weeks.

TONIC AND REJUVENATIVE HERBS

There is a whole class of tonic herbs in Ayurvedic and Chinese medicine, as well as several Western herbs of similar properties. These are the prime tonic and rejuvenative substances to take.

TONIC HERBS AND FORMULAS

Prime Ayurvedic Tonic Herbs	Ashwagandha, shatavari, amalaki, bala, kapikacchu, shilajit, white musali, vidari kanda, vamsha rochana
Ayurvedic Tonic Formulas	Chyavan Prash, Ashwagandha compound, Shatavari compound, Dhatupaushtic powder, Triphala
Prime Chinese Tonic Herbs	Ginseng, astragalus, fo ti, rehmannia, lycium, schizandra, dioscorea, dang gui, cuscuta
Chinese Tonic Formulas	Four Gentlemen, Four Materials, Women's Precious Pill, Major Ten, Rehmannia 6, Rehmannia 8
Prime Western Tonic Herbs	Licorice, comfrey root, marshmallow, slippery elm, Solomonís seal, saw palmetto, spikenard
Common Tonic Foods	Milk, ghee, lotus seeds, almonds, sesame seeds, cashews, dates, raisins

Tonic Herbal Preparations

MILK DECOCTIONS

Powerful tonic drinks can be prepared by cooking powdered tonic herbs like ashwagandha, shatavari, comfrey root or ginseng in raw milk, generally 1-2 teaspoons of the herb per cup of milk. To enhance the tonic effect, one or two teaspoons of ghee, or a little raw sugar can be added before drinking (note that honey and ghee should not be used in equal proportions, as this is thought to be unhealthy). A small amount of a spice like ginger or cardamom should be added as well to aid in taste and digestibility.

HERBAL JELLIES

Ayurveda has a whole class of medicated jellies, prepared with such ingredients as tonic herbs, ghee, honey, raw sugar and various spices. They work best as part of tonification therapy.

Chyavan Prash is the most famous Ayurvedic jelly. Its prime ingredient is the tropical fruit amla or amalaki. Amla is the highest natural source of vitamin C. It retains the vitamin C content because it is bound up with the tannins in the fruit. Amla is a powerful tonic and builds the blood and reproductive fluids and nourishes the heart, lungs and kidneys. It is usually taken 1-2 teaspoons morning and evening, preferably with warm milk for better tonic action.

Brahma Rasayana, another important herbal jelly, is prepared with gotu kola (brahmi). It is excellent for tonifying the mind and nerves and building the prana.

HERBAL WINES

Ayurvedic herbal wines have warming and tonifying properties that make them into strengthening foods. They help build tissues and also improve Agni. Many of them are prepared with tonic herbs, such as ashwagandha, whose properties they enhance.

Draksha is the main basic herbal wine prepared with raisins and spices. It is not only good for maintaining the strength of the digestive fire, but also helps restore vitality. It is generally taken in doses of one tablespoon along with meals. Other good herbal wines include Ashwagandha wine, Aloe wine and Bala wine. Ashwagandha herbal wine, taken 1-2 teaspoons morning and evening, is great for giving strength and countering debility.

MEDICATED OILS

Medicated oils are mainly for external application. They are essential for the external part of tonification therapy. Many are made with tonic herbs such as ashwagandha, shatavari and bala and can help rejuvenate the body through absorption via the skin.

MEDICATED GHEES

Tonic herbs prepared in ghee gain additional strengthening properties. Ghee builds Ojas and sexual vitality, gives strength to the nerves and the mind, and helps increase fat and muscle in the body, without being overly heavy. To make medicated ghees, the usual procedure is to decoct the herbs in water and then add the water to the ghee (in usually four times the amount of the ghee) and gradually boil the water away until only the ghee is left. Most easy to make is licorice ghee. For the mind, calamus ghee is best. Ashwagandha ghee is also very good. Almost any tonic herb can be made as a medicated ghee. These are usually taken in one teaspoon dosages along with food or in warm milk.

116

I.8
AYURVEDIC THERAPIES
The Methods of Reintegration 2
DETOXIFICATION AND PANCHA KARMA

REDUCTION THERAPY

There are many different forms of detoxification, purification or reduction therapies. Any therapy which aims at eliminating or reducing something, whether it is promoting sweating, urination, or excretion, or reducing a fever, weight or water falls in this sphere. All of these are used in Ayurveda.

Reduction therapy in Ayurveda has two parts called palliation and purification. Palliation, Shamana, means calming or pacifying. It is largely for reducing Ama, the undigested food mass, and calming the doshas so they can be dispelled from the body through purification therapy. The dosha may be mixed with toxic accumulations, which irritate it and make its symptoms more complex. This mass must first be separated from the dosha to enable us to work on it directly.

Palliation Therapy

Palliation has seven parts:
1. Herbs for burning up toxins
2. Herbs for stimulating the digestion
3. Fasting from food
4. Fasting from water
5. Exercise
6. Sunbathing
7. Exposure to wind

These methods strengthen the digestive fire, Agni, and destroy toxins. They cleanse the digestive tract and allow the toxins in the deeper tissues to drain into it so they can be eliminated.

Purification Therapy

Purification, Shodhana, is a special therapy to eliminate disease-causing doshas. It does not refer to any application or reduction methods, nor can it be done without the proper preparation. The power and efficacy of Ayurvedic purification therapy comes through its system for guiding the toxins to their sites for elimination. Merely to flush out various organs is not effective if the toxins are not located at these sites.

Ayurvedic purification therapy is indicated when the aggravated doshas are in the G.I. tract. If they are mixed with the tissues, waste materials of the body or with Ama, the undigested food mass, they cannot be directly eliminated. Palliation methods must first be applied instead.

Purification therapy consists of five parts known as Pancha Karma, the five cleansing actions. They are the most radical way to cleanse the body and eliminate once and for all the disease-causing doshas.

1. *Vamana*, Therapeutic vomiting
2. *Virechana*, Therapeutic purgation
3. *Basti*, Medicated enemas
4. *Nasya*, Nasal medications
5. *Rakta Moksha*, Therapeutic release of toxic blood

The patient should have some strength to undergo Pancha Karma because these methods can be strongly reducing. Some of these methods can be used as part of other therapies. Purgation, for example, can be used by itself to treat many diseases like gallstones or kidney stones. These methods are sometimes applied in acute diseases, for instance, the use of vomiting therapy to treat asthmatic attacks. They can also be part of constitutional measures, such as the use of vomiting therapy for high Kapha type obesity.

It is not the purpose of this book to explain Pancha Karma in detail. Pancha Karma is a clinical practice that requires the proper equipment and facilities. Ayurvedic nurses are trained to administer the therapy, including measuring the eliminated substances. Its methods are varied according to the individual, disease, season and culture. But its methods can be used in a general way as part of self-care and everyone should know about them.

TWO LEVELS OF DETOXIFICATION

Ayurveda delineates two levels of detoxification treatment. The first is what could be called preliminary detoxification, involving normalizing digestion and elimination as under palliation therapy. The second deeper level is removing the excess doshas from the body, what has been described as Ayurvedic purification therapy.

Palliation therapy is easier to do and does not require the preparation of Pancha Karma and its stronger purification therapy methods. It can be employed as part of a mild detoxification approach for those not needing to, or not able to, undergo the deeper cleansing therapies. Done over a period of time its methods can be as effective as deeper cleansing practices.

Western and Chinese medicine do not discriminate between these two levels of cleansing. They may combine a method of deeper cleansing, like purgatives, with a preliminary detoxification method, like spices to improve digestion. What they usually do is more like this first level of Ayurvedic cleansing. They do not have a system for distinguishing the doshas from other more superficial toxins that may need to be eliminated. In making this division, Ayurveda brings clarity into detoxification programs and helps guard against the side effects of excess or wrongly administered detoxification therapies.

DETOXIFICATION THERAPIES AND DIET

PRELIMINARY DETOXIFICATION/ REMOVING AMA

The first stage of most healing processes usually involves a preliminary detoxification program. Most of us suffer from an accumulation of toxins, undigested food particles or waste mate-

119

rials, called *Ama* in Sanskrit. Ama not only causes disease, but also blocks the assimilation of nutrients. Without first clearing this accumulation, the right herbs and foods cannot be absorbed properly.

Most diseases are Ama-caused or Ama-related, including chronic diseases like allergies, arthritis and cancer. Ama weakens the immune system, causes the body to attack itself, and imbalances the metabolism. Ama is opposite in qualities to Agni or the digestive fire. When the Agni is good, Ama will not be formed. When Agni is low Ama easily increases.

A preliminary detoxification approach, like any cleansing therapy, is best done in the warm months of late spring and summer but has more latitude in its application because its methods are not as strong. Late spring, the month of May in most regions, is the natural season for detoxification.

Almost everyone can benefit from a mild detoxification in the spring season, such as eating fresh greens, raw foods and cooling herbs to cleanse the blood. With the rising of heat and promotion of growth externally, internal toxins accumulated through the winter season gradually begin to surface. It is important to eliminate them at this time so that they cannot cause diseases through the summer season.

AMA CONDITIONS/BY-PRODUCTS OF WRONG DIGESTION

Ama conditions, the accumulation of undigested food or waste materials, differ according to the doshas. Ama conditions are called Sama (in Sanskrit 'sa' means 'with', 'sama' means 'with ama'). There are Kapha Ama conditions, called Sama Kapha (toxic water), wherein toxins combine with the predominant Kapha dosha. Similarly, we can have Sama Pitta (toxic fire) and Sama Vata (toxic air) conditions. An anti-Ama approach can be applied to any of the doshas or combined with any of the therapies for them.

- Sama Kapha is revealed by indigestion and constipation along with a difficult expectoration of thick phlegm.

120

- Sama Pitta shows up as indigestion, hyperacidity and diarrhea, along with fever or toxic blood conditions.
- Sama Vata occurs with indigestion along with abdominal distention, gas and constipation.

Ama is evidenced by a tongue-coating, bad breath and foul body odor along with poor digestion and feelings of heaviness and dullness. Anti-Ama therapies should be employed until these factors clear. In this process of detoxification, as toxins are released, headaches or other side effects may occur temporarily.

HERBS FOR DETOXIFICATION

Of the six tastes, three—sweet, salty and sour—increase Ama. They not only increase the bodily tissues but also feed toxins. Astringent taste is neutral in regard to Ama. Though it can help dry up Ama, it can hold it in the body by its contracting action. Pungent and bitter tastes are effective for eliminating Ama. Bitter taste reduces it and pungent taste destroys it.

The main herbal method to treat Ama is to burn it up with herbs to increase the digestive fire. As Ama is opposite in properties to the digestive fire, Agni, herbs that stimulate Agni counter the effects of Ama. Best are the hot spices like cayenne, black pepper, dry ginger, pippali, asafoetida and mustard. These can burn up Ama directly. Other helpful warm spices include cardamom, cumin, coriander, basil and fennel. These destroy Ama indirectly by stimulating Agni.

The best anti-ama formulas are Trikatu and Asafoetida 8. When these are not available, a good formula is equal parts of cayenne, black pepper and dry ginger. Take this in dosages of 1 gram of the powder in capsules or with honey 2-3 times a day.

These herbs are good for Sama Kapha and Sama Vata conditions. In Sama Pitta conditions they are helpful, but care must be taken that they do not aggravate Pitta by their hot nature. Combine them with equal amounts of bitters like gentian or barberry to balance them out.

Herbal bitters help scrape Ama out of the tissues and relieve the fever or infection that it causes. They are good when there is fermentation, heat, or inflammation and are specific for cleansing Ama from the blood. They are most effective in Sama Pitta and Sama Kapha conditions and are sometimes useful in small amounts in Sama Vata conditions when the condition is long standing. They are good for any Ama condition that has come about through eating too much sweet or fatty food.

Best are pure bitters like goldenseal, gentian, barberry and quassia. Chinese pure bitters are coptis, scute, phellodendron, gentian, and gardenia. Ayurvedic pure bitters include katuka, neem, and aloe. Ayurvedic formulas include Tikta and Mahasudarshan powder. When these are not available, a good formula is gentian, barberry and turmeric in equal parts, taken in dosages of 1 gram of the powder in capsules, or with honey 2-3 times a day.

FASTING

Fasting is an important part of any detoxification approach but requires some strength on the part of the patient, particularly fasting more than a few days. Fasting is often a good step for starting a detoxification diet: 3-5 days for fasting for Vata, 5-7 days for Pitta, and 7-10 days for Kapha.

It is best to fast on herbal teas or vegetable juices. A fruit juice fast is not advisable because sweet taste increases Ama. Lemon juice, however, is good, particularly mixed with ginger juice. A little honey can be used as well because of its special detoxifying properties. Fasting is often combined with herbs to improve the digestive fire, taking of pungent herbs or spice teas like ginger, cinnamon, cardamom, and fennel. Bitters can be helpful, like aloe gel, barberry or gentian.

Fasting is an important initial treatment for many diseases because it dispels toxins and enkindles the digestive fire. When the appetite returns, however, it is important not to continue the fast because continued fasting can suppress the digestive fire. Signs of proper fasting include a clear tongue coating, pleasant body odor, normalization of appetite and digestion, and feelings of clearness, lightness and lack of tiredness.

PURGATIVES, COLONICS AND ENEMAS

Cleansing the bowels is another route of detoxification that can be combined with fasting or detoxification diet. In Ayurveda, purgatives and enemas are part of deeper cleansing approaches (Pancha Karma), and have stronger effects as part of this process. However, they are sometimes used in a simpler way to cleanse Ama from the system.

Purgation is best when there is constipation or irregular bowel movements. If the stool sinks rather than floats, it indicates the presence of Ama in the system. Purgation is particularly useful for accumulated masses of undigested food in the colon. These can be found by palpation. They will be hard, irregular and usually not painful to touch. Purgation is also useful for food poisoning or toxic digestion conditions. However, it should not be employed where there is chronic loose stool, diarrhea, debility or emaciation, even when a tongue coating or other Ama signs exist.

As colonics are the strongest and most direct way to cleanse the colon, they can be helpful in detoxification. In this regard Kaphas can usually take more colonics, Pittas moderately, and Vatas, the least. In fact, we must be careful giving colonics to Vata types, who can be easily weakened by them. Colonics are not advisable for the weak, emaciated, debilitated, anorexic, tired, or those suffering from nervous system disorders or fear and anxiety. However, one or two cleansing colonics are usually good for the majority of people. They are best prepared with herbs, oil and salt, just like Ayurvedic cleansing enemas, to protect the mucus lining of the colon. Mere water colonics can wash away the lining of the colon and cause irritation. A colonic should be followed up with spicy herbs to promote digestion because it strongly reduces the digestive fire.

Although colonics are helpful to clean out deep-seated accumulations in the colon, Ayurveda prefers the primary Pancha Karma methods of emesis, purgation and enemas for a more direct and effective purification of the doshas. Enemas are often better (particularly for Vata) than colonics, as their action is not so drastic. The cleansing enemas of Pancha Karma are used mainly for this purpose.

Purgative herbs cleanse both the small and the large intestine, though their cleansing action is not as thorough as colonics. It is often helpful to take purgatives the first day of a fast. Additional purges may be taken every three days to a week during the fast, particularly if a strong evidence of Ama exists.

Demulcent and bulk laxatives such as psyllium and flaxseed are not advisable in many detoxification conditions because they can further clog or congest the system. Bitter purgatives like rhubarb root and aloe are helpful, along with hot spices like ginger to protect the digestive fire and burn up Ama.

TRIPHALA

Triphala, or the Three Fruits, consists of the fruit of three tropical trees, called myrobalan plums: haritaki, amalaki, and bibhitaki. It is the safest and most strengthening of the laxative herbs. The same results as with stronger detoxification methods can be achieved by taking the formula Triphala in moderate dosages over longer periods of time along with an anti-Ama diet. Enough Triphala, usually 3-10 grams, should be taken before sleep to ensure a normal evacuation upon rising. It can be taken as tablets or infused in warm water with a little honey (Triphala does taste bad and its taste is difficult to mask). The dosage can be adjusted based upon personal experience and can gradually be reduced over the period of time.

Triphala not only gradually cleanses the bowels of all toxins, but also improves the digestive fire. So it does not have the side effects of other purgatives. In addition, it has a strengthening and nutritive effect upon the deeper tissues of the bone, nerve and reproductive.

It is good to take Triphala along with digestive spices such as Trikatu. This gives a balanced approach for cleansing both the stomach and colon and makes for a good metabolic regulator. It is useful not only in Ama conditions, but also as part of a regular diet for preventing Ama from building up.

ALOE GEL

When Triphala is not available aloe gel can be used instead. Be sure to get the undiluted gel as it is often diluted with water

124

when called Aloe juice. Aloe gel is better for Sama Pitta or Sama Kapha. It cleanses the colon over a long period of time without overly reducing the digestive fire. Take 2-3 teaspoons 2-3 times a day, with a little spice such as ginger, black pepper or turmeric. Along with an anti-Ama diet or with regular diet to reduce the dosha, aloe gel is an effective method of cleansing the tissues and the digestive tract without any debilitating side effects.

DETOXIFYING OR ANTI-AMA DIET

According to Ayurveda, certain difficult to digest foods are likely to cause a build-up of toxins and waste materials (Ama) in the system. These are foods that are heavy, greasy, stale or old, like cheese, pork, and lard, white sugar and white flour products. Yogurt is sometimes included here as it tends to clog the channels.

Ama-forming foods are mainly Kapha (watery) in nature, so that an anti-Ama diet is much like an anti-Kapha diet. It is similar to the regular Western health food, mucus-free, live and raw food diet. Such a diet is used in Ayurveda but it is not given to everyone. It is mainly part of a preliminary cleansing treatment. It is not appropriate for those suffering from cold, debility or underweight.

FRUIT

For detoxification most fruit should be taken only in small amounts. Avoid sweet fruits and fruit juices, especially bananas, pears, persimmons, grape or cherry juice. Some sour fruit juices such as lemon, lime or grapefruit and astringent fruit like cranberry or pomegranate can be helpful.

VEGETABLES

Most vegetables are good detoxifiers. They are best raw but steamed is also good. Sprouts like alfalfa, sunflower, buckwheat, wheat, rice and barley are the first choice because they contain special enzymes that help digest Ama. Vegetable juices such as celery, parsley, cilantro and spinach are good but carrot is often too sweet, particularly by itself. Avoid heavier root vegetables, like potatoes and sweet potatoes, as well as mushrooms.

GRAINS

Most whole grains are all right for mild or long term detoxification approaches, but not good for short and radical action. In all cases of detoxification avoid breads and pastries, particularly those made with white flour. Sweet and heavy grains, wheat and oats, should be taken sparingly. Wheat can cause allergies in people with high Ama. Kicharee—equal parts long grain rice and split mung beans—is an excellent food for mild detoxification. Barley is also good, particularly as a soup.

BEANS

For detoxification avoid beans because they cause gas, which tends to produce Ama. Mung beans, however, are good for most Ama (toxic) conditions, particularly for Sama Pitta (toxic fire) and are an exception in this regard.

NUTS AND SEEDS

Most nuts, particularly when roasted or salted, are heavy and mucus-forming. They should be generally avoided in Ama conditions. Sunflower, pumpkin, sesame and other seeds are better but should not be taken in large amounts.

DAIRY PRODUCTS

Dairy is highly Amagenic (ama-increasing), particularly when pasteurized. Milk is very mucus-forming, as is yogurt, cheese and butter even more so. Generally avoid dairy, though buttermilk (not salted) can be taken. It is better to take acidophilus in pill form than to eat yogurt. Or to mix yogurt with equal parts of water and take with spices like ginger and cardamom.

ANIMAL PRODUCTS

Animal products strongly feed toxins. Animal fats, lard and red meat particularly, should be avoided. Pork is the worst. Fish, including shellfish, can be very mucus increasing, especially when not fresh. Chicken and turkey are the safest meats to take for mild detoxification diets, specifically the white meat. But it is better to avoid animal products altogether, including eggs, for any strong detoxification procedure.

OILS

Oils should be generally avoided as they are mucus forming. Ghee or clarified butter can be taken in small amounts. Drying oils such as mustard or flaxseed can be used in small amounts as well.

SWEETENERS

Avoid sweeteners, except a little honey. White sugar is the most Amagenic (toxin forming) of all foods and brown sugar is not much better.

SPICES

All spices are generally good for Ama conditions, including hot spices of all types. However, salt increases Ama and should be used sparingly, preferably rock salt, which is lighter and easier to digest than sea salt. Sour articles like vinegar, wine and pickles should be avoided because sour taste increases Ama and promotes fermentation.

BEVERAGES

Avoid cold drinks, especially those with ice. Spring water or distilled water is good, but always take water warm. Herbal teas are excellent. Hot spice teas like ginger, cinnamon and cardamom are best. Coffee should be avoided but a little black tea is all right if not prepared with much milk or sugar. A good method of detoxification is to sip hot water, or a hot spice tea like ginger or cinnamon throughout the day, taking a little every half hour or hour.

DIETETICS

The anti-ama is the most restrictive of the diets. Food combinations should be kept simple with only a few different foods per meal. Do not drink too much with meals and only take spice teas afterwards. The food should be taken raw or cooked fresh. Take several hours between meals and usually three meals a day should be taken. No food should be taken before 10 am or after sunset. The main meal should be at noon. Meals should be light and easy to digest. All overeating should be avoided.

CAUTIONARY NOTE

As this is a fairly reducing diet it should be implemented carefully. Vata people generally should not follow this diet more than two weeks. Pittas can handle it for one month. Kaphas can follow it for longer periods. It can be modified according to the diets for the three doshas, particularly when taken over a longer period. Pitta and Kaphas can take more raw food. Vatas do better on a general light diet.

Detox diets should not be given to those who are weak, emaciated, or devitalized, the very old or very young, nor should it be continued if the individual becomes debilitated. Signs of an excess detoxifying diet include insomnia, palpitations, low energy, fainting, absence of menstruation, and long-term loss of appetite. The Western raw food diet, which is similar, also has such side effects. Though it is a helpful tool, it has its limits and should not be turned into a panacea.

AYURVEDIC PURIFICATION THERAPY/ PANCHA KARMA

PRELIMINARY PRACTICES (Purva Karma)

PREPARATION

Palliation therapy, consisting of preliminary detoxification and Ama-reducing methods according to one's dosha, should usually be followed for a period prior to Pancha Karma. One week is the minimum time for this, one month an average time, and six months a long time. A patient should be ready for Pancha Karma and prepare for it for some time in advance.

128

Oleation and Sweating Methods

Application of oils, *Snehana*, also called 'oleation therapy' is an important therapeutic method in Ayurveda, with oils used both externally and internally. Steam therapy or therapeutic sweating, *Svedana*, is another important method. These two are significant parts of Pancha Karma but are also useful in themselves for treating various conditions and for health maintenance. They are the main preliminary practices of Pancha Karma.

After adequate detoxification, a period of daily oil application and sweating therapy should be followed for at least one week for health maintenance and three weeks for the treatment of severe diseases. Warm sesame oil is applied all over the body in large amounts, while the patient lays on a special Ayurvedic massage table. Special medicated oils (like Narayan or Mahanarayan oil) can be applied, particularly to specific disease sites. The skill in massage is not the issue here. Oleation therapy is concerned with the application of oil, not with body massage. Oils are taken internally at the same time, most commonly ghee (clarified butter).

Sweating is done a few minutes after oleation, generally using a special Ayurvedic sweatbox, often with the addition of the steam of diaphoretic herbs (camphor, eucalyptus, mint, or bayberry) for most patients, or with tonics (Dashamula and bala) for weaker types. Herbs can be decocted in a pressure cooker, to which a hose is attached at the top (called nadi sveda). The medicated steam is applied to specific sites in the body, such as swollen joints in arthritis.

Some people get the impression that oil and sweating therapies, Snehana and Svedana, are Pancha Karma, because they are its most obvious and frequently applied methods. Much of the skill of Pancha Karma therapy consists of preparing the toxins for elimination through oil and sweating therapies. The actual elimination methods can be done quickly once the preparation is made. However, if one stops with these preliminary practices, one has not actually done Pancha Karma.

Oil application and sweating therapy are designed to bring the aggravated doshas into the digestive tract for elimination.

They soften and liquefy them to direct them from the external disease pathway, the plasma and blood, to the internal, the g.i. tract. If one stops there, one has merely brought the aggravated doshas back to their site of accumulation, which will cause distress and disease. If they are not eliminated, they will be reabsorbed and go back to the tissues where they were lodged.

Heavy application of oils, also, will depress the digestive fire and cause loss of appetite or constipation. Hence, oil application should not be heavy, or it should be balanced out by taking ginger or other spicy herbs to improve the digestive fire. Many of the effects of short intense oil massage can be gained by mild daily application of oils over a long period of time.

Saunas, warm baths or showers or diaphoretic teas, such as cinnamon and ginger, can be used for sweating therapy. Many of the effects of short intense sweating therapy can be gained by regular usage of such sweating methods.

PRIMARY PRACTICES OF PANCHA KARMA
(Pradhana Karma)

1. THERAPEUTIC VOMITING (Vamana)

Therapeutic vomiting should be approached with care. If we strain ourselves to vomit, we can damage our nerve reflexes; therefore, this procedure is usually contraindicated for Vata constitution. However, with a little patience and practice it is possible to learn to do therapeutic vomiting ourselves. It can be done on a regular basis to cleanse the stomach and can be used as part of palliation therapy.

Strong teas of licorice, calamus, camomile or lobelia are used, generally about one ounce of the herb per pint of water, or simply a large amount of salt water can be used instead. A mild carminative tea like mint or fennel should be taken first in amounts of one pint. One should then apply a finger down the throat. Once the vomiting reflex arises one should follow it out all the way. It is easier to empty the stomach through one or two strong reflexes than through a series of weak ones. It is also less likely to produce side effects. It is important to empty the stomach thoroughly.

Vomiting is contraindicated for the weak, emaciated, anorexic, young, old, convalescent, for those suffering from dry cough. It is mainly for those with congestion of phlegm in the lungs and stomach, usually Kapha constitutions. The best season is spring, particularly late spring when the weather has warmed up. It should not be done during stormy or rainy weather. It gives better results if done around the time of the full moon. Best time is morning after sunrise.

Much of the effect of short-term emetic therapy can be gained through the long-term use of expectorant herbs like ginger, elecampane and calamus, and by formulas such as Trikatu and through following a strict anti-Kapha diet.

2. PURGATION

Purgation, Virechana, is the simplest Pancha Karma method and its effect is easy to observe. A strong purgative is given like rhubarb root, senna, aloe or castor oil. The following formula is excellent: Mix 4 parts rhubarb root with 1 part each of fennel, ginger and licorice. Take 2-5 grams of the powder before sleep with honey or warm water. Or two teaspoons of castor oil can be taken in warm milk with ginger. Triphala, a mild Ayurvedic purgative, is only strong enough if taken in large doses of 10-30 grams.

Purgative herbs are usually given in the evening, so that five to eight bowel movements occur the next day, flushing out the intestines. Late spring and summer are the best seasons.

Purgation is used to eliminate excess Pitta from its site in the small intestine. Note that purgation is not so much for treating the large intestine. This is because purgatives start their main action in the small intestine. This cleansing of the small intestine can weaken the digestive fire and so it is not always advisable for Vata types.

Purgation therapy can be used whenever we need to cleanse the intestines. It can treat constipation, old fevers, acute diarrhea, dysentery, food poisoning or any of the diseases of excess bile and toxic blood.

Contraindications for purgation therapy are for the very young, the very old, the weak, debilitated, emaciated, pregnant or those suffering from chronic diarrhea.

3. CLEANSING ENEMAS

Enemas (basti) are a mild therapy and can be used for many conditions. There are many different kinds of enemas, some of which are useful for tonification, others for reduction. Cleansing enemas (Niruha basti) are used in Pancha Karma to dispel excess Vata from its site in the large intestine. They are made with decoctions of anti-Vata herbs. Strictly speaking, tonifying or building enemas are not part of Pancha Karma but they are often given after the cleansing enemas as part of follow up practices and rejuvenation.

A typical cleansing enema can be made with 5 grams each of calamus, fennel and ginger along with 1-2 teaspoons of rock salt and 1/2 cup of sesame oil per quart of water. Without the addition of the oil or demulcent herbs like licorice, cleansing enemas are drying and depleting. The patient takes this mixture in the early morning or whenever the signs exist that Vata is ready for elimination. Cleansing enemas may be followed up with building enemas consisting mainly of sesame oil and warm water in equal proportions.

4. NASAL APPLICATION OF HERBS/ NASYA

Ayurveda has a whole variety of herbal preparations, including decoctions, oils and ghee, and the smoking of herbs for direct action on the nasal passage. This is called Nasya, literally, 'what relates to the nose,' in Sanskrit. For the purification action of Pancha Karma, cleansing herbs are given through the nose, either

132

as snuffs, decoctions or oils. Good herbs include calamus, bay-berry, sage, basil, and gotu kola.

Calamus, bayberry, sage or ginger powder can be snuffed to clear the sinuses. Calamus or gotu kola prepared in sesame oil or ghee can be applied in drops to cleanse the sinuses and nourish the brain. Cloves, calamus and bayberry can be smoked to cleanse the nasal passages. Different Ayurvedic doctors and companies have their special Nasya oils for the different doshas or for acute or chronic conditions.

Nasya is useful for many Vata and Kapha disorders. It allows for direct action on prana and the brain. It has strong decongestion action and allows a more specific application of expectorant herbs. It is helpful in some Pitta disorders, as well as any diseases of the head and nasal passages.

Oil massage to the head and face, along with inhalation of steam, helps dislodge toxins and makes the nasal treatment more effective. This is a more local form of oil and steam therapy, which is the preliminary treatment for Nasya. Such Nasya therapy can be done independently of Pancha Karma and as part of health maintenance.

5. THERAPEUTIC RELEASE OF TOXIC BLOOD

In the proper application of blood-releasing therapy, toxic blood is taken out of various sites in the body, usually along the back. The blood should be dark in color. Once it becomes bright red, the treatment should stop. The amount taken out is generally from two to eight ounces.

Some people recommend the donating of blood instead. While this does aid in new blood formation, it may not always be the toxic blood that is eliminated. This therapeutic bleeding therapy is not used as much in Pancha Karma as it once was, but it is still common in all systems of Oriental medicines. The use of alterative and blood-cleansing herbs has a similar affect over a long period of time, particularly spring cleaners like dandelion, sarsaparilla, sassafras, and comfrey leaf. Also good are blood-cleansing spices like turmeric and saffron.

FOLLOW-UP PRACTICES (Uttara Karma)

Pancha Karma treatment has several follow up practices. It is not an isolated therapy that can be done once and forgotten, but must be integrated into one's entire life-regimen. First, it may be necessary to repeat the whole process of Pancha Karma. More than one session may be needed to cleanse deep-seated toxins, particularly if shortened (week long sessions or less) versions of Pancha Karma are followed. Pancha Karma may be repeated after one to three months. It is good to do at least once a year for health maintenance purposes.

Second, after Pancha Karma, we should return to a diet and life-style in harmony with our constitution, or establish one if we have not done so already. Pancha Karma allows us to more effectively implement our life regimens, not to substitute for them. If we follow Pancha Karma with a return to bad habits, we may make our condition worse by suppressing the healing energy of our body that we have just developed.

Most important, if the treatment has been successful, we should be ready for a higher form of tonification therapy. Having eliminated the disease-causing doshas, we can now rebuild our damaged tissues on a new level of purity and strength.

May Vata (the life-force) blow to us the medicine that gives peace and happiness to our hearts. May it prolong our lives.

And Vata you are our father, our brother and our friend. Grant us the power of life.

Rig Veda X.186. 1-2

In the Waters are all medicines and Agni which gives health to all.
May the waters prepare the medicine that is a protection for my body, that I may long see the sun.

Rig Veda I. 24. 20-21

Part II
THE AYURVEDIC TREATMENT OF DISEASE

The following section lists diseases according to the bodily systems. First is an examination of the system as a whole, then its specific diseases. The diseases chosen are typical but not exhaustive. We have chosen not only common complaints but also conditions that are important from an Ayurvedic standpoint and its particular understanding of the disease process.

In examining any particular disease, please note the information provided on that system as a whole. These suggestions should be integrated with the life-regimens of Part I. For more detail on formulas and therapeutic treatments, Part III can be consulted. The goal is to provide a comprehensive yet simple method for treating disease through understanding the underlying doshic imbalance.

A being the size of the thumb dwells in the middle of our nature like a flame without smoke. He is the Lord of what has been and what will be. He is yesterday and he is tomorrow.
KATHA UPANISHAD, 2. 12-13

II. 1
DISEASES OF THE DIGESTIVE SYSTEM
The Stomach, Liver, and Small Intestine

AGNI, THE DIGESTIVE FIRE

There is a god or cosmic power that dwells within us, who determines how we function on a physical level. Without propitiating that deity, we must suffer from disease. That god is our own digestive fire, called Agni in Ayurveda, which means "the transforming will or force" and exists on higher levels as well as the power of discernment. It is important not only that we feed ourselves properly; the digestive fire must also be cared for so that it has the power to adequately extract our nourishment.

Most diseases arise from poor or wrong functioning of the digestive system. The digestive fire, Agni, is central to health. It is not only responsible for absorbing nutrients in food, but it also destroys any pathogens and renders the food acceptable to our systems. Undigested food becomes like a pathogen in the body, breeding toxins and upsetting the immune system.

When Agni is normal there is good digestion, circulation, and complexion; pleasant breath and body odor; adequate energy and strong resistance to disease. When Agni is abnormal there is poor digestion, poor circulation, bad complexion; offensive body odor, intestinal gas, constipation; low energy and poor resistance to disease. *Therefore, treating the digestive system—regulating Agni— is a radical (root) treatment for most diseases.*

Four States of the Digestive Fire
Agni has four states in Ayurveda:
    1. High 2. Low 3. Variable 4. Balanced

136

1. High Agni

Agni is usually high in Pitta (fire) types, with excessive appetite. Circulation is strong, but toxins in the blood and bleeding are more common. The stool will tend to be loose with some diarrhea. Resistance to disease is generally good, but when they do occur, diseases are apt to be sudden and severe (like febrile disorders or heart attacks).

2. Low Agni

Agni is usually low in Kapha types, with poor appetite, low metabolism and tendency to gain weight even without excess food consumption. There will be excess mucus and congestion. Circulation is poor and colds and flu are more common, but diseases are often not severe.

3. Variable Agni

Agni is variable in Vata types with periods of strong appetite, even extreme hunger, alternating with loss of appetite and forgetting to eat. Gas, distention and constipation are usually signs of variable Agni. Circulation is also variable, as is resistance to disease. More debilitating diseases and long-term derangement of the nervous system are more likely.

4. Balanced Agni

Signs of balanced Agni are a normal and regular appetite that is constant and easily satisfied with natural, not strongly spiced foods. Bowel movements will be regular and there will be little production of gas or bloating. Sensory acuity and mental clarity will also usually be strong.

HERBS FOR THE DIGESTIVE FIRE

Agni is increased by pungent, sour and salty tastes and decreased by sweet, astringent and bitter, though bitter taste in small amounts before meals can also increase Agni. Spices are usually the best thing for increasing Agni. The digestive fire has the same nature as spicy taste. It is hot, dry, light and fragrant. The right intake of spices is a major aid in the treatment of most diseases of the digestive system.

- When one's Agni is high, spices should generally be avoided but digestive bitters—aloe, barberry and gentian—can be taken (typically such formulas in Ayurveda as Tikta or Mahasudarshan churna). These lower the digestive fire without increasing toxins.
- When Agni is low hot spices can be taken—cayenne, ginger, black pepper (typically the Trikatu formula)—but all spices are good.
- When Agni is variable, spices and salts should be taken—asafoetida, ginger, cumin, rock salt (typically the Asafoetida 8 formula).
- When Agni is normal mild sattvic (harmonizing) spices—cardamom, turmeric, coriander and fennel—can be taken to maintain balance.

As a general formula for maintaining the digestive fire, particularly in low or variable states, Ayurvedic formula no. 1, the Digestive Tonic (an improved form of Trikatu) or Trikatu can be taken, 1 gram or 1/4 teaspoon a half hour before meal. Vata types can take it with warm water, Kapha with honey, Pitta with cool water or aloe gel as a vehicle.

Agni can also be increased by exercise, including yoga postures (asana), by deep breathing (pranayama), meditation, by fasting or light eating and by sleeping less. Staring at a ghee lamp is also helpful.

It is decreased by most damp, heavy, oily and sweet foods with the exception of ghee (clarified butter), which in small amounts increases it. Sedentary life-style, excessive sleep or too much sex are additional factors which weaken the digestive fire.

The Stages of Digestion

According to Ayurveda, digestion occurs in three stages.

1. Kapha dominates the first stage of digestion in the mouth and stomach. It includes the saliva and the alkaline secretions of the stomach lining. Here the water and earth elements are extracted from the food. Kapha types have an excess of these secretions with consequent nausea, bringing up of mucus, profuse salivation and poor appetite. Excess eating of sweet and salty foods will increase these secretions and also cause these symptoms.

2. Pitta dominates the second stage of digestion, with the secretion of acids in the small intestine. Here the fire element is extracted from the food. Pitta types suffer from hyperacidity and burning sensation in the stomach. Excess eating of sour and pungent substances increases these secretions.

3. Vata dominates the third stage of digestion in the large intestine with the formation of the stool. Here the air and ether elements are extracted from the food. Vata types suffer from gas and constipation. Excess eating of light, dry, bitter, astringent or pungent substances increases these symptoms.

THE SIX TASTES AND THE DIGESTIVE PROCESS

The six tastes mirror the digestive process in this order: sweet, sour, salty, pungent, bitter and astringent.

- Sweet taste is digested first, particularly sugars
- Salty taste is digested second and turns into sweet taste in the mouth and stomach.
- Sour taste is digested when the food enters into the small intestine.
- Pungent taste is digested when the food enters into the large intestine.
- Bitter and astringent tastes are digested last. They serve to close off the digestive process and help produce the stool.

Another important dietary factor is the order in which we eat our foods. A proper eating order may allow us to digest foods that we otherwise could not. By this logic salads are better at the end of a meal, and desserts are better at the start of meals or along with them.

Sweets should be eaten first. If eaten after other food sweets can stop the digestive process, allowing an undigested food mass to form and to ferment. It is good to have something sour like chutneys or yogurt, in the middle of the meal.

After meals it is good to have astringent teas such as regular black tea, alfalfa, raspberry leaf or strawberry leaf. If bitter and astringent tastes are eaten first (except bitter herbs in small amounts before meals) they will reduce the appetite and weaken the digestive process, restricting the assimilation of nutrients

Indigestion and Ama-Formation

Improper digestion results in the accumulation of an undigested food mass, or Ama. Ama formation is indicated when the stools are poorly formed, breath is unpleasant, appetite is abnormal and a coating appears on the tongue. This undigested mass stagnates and ferments and eventually, entering the bloodstream, moves to different parts of the body causing various diseases.

- For Kapha types, Ama accumulates along with phlegm in the stomach, and moves into the lungs and the lymphatic system causing Kapha disorders.
- For Pittas, Ama accumulates along with acid in the small intestine, and moves into the liver and the blood causing various Pitta disorders.
- For Vatas it accumulates with gas in the large intestine, and moves into the bone and the nerve tissue causing various Vata disorders.

TREATMENT OF AMA (THE BY-PRODUCT OF INDIGESTION)

Herbs that improve digestion and strengthen Agni also counter Ama. Spices are great for destroying Ama or inhibiting its formation, particularly hot spices like cayenne and ginger. Bitters are useful for reducing Ama in the tissues and help destroy it, particularly pure bitters like goldenseal or gentian. The drying and detoxifying action of combined pungent and bitter herbs is good for eliminating deep-seated toxins, like taking ginger and gentian together.

Astringent taste restrains Ama but can hold it in the body. Sweet is the strongest taste for increasing Ama. Salty and sour tastes cause Ama to ferment.

THE NEED FOR REGULAR EXAMINATION OF THE DIGESTIVE SYSTEM

Even a person who has no immediate disease problem should examine their digestion, including the tongue, breath, appetite and elimination, making sure that toxins are not forming. It is easiest to stop the disease process at its origin in the digestive tract. Once it moves into the tissues it becomes difficult. Thus, in treating all diseases and for disease prevention, we must first consider treating the digestive system.

THE DIGESTIVE SYSTEM AND MEDICATIONS

Always consider the strength of digestion for whatever herb that is given. Any herb not properly digested will, like undigested food, turn into a toxin. The same is true of minerals and vitamins. For this reason formulas for treating the digestive system are useful adjuncts for insuring the assimilation of other herbs.

DISEASES OF THE STOMACH

The stomach is the site of the first stage of digestion. Most digestive disorders either begin in the stomach or are first noted there. The stomach is a Kapha organ and diseases of Kapha, the biological water-humor, usually originate there. The condition of the stomach indicates the general state of Kapha in the body—our sense of contentment, nourishment and happiness. It is like the mother for the rest of the body. The stomach is a sensitive organ easily upset not only by wrong diet but also by emotional disturbances or worry.

Vomiting/Nausea

Vomiting is an excessive movement of the upward-moving air (udana). Nausea is a milder version of it. Vomiting can be brought about by accumulations of the doshas, by toxins or by psychological factors such as fright or repulsion. Its causes include bad food or water, bad food combinations, overeating and other dietary indiscretions. Vomiting can be involved with other digestive or respiratory system disorders, so care should be taken to find its cause. It is related to cough and asthma and can be treated by many of the same herbs and formulas. Excess use of emetic therapy or undue promoting of vomiting can cause it, as well as undue suppression of the digestive fire by any factors.

Nausea and vomiting occurs more frequently in Kapha types. Kapha accumulates as phlegm in the stomach, where it blocks peristalsis and causes udana, the upward-moving air, to rise up. Vomiting occurs to clear this Kapha out. Any excess eating of Kaphogenic foods like sweets, oils, dairy, meat, or just overeating can precipitate it.

TYPES OF VOMITING
- Vata type vomiting is dry or scanty vomiting with thirst, pain in the chest and sides, palpitations, anxiety and astringent taste in the mouth. It is often a nervous reaction.
- Pitta vomiting is the bilious variety with sour fluid, bitter taste in the mouth, burning sensation, thirst and a red face.
- Kapha type is watery or mucousy vomit with sweet taste in the mouth, excessive salivation, heaviness and labored breathing.

Vomiting can occur in stomach flu or with putrid food in the stomach. It is also common during pregnancy (morning sickness) as an hormonal imbalance.

In Chinese medicine, vomiting, like cough, is caused by rebellious chi or adverse chi rising. It is treated by herbs and to regulate the chi like cardamom or fresh ginger. This condition and its treatment resembles the Vata type in Ayurveda. Other factors

142

include accumulation of dampness and internal cold, which is like Kapha. The herbs used for it are mainly hot spices. Another causative factor for it in Chinese medicine is heat in the stomach, which is much like Pitta and treated by bitter herbs.

GENERAL TREATMENT OF VOMITING

Anti-emetic herbs are administered to stop vomiting. Mainly spicy herbs have this special potency. As it is mainly an acute condition, treatment is usually symptomatic.

However, the patient should first be examined to see if it is a condition of toxins or food poisoning. If so, vomiting should be encouraged by using emetic herbs such as calamus, licorice and salt (the latter two in large amounts). Often a good old 'finger down the throat' will do, but first take mint tea or warm water, up to one pint, to make the vomiting easier. The favorite Western emetic is lobelia (with a touch of cayenne). The Chinese prefer the calyx of the persimmon fruit.

If there is a severe Kapha condition of mucus and congestion, it may also be better to promote vomiting. Otherwise the mucus may be trapped in the stomach and lungs and continue to depress their functions.

Many common spices are good to prevent vomiting. Among the best are fresh ginger, fennel, basil, nutmeg, cardamom and cloves. A good simple formula is cardamom and fennel in equal parts, 1 teaspoon infused in a cup of warm water with a little honey. This stops almost any kind of vomiting. Lemon juice with a little honey or sugar is also good.

The typical Ayurvedic formula is Cardamom combination, which is particularly good for Kapha and Vata. Chinese formulas include Minor Pinellia and Hoelen combination, good for almost any kind of vomiting.

SPECIFIC TREATMENT FOR VOMITING

For Vata, an anti-Vata regimen is indicated. Sleep, relaxation, calm and meditation are important because the causes are usually psychological (hypersensitivity of the mind and nervous system).

143

Cardamom compound can be taken with warm milk, or cardamom and fennel can be added to honey or warm milk (1/2 tsp. of the powder of each).

For Pitta, an anti-Pitta regimen should be followed. Mild herbal bitters will be helpful, such as barberry or aloe gel, along with the anti-vomiting herbs coriander, cardamom and fennel. Strong bitters—aloe powder or rhubarb root—tend to aggravate nausea and vomiting. The main Ayurvedic formula is Avipattikar powder.

Kapha vomiting is due to excess mucus, which should be cleared up with expectorant herbs. An anti-kapha regimen is indicated. Cardamom by itself is often excellent. Trikatu is the best common formula, or Clove combination, taken with honey.

Hyperacidity

Acid or sour taste is a sign of Pitta disorders, usually indicating high Pitta in the small intestine. There will be heartburn, belching of sour fluids, perhaps nausea and vomiting.

The causes are mainly dietary: too much spicy or sour food, too much greasy food, alcohol or overeating in general. Excess intake of sweets, including pastries, cakes and pies can also cause hyperacidity. Sugar causes fermentation and acid production in the stomach, particularly if wrongly combined with other food types.

TREATMENT OF HYPERACIDITY

An anti-Pitta diet is prescribed, with antacid food such as milk or ghee and an emphasis on whole grains like basmati rice. Bananas should be avoided as they have a sour post-digestive effect. Sour taste, as in pickles, yogurt, wine and vinegar should be avoided.

Good herbs are aloe gel, shatavari, amalaki, licorice, marshmallow, gentian, barberry, and conch shell—herbs with mainly demulcent and bitter properties. Antacid formulas include Conch shell combination (Shankha bhasma) taken with cool water or aloe gel. The Antacid formula (no. 12) is specific to this condition.

144

A good Chinese herb is oyster shell, which is also antacid.

Hyperacidity can also occur with weak digestion. Food will sit in the stomach and ferment, producing a burning sensation. This is more common in Vata and Kapha types. Typical formulas for improving the digestive fire are indicated such as Asafoetida 8 and Trikatu.

Mineral herbs such as oyster or conch shell (and most antacid medicines or baking soda) tend to depress the digestive fire and should be used with care or combined with the appropriate spices for weaker digestions.

Ulcers

Ulcers are an inflammation of the mucus lining of the stomach. They involve pain, a burning sensation and, when severe, result in bleeding. If perforated, they can be life threatening. They are usually due to psychological factors such as stress, worry or overwork. However, there are many dietary causes as well, including too much spicy or sour food.

Ulcers related to hyperacidity are most commonly a Pitta condition. Excess acid from the small intestine accumulates in the stomach and burns through the lining, causing inflammation. Yet it is not always an excess of stomach acid that causes ulcers. Some ulcers may be due to high Vata and its characteristic excessive thinking and nervous sensitivity. This causes an irregular appetite and digestion, specifically untimely secretions of acid that leads to ulcers. Vata types who are prone to worry often come down with ulcers. Sometimes there is a deficiency of the mucus (Kapha) secretions of the stomach. This allows a normal or even low amount of acid to burn through. Ulcers can even be caused by a deficiency of stomach acid; the food stays in the stomach too long and eventually burns through what may be a thin stomach lining.

GENERAL TREATMENT OF ULCERS

A bland diet is indicated, with whole grains and other easy to digest foods. A milk fast may be advisable, taking three or four glasses of warm milk every day for a few days until the ulcer gets better. Alcohol and smoking should be avoided. Spices, pickles, vinegar and other strong-tasting substances should be eliminated from the diet until the condition improves. Bananas and night-shades should be taken with discretion. The therapies are similar to those for hyperacidity but should be followed more strictly.

Demulcent herbs for soothing the stomach lining are indicated—aloe gel, shatavari, licorice, marshmallow, comfrey root, or slippery elm. Aloe gel is the simplest and most effective home remedy. The Antacid formula (no. 12) is generally good as it regulates stomach acidity and protects the mucus membranes.

PITTA TYPE ULCERS

The general treatment prevails. A bland anti-Pitta diet should be taken. Bitters are good such as aloe, barberry, gentian, chiretta, and katuka. Formulas are Sudarshan powder and Mahasudarshan powder, as well as Shatavari compound.

Good Chinese herbs are coptis, scute, gentian, and gardenia. Formulas include Coptis and Scute combination. Western herbs are goldenseal, gentian, and barberry. An excellent simple formula is equal of parts gentian, barberry and licorice, 1 teaspoon of the powder infused in a cup of warm water before meals.

VATA TYPE ULCERS

Excess dry, light or spicy food can cause an ulcer. Too much cold or raw food can also cause it by disturbing the digestive fire. Forgetting to eat or irregular or inadequate food intake can cause variability in acid production, making it too low at some times and too high at others. General Vata stress and anxiety are the psychological factors.

Vata ulcers involve more pain and less burning sensation. The person feels cold, light headed or anxious. Application of heat to the stomach will give relief (if not, it is probably a Pitta condition). Other Vata symptoms will prevail like palpitations, insomnia, abdominal distention, gas or constipation. Until regular eating habits are firmly established Vata type ulcers are unlikely to be cured, regardless of the herbs taken.

146

Treatment requires, at first, a bland diet but mild spices can be safely used. Take a simple diet of Kicharee (equal parts mung beans and basmati rice) along with a little ghee, salt and a little ginger. You may need to follow this for a month in order to correct the main symptoms. A milk fast or warm milk after meals can help as well.

Typical anti-Vata digestive formulas can be helpful like Asafoetida 8, Lavanbhaskar powder or Trikatu, but use with care if the tongue is dry, cracked or red in color. They should be taken with warm milk or ghee.

KAPHA TYPE ULCERS

Kapha people seldom get ulcers as they seldom worry. Kapha ulcers are characterized by phlegm and nausea, lack of appetite, dull pain and heaviness. They may be caused emotionally by grief, greed or attachment. The main dietary cause is overeating or eating too much sweet or oily food.

To correct a Kapha type ulcer a light, anti-Kapha diet is necessary. Strong digestion promoting spices are indicated including cayenne, dry ginger, black pepper, cloves or formulas such as Trikatu. Demulcents may aggravate the condition.

A cautionary note: if there is any uncertainty as to whether Pitta is involved, or any kind of burning sensation is noted, hot spices should not be used but the general anti-Pitta therapy should be followed instead.

DISEASES OF THE SMALL INTESTINE

In Ayurveda, the small intestine is the seat of Agni, the digestive fire. Its main treatment is to improve Agni with spicy digestive stimulants, as listed under the digestive system generally. The digestive fire has two actions: primarily, it grasps the essence of nourishment from the food, but secondarily it kills any bacteria or pathogens in the food. When it dysfunctions not only will digestion be hindered, but toxins will enter the body through the digestive tract causing low resistance and poor immune function.

The small intestine is called *grahani* in Sanskrit, meaning 'that which grasps things'. When the small intestine is not functioning properly the food will not be adequately assimilated or absorbed. There will be chronic indigestion and poor elimination, almost no matter what we may eat. We will be plagued with digestive system dysfunctions such as constipation, diarrhea, gas, lack of appetite, excessive appetite, or any alternation of these. We may live with this dysfunction because it may not result in severe diseases, but we will seldom feel really good or healthy.

Such digestive dysfunctions are related with other diseases such as hypoglycemia, candida, food allergies, chronic diarrhea or dysentery, and chronic gastritis or intestinitis. Often these are only complications of the poor functioning of the small intestine. Sometimes medical doctors dismiss such digestive dysfunction as a mental condition if nothing physically wrong exists in the patient. The Ayurvedic view brings such maladies together as small intestine disorders, making understandable otherwise difficult conditions to diagnose, with contradictory symptoms.

Malabsorption

Weakness of the small intestine creates what Ayurveda calls 'malabsorption syndrome.' It has been equated with 'sprue syndrome', a condition of chronic poor digestion usually occurring in the tropics where the body is unable to deal with the high bacterial content of the environment. However, this syndrome also occurs as part of the general deterioration of our natural environment today. We are seeing more pollution and new strains of bacteria and viruses to weaken our digestive systems. Probably at least half of us will have a malabsorption condition at one time or another.

From a dietary standpoint, malabsorption can be caused by any dietary extremes. These include too complex or too irregular a diet, food that is too hot or too cold, too much raw food or too

148

much over-cooked food, too much sweet food, overeating, or too much fasting. Eating canned food, junk food or an otherwise devitalized diet can also bring it about. Such foods imbalance the digestive fire, particularly if we change quickly from one such indiscretion to another. Not surprisingly, dietary extremists frequently end up with this condition.

Malabsorption occurs as a result of chronic digestive system disorders such as diarrhea, dysentery, and constipation. It is brought on by excess use of purgatives and colonics and by medicinal or recreational drugs, stimulants and antibiotics. Individuals who are overly stressed or hypersensitive are especially at risk for it.

Symptoms of malabsorption are variable appetite, unpredictable digestion, poorly formed stool with undigested food particles and foul smell, alternating constipation and diarrhea, and abdominal pain centered in the umbilicus. Spots or ridges on the fingernails are common. Malabsorption often results in emaciation, no matter what the individual may eat. There will be debility and weakness of the muscles and bones, and a tendency to low-grade infections. Unlike diarrhea and dysentery, there will be no dehydration. Colonics, purgatives and enemas make the condition worse.

Many of these conditions are classified in Chinese medicine under 'chi' (primary energy) disorders, primarily spleen chi deficiency but sometimes as complicated with chi stagnation. Symptoms are weakness, fatigue, lack of strength, shortness of breath, lack of appetite, poor assimilation, chronic diarrhea, and poor resistance.

TYPES OF MALABSORPTION

While malabsorption can occur in any of the three doshas, it is more common in Vata types given their irregular habits.

• Vata type malabsorption syndrome is characterized by intestinal gas, abdominal distention and migrating pain, dry skin, cracked tongue, anal fissures, hemorrhoids, chronic

149

low weight and a tendency towards arthritis. The stool will be watery, frothy and passed with noise or gas alternating with hard, dry stool. Palpitations, anxiety and insomnia will occur, with feelings of faintness, ungroundedness and depression.

• Pitta type malabsorption is indicated by inflammation, ulceration or a burning pain in the intestines. Diarrhea of yellow color will be common along with anemia and emotional symptoms of anger and irritability.

• Kapha type symptoms include mucus in the stools, dull aching pain in the abdomen, heaviness, congestion in the lungs, less weight loss, and a tendency towards edema and diabetes.

General Treatment of Malabsorption

The best food generally is buttermilk (takra). It is best to prepare one's own, as most commercial buttermilk is overly salted. To make Indian buttermilk take fresh yogurt, not too sour, add an equal amount of water and blend for a few minutes. This creates the kind of buttermilk which Ayurvedic medicine prescribes. The whey or liquid part left over from yogurt or curds is also good and can be used in cooking. Take a buttermilk fast for three to five days, ingesting three to six cups a day along with some mild spices like ginger, cumin, coriander or asafoetida.

Then proceed to a kicharee (basmati rice and mung bean) diet for an additional three to five days. Gradually add other foods starting with root vegetables like carrots, yams or potatoes cooked in kicharee. Following this procedure you can re-program your digestive system and restore it to normal functioning. Many simple starches are good to help restore absorption including kudzu (pueraria starch), basmati rice, lotus seed flour and potatoes.

Spices to improve absorption usually combine pungent and astringent tastes. These include nutmeg, cardamom, pippali, cloves, fresh ginger, cinnamon, fennel, cumin, bayberry, cyperus, haritaki, and chitrak. Herbal wines such as Draksha or Cyperus compound wine are excellent. The Herbal Absorption formula (no. 9) is devised for this purpose, and should be taken with buttermilk. Pitta types, having malabsorption and acidity, can take it with aloe gel.

SPECIFIC TREATMENT OF MALABSORPTION

Vata types should follow an anti-Vata diet with the spices mentioned above. Whole grains and Kicharee are good; avoid cold or raw food and raw juices. Or take buttermilk with fresh ginger or nutmeg. Draksha or a little red wine can be taken with meals. Formulas include Nutmeg compound, Cardamom compound or Garlic compound, as well as Vata's standard digestive formula of Asafoetida 8. These can be taken with buttermilk.

Pittas should follow an anti-Pitta diet avoiding all fried and greasy food. Buttermilk can be taken with fennel and coriander, with herbal bitters or with formulas such as Tikta or Avipattikar powder.

Kaphas should follow an anti-Kapha diet, avoiding cold water, ice cream, cheese, and pastries. Buttermilk should be taken with dry ginger or such formulas as Trikatu or Clove compound.

In chronic and debilitated conditions, tonics such as ashwagandha, bala, ginseng and astragalus are necessary. Chinese Chi tonics, the Four Gentlemen for mild conditions, or Saussurea and Cardamom compound for severe conditions, can be helpful. Chinese ginseng itself is excellent.

DISEASES OF THE LIVER AND GALL BLADDER

The liver is a Pitta (fiery) organ and the site or origin of many Pitta (infectious and inflammatory) disorders. Most liver disorders such as jaundice and hepatitis are typical Pitta diseases. Such Pitta disorders as ulcers and hyperacidity have their origin in wrong function of the liver and gall bladder. Pitta literally means bile. Excessive bile production or congestion in the flow of bile usually indicates high Pitta. In Ayurveda, the liver is the seat of fire and easily heats up, causing various inflammatory diseases. The subtle enzymes, the *bhutagnis*, are located in the liver. They transform digested food particles into the forms of the five elements needed to build up the tissue for the five sense organs in the body.

Moreover, the liver is the site of most Pitta (fiery) emotions. Negative Pitta emotions are irritability, anger, jealousy and ambition; positive ones are courage, confidence, enthusiasm and will power. Disturbances in these emotions can cause liver dysfunction.

These factors relate mainly to the solar plexus and to the navel chakra. Pitta constitution individuals, and those prone to liver disorders, should keep the navel center both clear of blockages and not overly active. This can be done by surrendering one's personal will to the higher creative and spiritual will in the heart.

Care of the Liver

There are many good, generally bitter, herbs for promoting the flow of bile, cleansing the blood, detoxifying the liver and relieving high Pitta. These include common Western herbs like gentian, barberry, dandelion and goldenseal. Europeans commonly take digestive bitters to counteract their generally Pitta diets (alcohol, red meat and generally hot, greasy, oily, heavy or overly sweet foods) that can impair liver function.

Turmeric and barberry in equal parts are very good for clearing liver energy and preventing emotional stagnation. Adding gotu kola to them calms the liver and mind as well, and helps counter addictions to sugar, fat, and alcohol, which impair liver function. Aloe gel is an excellent liver tonic. Take 2-3 teaspoons, 2-3 times a day. It has both cleansing and building properties. The Liver Tonic (formula no. 8) is excellent.

The Chinese herb bupleurum is also specific for liver care. Many Bupleurum formulas exist in their system for harmonizing the liver including Major and Minor Bupleurum.

The most specific Ayurvedic herb for the liver is Bhumyamalaki (Phyllanthus niruri). Modern clinical studies both in India and the West show that as a single herb it is effective in most liver disorders. So far it appears to be the only substance that can treat hepatitis B in carriers, thus arresting the spread of the disease.

Mild spices such as coriander, fennel, cumin, turmeric, cyperus, mint, lemon and lime help promote liver energy and improve appetite in conditions of sluggish or congested liver. They can be used as spices in cooking or taken as teas before or after meals. Many green herbs—dandelion, nettles, chickweed, and comfrey leaf—are good for cleansing the liver; chlorophyll in general is good for this purpose. Cooling nervine herbs such as gotu kola, skullcap, passion flower, sandalwood and bhringaraj are best for lowering the liver-deranging fiery emotions.

In terms of diet, the liver is best cleansed with an anti-Pitta approach, emphasizing raw vegetables and green vegetable juices. Sugars, fats and oils should be avoided, except for ghee. Ghee is the easiest oil for the liver to digest and helps restore its enzymatic function. It is a good vehicle to take bitter liver-cleansing herbs.

A liver-cleansing regimen is helpful in the spring as part of a general detoxification and blood purification approach. At this time wild green herbs and green vegetables with anti-Pitta properties are easily available.

Hepatitis/Jaundice

Hepatitis, an inflammation of the liver, is originally an infectious disease, but wrong diet and other mainly Pitta provoking factors increase the possibility of contracting it. The viral form is the most dangerous and has a more rapid onset. The bacterial form is not as easily transmittable or as quick to show symptoms, but has long-term debilitating effects. Bad food and water and lack of sanitation mainly cause this disease. When severe, it results in jaundice, with yellow discoloration of skin, eyes, urine, feces and mucus.

Symptoms of hepatitis are fever, loss of appetite, nausea and vomiting, pain and tenderness in the liver area or hypochondriac region, yellow discoloration of skin, eyes, nails and waste materials, fatigue, and diarrhea.

Provoking factors include too much oily, greasy food, meat (particularly red meat), or sweets. As the liver is responsible for sugar and fat metabolism, these foods tax its powers. Smoking, drinking alcohol and the use of recreational drugs (marijuana, amphetamines) are also very damaging to the liver. A history of infectious diseases such as herpes or mononucleosis also makes one susceptible. Psychological factors are anger, resentment, depression and suppressed emotions.

Herbal medicines are helpful in both acute and chronic hepatitis, particularly the latter. Western medicine has little to offer for hepatitis except bed rest. This is recommended under the herbal therapies also, sometimes for a period of several weeks.

TREATMENT OF HEPATITIS

For acute hepatitis, treatment is strongly anti-Pitta. Follow an anti-pitta diet, avoiding hot, spicy, sour and salty food as well as meat, fish, cheese, oils, fried food, and pure forms of sugar and concentrated sweets. Even milk and ghee should be avoided in acute conditions. Raw green vegetables and sprouts can be taken to cleanse the blood. Mung beans are the best staple food for strengthening liver function. A monodiet of mung beans can be followed for a week or two to reorient the liver. Then basmati rice can be added to make Kicharee, along with turmeric, coriander and other liver-cleansing spices. Complete rest is recommended and strong exercise, travel or sexual activity should be avoided. Treatment should be followed for at least three months to prevent the condition from becoming chronic.

Mainly bitter herbs are indicated, with bile clearing, blood cleansing and mild purgative action. Aloe gel is the best general herb, particularly with small amounts of turmeric and coriander, 1-2 teaspoons before meals. Aloe herbal wine is excellent in most conditions, chronic or acute.

Ayurvedic herbs are phyllanthus, katuka, aloe, barberry, nishot, guduchi, gotu kola, bhringaraj, and chiretta. Additional formulas are Tikta 1 teaspoon twice a day, Guduchi extract 1-2 teaspoons twice a day; Sudarshan powder 1-4 grams twice a day; or the Liver Tonic (no. 8). Phyllanthus by itself is excellent and is available in pill form in this country, 1 gram before meals. Triphala can be taken as a laxative. Take these herbs with aloe gel or aloe juice as the vehicle. Isatis (in Sanskrit nila) is an important Ayurvedic and Chinese herb with proven antibiotic properties for infectious hepatitis. Dosage is one ounce of the root or leaves daily, preferably with other liver-cleansing herbs.

Good Chinese herbs include coptis, gentian, rhubarb root, and bupleurum. Formulas include Gentian combination (strong type), Capillaris combination (for acute jaundice), Rehmannia 6 (weak type). Western herbs include goldenseal, barberry, rhubarb root, cascara sagrada, yellow dock and dandelion. Dandelion leaf has better detoxifying properties in acute stages; the root is more useful in chronic conditions.

For chronic hepatitis the best herbs are tonics like aloe gel, guduchi extract, amalaki, shatavari and formulas such as Chyavan Prash and Shatavari compound. Oils for rebuilding the liver (once it can digest oil) are important like sesame, olive and avocado. Chronic hepatitis usually involves anemia and becomes a wasting disease; so iron supplements or Ayurvedic iron preparations are necessary. For cirrhosis, bhringaraj is the best Ayurvedic herb.

Phyllanthus, again, is excellent, specifically for hepatitis carriers who may otherwise not exhibit symptoms. It has proven effective in chronic hepatitis conditions when all other medicines have failed. Take 1 gram of the powder in a teaspoon or two of aloe gel before meals. Chinese herbs for rebuilding the liver are dang gui, rehmannia, lycium and he shou wu (fo ti) and formulas like Rehmannia 6. They have similar long-term tonic action.

Gallstones/Choleocystitis

Congestion and obstruction in the flow of bile cause gallstones. They occur along with choleocystitis or inflammation of the wall of the gall bladder. There is often acute pain in the liver and gall bladder region along with swelling and tenderness.

The condition, particularly with pronounced inflammation, is mainly due to Pitta, which literally means bile. Pitta type gallstones are yellow, green or red in color, with sharp angles. Vata type are black or brown, and dry or rough. The pain will be severe but inflammation and fever will not be pronounced. Kapha type are round, soft, whitish, like phlegm, and seldom involve significant pain.

TREATMENT OF GALLSTONES

In acute cases an initial purgation with liver cleansing herbs is good—aloe, rhubarb root, senna, or cascara sagrada. Usually, the more acute the pain and the higher the fever the stronger the purgative action that can be used. However, such acute cases generally require clinical care. Purgatives should be followed with the liver cleansing and clearing herbs under the hepatitis section. In chronic conditions, the treatment is like that for chronic hepatitis, and strong purgatives should not be used.

Special herbs with stone-removing (lithotriptic) properties include Ayurvedic herbs pashana bheda, gokshura, and katuka; Chinese desmodian and lygodium; and Western herbs corn silk, uva ursi, and gravel root. Corn silk tea, 1 ounce per pint of water along with 1 teaspoon of coriander taken daily is effective in milder cases. Most herbs for urinary-tract stones help clear gall stones if taken with an herb to conduct the action to the liver area, like coriander or lemon grass.

A good common formula is turmeric, barberry, gravel root, corn silk and coriander in equal parts. The diet should be as per the constitution, but in acute cases avoid all food the liver has trouble digesting (sweets, oils, and fats). Liver-harmonizing formulas such as the Liver Tonic (no. 8) can be taken with strong teas of these stone-dispelling herbs as their vehicle.

ADDITIONAL DIGESTIVE DISORDERS

Food Allergies

Allergens are subtle, high energy particles that can irritate the nervous system. Food allergies may result initially from overexposure to these allergens. In the long run, however, allergic reactions are usually due to a hypersensitivity of the nervous system and indicate some internal weakness. Their causes are often emotional including stress, anxiety and worry. Allergies also result from our toxic environment, junk food, bad air, noise and other forms of environmental pollution. Food allergies indicate we are not able to assimilate these particular foods, so it is largely a kind of malabsorption syndrome.

Allergies occur when the immune system is depressed. Taking drugs and antibiotics or exposure to chemicals lowers our immune function. Poor nutrition as a child creates a weakened immune system. The immune system is transferred through the mother's milk. If children are not breast fed at all, weak immune systems and allergies become more common.

Food allergies are more common in Vata types because they possess the most sensitive nervous systems. Allergies show that, on some level, the individual is rejecting food and does not feel properly nurtured in life. Food allergies are also more common where there is low vitality; the energy is not sufficient to give adequate resistance to environmental forces. Food allergies are not uncommon in Kapha types with their low state of the digestive fire.

Symptoms of food allergies include bloating, gas, indigestion, diarrhea or constipation, congestion, headaches, and skin rashes. These usually occur after eating various 'provoking' type foods such as milk, wheat, soy, corn, nightshades (tomatoes), peaches, or strawberries. These foods may be either generally hard to digest (like milk and wheat), or contain various hard to digest substances, such as the alkaloids in the nightshades.

- Vata people most commonly become allergic to Vata-aggravating foods like beans, soy and corn.
- Pitta people most commonly become allergic to tomatoes and other nightshades and to sour fruit such as peaches and strawberries.
- Kapha people have more allergies to Kapha-increasing foods such as dairy products and wheat.

GENERAL TREATMENT OF FOOD ALLERGIES

Contact with allergens should be limited by avoiding the pro-voking food items, but the immune and digestive systems should be strengthened as well. It is not always possible to identify the exact foods causing the allergic reactions. If they can be identi-fied, it is not always possible to avoid them altogether. Some people are so sensitive they can be allergic to almost anything.

Initially a strict diet according to one's constitution should be followed, avoiding all known allergens as much as possible. It is important, however, not to become overly self-protective in avoiding allergens because emotions are often as damaging to the immune system as particular foods. Be watchful rather than fear-ful. A positive attitude in life is one of the best treatments for this condition.

Herbs and formulas to increase the digestive fire and to regu-late digestive function are indicated. These are the same as those for improving digestion for each dosha—Asafoetida 8 for Vata, Avipattikar or coriander and turmeric for Pitta and Trikatu for Kapha.

Treatment for this condition is similar to that for the Malabsorption syndrome. Spices like nutmeg, cardamom, bay leaves, fennel, cumin and ginger are good, as is the Absorption formula (no. 9). For Pitta, herbal bitters or Ayurvedic herbs like guduchi are excellent.

Long-term treatment, once the allergic sensitivity is relieved, consists of tonification with such herbs as ginseng, ashwagandha and shatavari. In avoiding the foods that we are allergic to, we must be careful not to follow a too-reducing diet, as the long-term treatment requires that we build up our strength.

Candida

Candida is an infestation of the candida albicans yeast. It usu-ally starts in the g.i. tract but can enter the blood and lodge itself in various organs. Its treatment is similar to parasitical conditions below. The symptoms include chronic low energy, low-grade fevers, variable digestion, weak immune system, and food allergies. Many signs of candida are common to weak digestive system complaints or to other immune disorders. It is helpful to have a medical test to check for the existence of the pathogen.

Candida is usually caused by weakness of the digestive fire. It is usually an Ama or toxic condition brought about by the accumulation of an undigested food mass in the intestines. As yeast requires water in which to grow, Kapha people more commonly come down with this condition. However, dampness in the digestive tract can also occur as the result of poor absorption of water. This can allow candida to grow in Vata or Pitta types who otherwise may suffer from dry skin or even dehydration.

Causative factors behind candida are eating too much sugar, taking stimulants or drugs, excess use of antibiotics, depressed immune system, frequent colds, flu's or yeast infections, hypersensitivity, emotional factors such as worry and fear, as well as the general toxic state of our environment.

GENERAL TREATMENT FOR CANDIDA

According to Ayurveda, conditions such as candida are symptomatic of an internal weakness or disharmony. The treatment principle is not merely to kill off the pathogen (in this case the yeast), but to strengthen our internal energy. This involves normalizing digestion and then taking herbal tonics to fortify the immune system. Such tonic herbs include ashwagandha, bala and kapikacchu in Ayurveda or ginseng, astragalus and schizandra in Chinese medicine.

While it is initially important to avoid yeast-containing foods and to take anti-fungal herbs, this may not take care of the internal weakness and can have long-term side effects similar to those of antibiotic drugs. It can further weaken the immune system. It is particularly dangerous in Vata constitutions because reducing diets aggravate Vata. Such treatment methods are still based on a view of the problem as external in origin. Though the methods are naturalistic, the way of thinking is still allopathic.

An anti-Ama or detoxifying diet is indicated, mainly the avoidance of heavy, damp and mucus-forming foods including sugar, dairy, breads and fruit. Cold water, ice, and cold or raw foods should also be avoided.

Hot spices with anti-parasitical powers are necessary, such as cayenne, asafoetida and prickly ash. Garlic alone, 3-5 cloves a day, can work wonders. Garlic not only helps destroy the yeast but also protects and builds up the digestive power. Spices like cardamom, bay leaves and calamus that help digest sweet and mucus-forming foods are important, or take the formula Trisugandhi powder.

Special anti-fungal herbs and anti-parasitical herbs are useful, such as valerian, wormwood, mugwort, saussurea, vidanga or the special anti-candida herb from South America, pau d'arco. They work well when balanced with spicy herbs.

SPECIFIC TREATMENT OF CANDIDA
Vata Type Candida

Symptoms are insomnia, lower back pain, dry skin, nervousness, restlessness, feeling spaced out, ringing in the ears, depression. There will be chronic gas, abdominal bloating, and constipation, with erratic or variable energy.

An anti-Ama (detoxifying) diet can be followed initially for two weeks or so. For the long run a predominately anti-Vata diet is indicated, with emphasis on complex carbohydrates like whole grains, including Kicharee. Sugar, including sweet fruit juices, and yeast foods should be avoided. Food should be cooked with spices or curried. Dairy should be avoided except for buttermilk and ghee. Salads and raw food should not be taken. Beans, cabbage family plants and mushrooms also should be avoided. The best spices are asafoetida, garlic, basil, ajwan, and cayenne. Formulas to take include Asafoetida 8 and Garlic compound tablets.

Pitta Type Candida

Indications are fever, thirst, burning sensation, hyperacidity and acute infections. The treatment involves an anti-Pitta diet but avoiding sugars. Raw food and greens will be particularly good, as is chlorophyll juice. Bitter detoxifying herbs are indicated—aloe, katuka, chiretta, neem, and barberry. Chinese bitters—coptis, scute, phellodendron and gardenia are similarly useful, as are Western bitters like goldenseal, barberry, gentian, wormwood and pau d'arco.

Formulas include Tikta, Sudarshan powder and Mahasudarshan powder. As the liver is involved, the Liver Tonic (no.8) and other liver-regulating herbs like gentian or guduchi are important.

Kapha Type Candida

There will be accumulation of phlegm, frequent colds and flu, swollen glands, edema, heaviness, dullness and excessive sleeping. Take an anti-Kapha diet avoiding all heavy, oily or greasy food such as meat, fish and dairy, as well as all sweets. Whole grains—corn, millet or rye—are good, as is mung beans.

All hot and spicy herbs listed above are good, particularly hotter herbs like cayenne and black pepper. Formulas include Trikatu and Clove compound taken with warm water (not honey). Trisugandhi formula is also good or cardamom, bay leaves and dry ginger in equal proportions.

Obesity

Modern western culture values thinness (a Vata or air type frame) as the ideal and most attractive of all body types. It makes anyone who does not fit this model feel overweight, even if their weight is normal for their physique. Many eastern and traditional cultures value a hefty physique and holding of some fat (a Kapha or water type frame), indicating affluence or plenty to eat. The right weight for a person should be judged by their body type, not cultural standards of beauty that may not be appropriate to the person's natural build.

The ideal Kapha body type is not going to be thin, but must have a good development of flesh and body fat—a round or stocky build. The ideal Pitta type will be average in build but often does better with a little extra weight. The ideal Vata type requires enough body fat to cushion the tissues and provide for support and resistance to disease. As people get older, particularly over forty, they naturally take on a little more weight as well. They should not be held to the standard of youth. Similarly, women naturally take on weight during pregnancy and can hold some of that after childbirth, particularly Kapha types.

We should discriminate overweight as a cultural condition from obesity, which is carrying too much weight than is healthy for your constitution. Obesity usually involves holding about twenty percent more weight than what is normal for your body type. It is not simply overweight relative to the existent cultural norm. Attempts to stay artificially thin may be unhealthy and can aggravate Vata, not to mention the emotional distress that they can cause. Overweight only truly becomes a disease when the extra weight held is high for the body type and leads to other health problems like hypertension, diabetes or arthritis.

Still, according to Ayurveda, it is generally better to be too thin than too heavy for your type. It is easier to build up a person who is too thin than it is to reduce one who is too heavy. A heavy body is a good breeding ground for toxins (Ama) and may reduce the life expectancy.

Causes of obesity include overeating, eating too much heavy or cold food, too frequent meals, excessive sleeping, and lack of exercise. Hormonal imbalances complicate the condition. Emotional factors include attachment, sentimentality and grief. Lack of self-esteem or low sense of self-worth can be an important factor. Sometimes the extra weight is a security factor, put on for greater protection in dealing with the world. Generally, the digestive fire will be weak in this disease of low or slow metabolism. It is usually a Kapha condition as Kapha types easily put on more weight.

Weight-reducing and appetite-suppressing drugs also suppress the digestive fire and long-term can further weaken the metabolism. They increase Vata and aggravate nervous-type obesity.

GENERAL TREATMENT OF OBESITY

First determine your normal body weight and see how obese you really are. If you are significantly overweight then proceed with the anti-obesity remedies. If the problem is more cosmetic, wanting to be a little thinner, then try a few simple measures like taking more spices in your diet, avoiding eating early in the morning or late at night, increasing your exercise and doing some fasting occasionally.

Obesity requires a lightening (langhana) or reducing method, with a long-term light diet both in terms of food quantity and quality. Not only eat less but also avoid heavy, greasy, fried or fatty foods. Learn the joy of fasting, fasting one day a week or one week a year. Add spices to your diet and drink warm and spicy teas regularly to improve your digestion. Use mild laxatives like Triphala to keep the bowels clean. Strong reducing therapies should not be started in the winter season, as they can lower body heat and resistance to disease. Usually long-term mild reducing therapies will be more successful than short-term crash methods.

Guggul and myrrh are good general herbs, as is shilajit. Take 1 gram of guggul or 1/2 gram of shilajit 2-3 times a day with ginger and honey. Aloe gel with a little ginger or turmeric is another good combination. Take 1 teaspoon of aloe gel with 1/4 teaspoon each of ginger and turmeric powders before meals. Nervines are useful to calm the tendency towards excessive eating. The best is gotu kola but skullcap and jatamamsi are also good.

A good combination for obesity is taking Trikatu, Triphala and gotu kola with aloe gel or juice. The Herbal Weight Reduction Formula (no. 15), taken with honey, is a specific formula for this condition. A special herb for weight reduction in Ayurveda is Garcinia camboja. This single herb taken 1 gram before meals is excellent for lowering excess body fat and improving the metabolism.

Pranayama is excellent, particularly right nostril breathing or bhastrika, for raising the digestive fire and increasing the metabolism. Gems for Saturn, such as blue sapphire or amethyst, are good for weight reduction, while gems for Mercury like emerald, peridot and jade help calm the nerves and reduce cravings. Ruby or garnet for the Sun can be helpful when the condition is due to chronically low digestive fire.

163

KAPHA TYPE OBESITY

Obesity is more common in Kapha constitutions with their earthy and watery constitutions. Their appetite is continuous and they often eat as a means of relieving stress or tension. They can become attached to or addicted to the joys of cooking and eating. In addition, they may suffer from hypothyroid or other hormonal conditions that cause them to hold weight.

Their excessive weight consists largely of water and fat. It is related to weak function of the pancreas and kidneys, and the pulse and energy level may be low. The individual is generally flabby, pale in complexion and has moist skin. There will be excessive phlegm or saliva. Subcutaneous fat deposits may develop along with benign tumors.

The treatment is like the general treatment, primarily dietary, following an anti-Kapha diet for an extended period of time. All cold drinks should be avoided. Sugar and sugar products should be avoided as much as possible. Salt intake should be strongly reduced. Dairy, sweet fruits, breads, pastries, meats, fish and oily foods should be taken as little as possible. Take sprouts, yeast and other enzymatic agents as digestive aids. Eat more vegetables, preferably steamed without much oil or salt, beans and whole grains, and less of the heavier foods. Mung beans are excellent as a staple food.

Food should not be taken before 10 AM or after 6 PM. Consume hot spices like cayenne, ginger or Trikatu to raise the metabolism. Fasting one day a week is excellent, unless there is debility. For liquids during fasts use spice teas or vegetable juices, but not fruit juices. As the condition is a long-term metabolic imbalance that the system has become accustomed to, such measures should be employed gradually, allowing a slow, natural speeding up of organic functions that will not shock the system.

Excessive sleeping, or sleeping during the day, should be avoided. Exercise, particularly of an aerobic nature, should be undertaken. However, if the person is weak, exercise should not be taken to the point of strong sweating, shortness of breath or fainting.

164

Herbs include: hot spices to increase the metabolism—cayenne, black pepper, ginger, garlic and turmeric—and bitter herbs to reduce fat—katuka, barberry, gentian, and myrrh. Barberry is a rejuvenative for fat tissue, both eliminating excess fat and producing better quality tissue. The usual combination of turmeric and barberry is also useful here for obesity. Guggul or myrrh (preferably as a tincture) is specific and can be taken along with spices or bitters.

Ayurvedic formulas include Trikatu, Triphala, the Digestive Stimulant (no. 1) or the Weight Reduction formula (no. 15). Mild laxatives such as the Ayurvedic Triphala, aloe gel or cascara sagrada are helpful. Strong purgatives are not good because they can lower the metabolism further. Trikatu and Triphala together with honey are excellent, 1 gram with meals.

Mild diuretics—plantain, corn silk or gokshura can be helpful, as well as herbs or formulas for improving kidney function such as shilajit or gokshura. Nervine herbs such as gotu kola and calamus combined or skullcap counter the habit side of the disease.

Chinese formulas include Citrus and Craetagus, which is good for overeating and food stagnation (Ama) conditions generally. Additional Western herbs are alfalfa, dandelion and chicory.

VATA TYPE OBESITY

Vata caused obesity is characterized by irregularity in weight. Periods of overweight fluctuating with periods of normal weight, or even underweight, may occur. Weight gain or weight loss may be sudden or unpredictable. Appetite will also be variable. Excessive amounts of sugar or carbohydrates taken to help calm the nerves will contribute to obesity. Psychological factors are fear, anxiety, worry and nervousness. Extra weight will give greater feelings of security or stability.

The most difficult form of obesity is a combined Vata-Kapha type with a nervous mind (Vata) and a slow metabolism (Kapha). Mental habit and physical weakness combine in ways that are difficult to counteract. Under such conditions it is better to aim at

165

reducing Vata (calming the nerves) than simply reducing Kapha (applying restrictive diet). Or take anti-Vata herbs like ashwagandha along with an anti-Kapha diet

The treatment involves an anti-Vata diet but with emphasis on complex carbohydrates (from natural sources, however, not artificial carbohydrates). Take whole grains and starchy vegetables, with beans such as mung or black beans. Avoid pure sugars and overeating. Use fewer of the hot spices (pepper and cayenne) and more of the spicy-sweet ones (fennel, cardamom, and coriander).

Ayurvedic formulas include Asafoetida 8 and Trikatu. Herbs to calm the mind and allay nervous habits are good, including gotu kola, calamus, jatamamsi, nutmeg and valerian or formulas like Sarasvat powder. Guggul or myrrh are helpful here also.

PITTA TYPE OBESITY

Obesity in Pitta types is usually caused by overeating. Their appetite is high and their digestion is usually good, so they can eat a lot. As they can easily digest sugar, they can also become addicted to it. They also often like meat. Their weight involves a good development of muscle and is usually not just flab.

The treatment involves an anti-Pitta diet. Meat, fish, oily or greasy food should be avoided, as well as sugars and pastries. One should take raw salads along with green herbs and chlorophyll. Digestive bitters like gentian are specific, as well as bitter laxatives.

Ayurvedic herbs include aloe, katuka, barberry, and turmeric. Formulas include Sudarshan powder, the Liver Tonic (no. 8) and other liver-regulating formulas. Chinese formulas include Major Bupleurum combination. Helpful Western herbs are barberry, gentian, dandelion, and cascara sagrada.

Underweight

Underweight can also be a disease, though our culture does not always recognize it as such. Lack of body weight can cause poor resistance, low vitality, nervousness and insomnia. There will be lack of appetite, depression, malaise, and psychological instability. There may be wasting away of the tissues including loss of hair, teeth falling out, weakness of the bones and lack of sexual vitality, as well as other signs of premature aging.

Causes are frequently constitutional: suppression of the digestive fire, too much fasting, dieting, eating of light, cold or raw food, or irregular eating habits. Other factors include overwork, too much exercise and excessive sexual activity. Psychological factors are worry and grief (often following loss of a loved one), excessive study or too much mental activity. Low weight may be involved in convalescence from a severe disease that has depleted the body tissues. It occurs more commonly in the elderly or in children.

Underweight is usually a Vata condition, as air types tend towards lightness. Vata individuals forget to eat or their irregular eating habits cause long-term suppression of the digestive fire. Use of stimulant drugs such as amphetamines can bring this condition about also.

TREATMENT OF UNDERWEIGHT

The treatment starts with an increasing or tonification therapy. An anti-Vata diet is usually best. Take heavy foods like root vegetables, whole grains, nuts, dairy products, oils and natural sugars. Meat or bone marrow soup may be necessary in the beginning or a mild starchy grain gruel (rice, mung beans or oats). Spices are indicated, but mild at first, such as cardamom or fresh ginger. The hotter spices like cayenne may cause further depletion of vital fluids by their drying nature, and overstimulate what is usually already a hypermetabolism.

Tonic herbs are essential—ashwagandha, shatavari, bala, or licorice prepared in milk, generally 1/2-1 teaspoon of the powdered herb per cup. Ayurvedic formulas are Ashwagandha compound, Shatavari compound, Dhatupaushtic compound, and Chyavan Prash. These can be taken with milk or with draksha.

Additional Western herbs include comfrey root, slippery elm, marshmallow, and saw palmetto. Chinese herbs are ginseng, astragalus, dang gui, and rehmannia. Chinese formulas include Ten Major Herbs and Woman's Precious Pill.

In underweight gems for Jupiter such as yellow sapphire, yellow topaz or citrine are best, along with gems for Mercury such as emerald, peridot and jade. Green color, which relates to the Mercury, is good for regulating metabolism—for increasing weight in those too thin and for decreasing it in those too fat.

PITTA TYPE UNDERWEIGHT

Underweight can occur as a high Pitta condition in which Pittas literally burn themselves up. Often there is high fire in the mind with excessive thinking and an overly critical nature. The condition may follow a severe febrile disease, blood loss or hepatitis. Anemia and poor liver function are usually involved.

The treatment is similar to that for Vata with an anti-Pitta diet that emphasizes building-type foods. All spices are to be avoided. Salads and raw vegetables should not be taken in excess, as they are not strengthening enough, but all manner of cooked vegetables are good. A milk fast may be advisable in the beginning, taking only warm milk with a little sugar three times a day for a week. Whole grains like wheat and rice are good and mung beans are probably the best food. Raw sugars may be used in moderation. Ghee is excellent in the diet.

Ayurvedic herbs include aloe gel, gotu kola and shatavari. Guduchi is excellent. Formulas include Chyavan Prash, Brahma Rasayana, Shatavari compound.

Chinese herbs include he shou wu (fo ti) and formulas include Women's Precious Pill (can be used by men also). Additional Western herbs are comfrey root, marshmallow, slippery elm, American ginseng, and licorice.

Anorexia

Anorexia can become a severe condition connected to overdieting and underweight. The digestive fire may be suppressed to the point where no food can be held in the stomach. There can be repeated vomiting to the point of dehydration. Causes are usually nervous sensitivity, emotional traumas or chronic under eating.

While nausea, vomiting and mild anorexia are usually symptoms of a Kapha disorder, severe anorexia with pronounced weight loss is mainly a high Vata condition involved with fear, nervousness, insomnia, pain in the chest and abdomen and palpitations. There may be a feeling of constriction in the throat, along with difficulty swallowing, possibly with a feeling of choking.

Even Vata people can become anorexic or lose their appetite if they eat too many sweet or Kaphogenic foods, particularly at the beginning of meals, like sugars, ice cream, milk, cheese or yogurt. Vata types like the calm they feel by excess eating of sugars and carbohydrates but it can derange them further. Periods of overeating of carbohydrates may alternate with periods of lack of appetite and under eating, thus deranging the whole digestive process and leading ultimately to severe anorexia.

TREATMENT FOR ANOREXIA

Spices to regulate digestion and stop vomiting are required, particularly cardamom, fennel and fresh ginger. Take regular teas of such herbs, particularly after eating. Ayurvedic formulas include Cardamom compound or Asafoetida 8, but remember that the taste of asafoetida may be hard to take.

A mild bland diet is best such as Kicharee (equal parts rice and mung). Coffee, tea and all drugs and stimulants must be avoided. The rest of the treatment is like that for underweight, with tonics like Chyavan Prash and Ashwagandha compound.

In addition, take calming and grounding nervine herbs such as valerian, nutmeg, jatamamsi or sandalwood. Adequate rest and a calming and supportive environment are required. A good herbal formula for anorexia is 2 parts ashwagandha, 1 part gotu kola, 1 part of cardamom and 1 part fennel. Take 1-2 teaspoons of the powder infused in a cup of water with a little honey, sipped every 2-3 hours until the system is calmed.

169

Sesame oil massage is very helpful, particularly to the head and feet (but not to the abdomen). Putting a little sandalwood oil to the head restores balance and calm.

II.2
DISEASES OF THE LARGE INTESTINE
The Importance of the Colon in the Disease Process

The large intestine governs the elimination of waste material from the body, the undigested portion of the food that we have taken in. As such it is perhaps the body's most important organ of elimination, removing waste matter from the entire digestive tract, including the left over bile and other digestive secretions.

However, the stool does serve a purpose in the large intestine. The bulk of the stool maintains the tone of the large intestine. It also functions as the earth element in the body to ground us. It supports not only the digestive system but gives stability to the prana and mind as well. Without the proper amount of stool in the large intestine our energy easily gets imbalanced or erratic as Vata becomes aggravated.

In addition, the large intestine is an important organ of digestion and assimilation. Its membrane absorbs the energy and the nutrients that build up the bones and the deeper tissues of the marrow, nerve and reproductive. It takes in the prana or deeper vitality from our food that provides deeper reserves of strength and Ojas.

Our pattern of elimination shows the final product of our digestion. Proper management of the colon is the foundation for treating the digestive system. For this reason, disorders of the large intestine are crucial in all digestive system disorders.

As the large intestine relates to Vata, which governs prana or vitality as a whole, its disorders are involved in most diseases. *In any disease condition we should always examine the large intestine and make sure to bring its functioning back to normal as one of the first steps of treatment.*

DISORDERS OF THE COLON

Diarrhea initially is the body's attempt to throw off toxins, but long-term diarrhea results in a lack of absorption of proper nutrients. Constipation indicates retention of waste materials in the body. These are the two main disorders of the colon, and other colon diseases like colitis or diverticulitis can be treated through them. Both constipation and diarrhea are due to an excess or accumulation of Apana Vayu, the downward moving air. Constipation is an excess of its dry attribute, whereas diarrhea is an excess of its mobile attribute.

A stool that is poorly-formed, has a strong unpleasant odor, or sinks quickly in water indicates indigestion and the formation of Ama (toxins). Such Ama must result in eventual health problems. It is as important to be aware of our pattern of elimination as of the state of our appetite.

Colon disorders relate to the first or root chakra. They are based on fear, the need for security and support, lack of groundedness and other first chakra emotional disharmonies. In their treatment we must also take care of our emotional root in life.

Many spices are good for strengthening absorption in the colon. These include ginger, cayenne, and black pepper, and especially, asafoetida, basil and nutmeg. In taking spices for our digestive fire, we should consider those for the colon as well. The prime Ayurvedic formula for colon digestion is Asafoetida 8 (Hingashtak), 1-2 grams of the pills or powder after meals. It alleviates gas and bloating, improves absorption, and stimulates and strengthens colon function in general.

CONSTIPATION

Constipation is the main digestive system disorder and reflects any problems in the digestive tract. Only if our elimination is proper can we be healthy, fit and energetic. For this reason the section on constipation is the most detailed of the disease treatments.

According to Ayurveda, normal and healthy colon function is indicated by a lack of tongue coating (except for a normal thin white coating). One should have an easy bowel movement the first thing in the morning. The stool should float (if it sinks it indicates Ama, poor digestion and the accumulation of toxins).

Almost everyone suffers from an accumulation of toxins in the colon, evidenced by a coating at the back of the tongue. Toxins in the colon and constipation, however, cannot always be simply treated with purgatives or colonics. These can weaken the tone of the colon and breed dependency. Their action on the system is strong and often traumatic; it can unbalance other organ functioning and, particularly, aggravate Vata, the biological air humor. Symptoms of excessive use of colonics and purgatives include lack of appetite, excessive weight loss, insomnia, diarrhea or continued constipation, palpitations, anxiety and vertigo or feeling faint.

The main cause of constipation on a physical level is dietary — eating food that is difficult to digest. It may also occur as the complication of a fever or infectious disease. Other factors include sleeping late in the morning, or not heeding the urge to go. Our American life-style of getting up quickly and rushing off to work tends to block the natural urge towards elimination. Sex in the morning causes apana, the downward moving air, to be weakened and can aggravate the condition. Coffee or tea in the morning may promote constipation, as they tend to be diuretic (drying). Our sedentary life-style and lack of exercise are additional aggravations.

Psychological factors behind constipation are insomnia, nervousness, stress, worry, grief and fear, as well as any excess stimulation of the nervous system (like too much television). Medical factors such as being bedridden or taking too many drugs or medications (particularly diuretics) have their effect as well.

General Treatment of Constipation

For any form of constipation that is not severe, first improve the digestion with the right use of spices in order to normalize the Agni or digestive fire. Ginger is excellent in this regard but almost all spices can be helpful. Laxatives that tonify the colon or improve colon function, like psyllium or Triphala are safer and often preferable to short-term quick purgatives. Castor oil, though its taste is hard to take, is probably the best herb for severe consti- pation because it is not as drying to the colon as bitter purgatives. It works well with ginger tea to balance digestive functioning on all levels. Laxative salts can also be helpful much like castor oil.

Strong bitter purgatives like senna and rhubarb root are better for acute or severe conditions. Acute constipation is evidenced by fever, thick tongue coating, severe bloating, gas, and severe abdominal pain on palpation. It usually indicates Ama, toxemia or some kind of food poisoning (which may be caused by bad food combinations). With these herbs fasting or a light diet should be followed for a few days. Care should be taken, however, if the pain is in the lower right abdomen. This can indicate appen- dicitis, in which case purgatives, though sometimes helpful, can be quite dangerous. In the case of women note any menstrual complications, which can also cause lower abdominal pain.

For chronic constipation, particularly in the elderly or in Vata types, make sure that the diet has an adequate intake of oily or bulk foods. These include dairy products, nuts, whole grains, and bran. Raw fruit and raw vegetables are ok if the digestive fire is strong. Many fruit juices are good, particularly prune, grape, and cherry, but not apple or cranberry, which can cause constipation. More oils or fats may be needed in the diet. Sesame oil is excellent, as is olive oil.

FORMULAS—TRIPHALA

The famous Ayurvedic compound Triphala is specific for chronic constipation. It is excellent for constipation in any of the three doshas, though not always effective in acute conditions. It is a great colon cleanser as well as a tonic and rejuvenative (ras- ayana) for the colon. Moreover, it nourishes the bones and nerves and improves the appetite. As a metabolic regulator, it will reduce fat in overweight conditions, while building the blood, muscles and nerves in underweight conditions. Dosage is 5-15 grams once a day in warm water before sleep.

174

Triphala ensures proper absorption of the prana, or life-force, from the food, which according to Ayurveda occurs in the colon. The colon is not just an organ of elimination but also one of digestion. Its proper function is necessary to provide adequate nutrition to the deeper tissues of the bone, nerve and reproductive. According to Ayurveda the membrane of the colon (puri-shadhara kala) takes in the prana or vital force from the food, if it is functioning well, but takes in the apana or waste gases, if functioning improperly. Proper regulation of the colon, which occurs through Triphala, is one of the keys to health and longevity.

OTHER HERBS FOR CONSTIPATION

Aloe gel, 1-2 teaspoons 3 times a day, is another good general treatment for most types of constipation. Aloe possesses both cleansing and lubricating actions, though it is not as tonifying to the colon as Triphala. It is particularly good for constipation that occurs along with fever or along with delayed menstruation.

The Colon Tonic (no. 5) is an improved form of Triphala, with a higher dosage of the main laxative in the formula, hari-taki. It has a broad spectrum usage—with honey for Kapha types, with cool water or ghee for Pitta and with warm water for Vata.

In terms of life-style, it is important to arise at dawn (Vata time and colon time) and to empty the bowels. Often a glass of warm water or warm herbal tea will stimulate peristalsis. Yoga postures or a mild massage of the lower abdomen are helpful. Squatting, rather than sitting on the toilet, is a more natural position for elimination and helps relieve blockages and spasms in the intestines that may inhibit normal evacuation.

A good breakfast, particularly of oily or laxative foods, such as oatmeal with milk or ghee, may bring about normal evacuation if it has not occurred by that point. Or taking prune or grape juices may do the job. Cold food, like cold cereals with milk, can block normal elimination.

TYPES OF CONSTIPATION

Ayurveda recognizes three states of the colon: mild, medium and hard according to our constitutional condition as Pitta, Kapha or Vata.

- Those with a mild state of the colon tend to have a loose or oily stool. If they become constipated, any mild laxative, such as warm milk or psyllium, will usually be sufficient. Constipation seldom becomes chronic. This is more characteristic of Pitta constitution as Pitta tends towards oiliness.
- Medium state of the colon characterizes Kapha. Stronger laxatives may be needed or more long-term usage of moderate laxatives, particularly combining Triphala, Trikatu (hot spices) and some use of bitter laxatives.
- Hard or difficult state of the colon characterizes Vata. Constipation is often chronic and difficult to remedy. Strong laxatives like castor oil may be necessary short-term, with a long-term taking of milder laxatives like Triphala. Major dietary changes may be required.

Constipation is usually a Vata disorder, particularly when it is a long-standing condition or in the elderly. It may also be due to high Pitta (heat which dries out the stool) or high Kapha (mucus congestion clogging the colon). Not uncommonly, it is an Ama or toxicity condition. Ama, undigested food, accumulates in the small intestine and is retained in the large intestine owing to blockage of the downward moving air (apana).

CHINESE VIEW OF CONSTIPATION

In Chinese medicine, acute constipation is related to fever and high fire that dries out the stool. It is similar to Pitta constipation in Ayurveda and similarly treated with bitter purgatives. Chronic constipation is related to deficiency of body fluids with progressive dryness in the colon. It is treated with bulk and lubricating laxatives, such as cannabis seeds, and is like the Vata type.

Specific Treatment of Constipation

Vata Type Constipation

High Vata is characterized by dryness in the colon, intestinal gas, abdominal distention and constipation. The tongue usually has a brownish coating at the back. There may be bad breath or the passing of gas, along with pain, tenesmus and anxiety. Headaches and light-headedness may occur.

Causes are wrong diet with too much dry or light food, irregular eating habits, smoking, taking of drugs, excessive thinking, worrying, fear and anxiety, over stimulation of the nervous system, and old age. Constipation is involved in many Vata disorders including arthritis, neurosis, epilepsy and paralysis. Treating constipation is a root treatment for many nervous system disorders.

TREATMENT

An anti-Vata diet should be followed with proper spices for balancing digestion. Include adequate oils in the diet—sesame oil, olive oil or ghee—to insure lubrication of the colon. Adequate bulk should be taken as well, such as whole grains (oats is best) or bran. Beans, dry grains, cabbage family plants, mushrooms and other light or drying food should be avoided.
Spices to balance digestion, particularly asafoetida and ginger should be taken with food to alleviate gas and promote the downward movement of Vata.

Apply sesame or almond oil externally to the skin, with regular oil massage of the body, but not if there is severe bloating or distention. Sesame oil will lubricate the lungs through the skin and the large intestine through the lungs. Warm milk with a teaspoon of ghee can be taken as a laxative before sleep for mild conditions.

Take Triphala, 5-15 grams (1—3 teaspoons) in warm water before sleep. For stronger laxative action, the amount of haritaki can be doubled or Triphala fried in castor oil can be used. For more obstinate constipation, particularly with disturbances of the nervous system, 1-3 teaspoons of castor oil can be taken before sleep.

Laxative salts like Epsom salt are good, 1-2 teaspoons before sleep. They moisten the stool and ease elimination. Lavanbhaskar powder is a good Ayurvedic formula using various salts, as it increases Agni and promotes elimination. Asafoetida 8 (Hingashtak) regulates peristalsis and has a mild laxative action.

Bulk laxatives like psyllium and flaxseed are excellent for mild conditions of Vata constipation. Psyllium husk powder, 1-2 teaspoons in warm water before sleep, is the best and seldom causes griping. Aloe gel is also useful as a lubricating laxative for Vata. It may be a little cold for many Vata types so a small amount of ginger juice or powder should be added to it. Bulk laxatives are heavy and should be balanced by spices (asafoetida or ginger), so they do not cause congestion.

Typical Chinese formulas include Cannabis Seed combination as a bulk laxative and Major or Minor Rhubarb temporarily for severe constipation.

ENEMA THERAPY

Enema therapy (basti) is the main method for calming Vata and is specific for constipation. First a cleansing enema is given, particularly when foul-smelling gas occurs. Use Vata-reducing herbs—Triphala, fennel, cardamom, or calamus—along with a smaller amount of demulcents like licorice or sesame oil. Prepare about half an ounce of such herbs in a quart of water for the enema and administer it slightly warm in temperature. Follow with an oil enema consisting of 1/2 cup sesame oil in 1/2 cup warm water, held for a minimum of twenty minutes.

When constipation is accompanied by general debility or by the weakness of old age, tonic herbs can be taken as nutritive enemas. These herbs include ashwagandha, bala, calamus and shatavari. They can be taken in oil, like sesame oil, or as milk decoctions, retaining one cup of the mixture for at least twenty minutes like the oil enemas.

CAUTION

The presence of the stool in the colon upholds the earth element in the body, which is necessary for keeping the air element from rising too high. Excess purgation therapy can cause anxiety, insomnia, palpitations, fainting, heart pain and other symptoms of high Vata. Again, one should proceed gently with Vata.

Pitta Type Constipation

Pitta constipation often occurs during the course or towards the end of a febrile disease. In Ayurveda, purgatives are contraindicated in new fevers but prescribed in old fevers. They are given after the fever is gone to clear out residual heat and toxins.

In Chinese medicine, purgatives are given during high fevers, as another method of draining the fever, but care is taken that the fever is 'ripe'. Indications of a ripe, or firm, fever are constipation, distention, gas and strong abdominal pain.

Pitta constipation involves irritability, anger, thirst, sweating with body odor, and burning sensations in the rectum. It is characterized by a red tongue with yellow coating and bad breath. The face may be flushed or red. There may be headache or insomnia with violent dreams.

Causes include too much spicy, sour or salty food, and too much meat or greasy food. In constipation the hot attribute of Pitta is aggravated. Hot food, exposure to the sun or heat, or an inadequate intake of fluids are the main aggravating factors. Pitta type constipation often involves liver dysfunction with congestion or obstruction of the bile. It is not simply a colon problem as it usually is with Vata. Detoxification of the liver may be necessary as well.

TREATMENT

An anti-Pitta diet should be implemented, avoiding too many oils, fats or sweets, which can overtax the liver. Release of anger and letting go of stress is necessary if constipation is due to emotional causes. Often warm milk and ghee or licorice tea will be enough to stimulate evacuation. In India a rose confection is used for this purpose. Only when accompanied with high fever and thirst will constipation be severe in Pitta constitutions.

Most bitter laxatives like rhubarb root and senna can be used safely when this condition is acute. They also cleanse the liver. Otherwise bulk laxatives may be sufficient. Aloe gel combines both properties and can be taken 1-2 tablespoons before sleep. Taken on a regular basis, 1-2 teaspoons 2-3 times a day, aloe gel will usually prevent constipation in Pitta individuals. In severe cases, take aloe powder 1-2 grams before sleep, to which a little coriander or fennel can be added to stop griping.

Ayurvedic herbs include aloe, amalaki, rose, and psyllium. Formulas include Triphala (taken with ghee or aloe juice) and aloe herbal wine. For most chronic or mild conditions 1-2 teaspoons of psyllium husk powder in warm water before sleep is sufficient.

Chinese herbal formulas include Major or Minor Rhubarb decoction, according to whether the condition is strong or moderate. Typical Western herbs include rhubarb root, senna leaf (strong action) and barberry, yellow dock, cascara sagrada (mild action).

PURGATION THERAPY

Purgation therapy (virechana) is the main treatment for high Pitta (fire), because it cleanses heat from the small intestine and liver, as well as the colon. But, for this therapy to work, Pitta must first be drawn into the gastrointestinal tract by the appropriate diet, herbs, oil massage and sweating therapy. Otherwise purgation may not be helpful.

Purgation is an important way of eliminating heat and toxins from the body. It purifies the blood as well as the digestive tract. It drains down the excessive fire rising upwards that occurs in infectious or delirious conditions of the head and brain.

Kapha Type Constipation

Kapha constipation is usually due to the system being clogged with mucus. There will be heaviness, lethargy, tiredness and other signs of high Kapha. Stools will be copious, whitish or with phlegm. The tongue will be pale and fat with a white or mucus

180

coating. The abdomen may be bloated, along with a feeling of dull pain and there may be edema in the lower abdomen as well.

The main cause is sluggishness or congestion of the colon. Provoking factors include too much heavy or mucus forming foods, excessive sleeping, sleeping during the day, sedentary life style, and other Kapha increasing actions. It can also occur as a complication of Kapha (phlegm) disorders in the upper body—stomach and respiratory disorders with excess mucus draining down through the digestive system. Hence while treating the constipation, other anti-Kapha therapies like expectorant or emetic therapy should be considered as well.

TREATMENT

Follow an anti-Kapha diet by avoiding heavy, constipating food including sugar, cheese, yogurt, bread, pastries, potatoes and pork. Fasting is good, for one to three days or longer. Increased physical and mental activity is needed, more aerobic exercise and less sleep.

Light laxative and purgative herbs are indicated. Bitter laxatives can be used in acute conditions like aloe, rhubarb root and senna. Such herbs also help remove fat and reduce weight. Hot spices, ginger, cayenne and black pepper are needed. A good formula is 3 grams of powdered rhubarb root along with 2 grams of dry ginger, taken in one cup of warm water before sleep.

Bulk laxatives and laxative oils should not be used as these increase Kapha and will promote stagnation. Cleansing enemas with spicy and expectorant herbs such as ginger, calamus and bayberry are also helpful.

Ayurvedic formulas include Triphala 2-6 grams along with Trikatu 1-3 grams, taken with aloe juice or warm water before sleep, or the Digestive Stimulant (no. 1) with the Colon Tonic (no. 5).

INTESTINAL GAS, BLOATING AND COLIC

Intestinal gas or colic pain indicates poor digestion and the formation of Ama. It is characteristically a high Vata condition but can be brought about by any of the doshas. It usually involves some bloating or distention, along with abdominal sensitivity or migrating abdominal pain. Most abdominal pain is related to gas or indigestion.

The causes are mainly dietary, eating foods that are difficult to digest, though nervous and emotional upset can trigger it as well. Such gas-forming foods include beans, cabbage family plants and raw onions which are too dry, and sweets like ice cream or oily foods which are too heavy. Other factors are wrong food combinations such as eating sweet foods or juices with starchy, salty or protein meals, or by combining dairy products with sour fruit or with bread, meat or fish. Overeating will cause it as well. Our cultural habit of eating sweet desserts after meals causes fermentation and gas. Psychological factors are mainly excess worry, strain and stress.

Gas and distention is a secondary condition or precursor of constipation or diarrhea. The downward moving air (apana) is obstructed. It usually indicates poor functioning of the digestive fire as well.

General Treatment of Gas and Bloating

Simple and moderate eating is required: not eating too much, too frequently, or combining too many foods at the same meal. Sweet taste should be avoided or taken in moderation by itself. Spicy, carminative (gas-dispelling) herbs are indicated. These include cardamom, fennel, ginger, peppermint, orange peel, bay leaves and most cooking spices.

Cardamom and fennel in equal parts are excellent for most indigestion, gas and abdominal pain, 1/2 teaspoon of the powder infused in one cup of water taken before meals. Asafoetida, valerian, jatamamsi, nutmeg and camomile have analgesic properties for intestinal pain. Castor oil, with a little cayenne or asafoetida, can be applied externally to the abdomen and will give quick relief. Ajwan, Indian wild celery seed, is very good, along with a little rock salt. Most digestive formulas are good, like Trisugandhi, Trikatu and the Digestive Stimulant (no. 1).

Specific Treatment of Bloating

Vata Type Bloating

Indications are gas and distention, with variable appetite, constipation, insomnia, palpitations or nervousness. There may be severe or migrating abdominal pain and discomfort. Too much light or dry food can produce this condition—beans, cabbage, raw onions, potato or corn chips, peanuts, or excess salads. Dry pastries, cookies, and dry fruit also aggravate Vata by their dry quality. But improper food combinations and irregular eating habits are the main thing. Worry, fear, anxiety and other Vata psychological factors are usually present. Travel and exercise may aggravate the condition.

Treatment consists of an anti-Vata and anti-Ama diet, closely watching proper food combination and regular timing of meals. The best herbs are spicy, carminative herbs—asafoetida, ajwan, ginger, fennel, cumin, cardamom, and calamus. Vata types should at least regularly take ginger tea if they have bloating problems.

Typical Ayurvedic formulas are Asafoetida 8, Lavanbhaskar powder or Trisugandhi powder, 1-3 grams before meals with warm water. Asafoetida 8 is usually the best. These herbs can be taken after meals as well, for overeating.

Chinese herbs include perilla leaf, magnolia bark, ginger, and citrus peel. Typical Chinese formulas include Magnolia and Ginger combination. Many common Western cooking spices are good for this condition including mint, sage, basil, bay leaves, oregano and thyme. Camomile and valerian help relieve pain and cramping.

Pitta Type Bloating

Symptoms of high Pitta such as hyperacidity, heartburn, diarrhea and irritability occur along with gas. The treatment begins with an anti-Pitta diet and avoiding hot and oily food. Carminative (gas-dispelling) herbs and formulas should be combined with bitters. Cooler carminative herbs are indicated like fennel, coriander, cumin, mint, and saffron. Good bitters are gentian, barberry, goldenseal, and katuka.

The typical Ayurvedic formula is Avipattikar powder but most bitters are good, particularly if combined with a small amount of dry ginger. The Antacid formula (no. 12) is also helpful. A simple and pleasant formula is coriander, fennel and cumin in equal parts. Take these herbs as a powder, 1/4 teaspoon before meals.

KAPHA TYPE BLOATING

Symptoms of high Kapha will prevail with phlegm, congestion, nausea or vomiting. Avoid overeating and eating late at night. Avoid sugars, desserts and greasy food in general, following strictly the anti-kapha diet. The herbs and formulas for Vata can be used with emphasis on the hotter herbs—cayenne, dry ginger, ajwan, calamus and cloves. Trikatu formula is indicated, with warm water, not honey in this instance.

DIARRHEA AND DYSENTERY

Diarrhea is a condition of frequent, loose or watery stools. If it becomes severe, dehydration can occur along with a collapse of energy and vitality. Diarrhea may be due to exogenous factors such as heavy meals or difficult to digest foods. These are foods that are too oily, too watery, too dry, too hard, too hot or too cold. Wrong food combinations, such as taking milk with meat or fish; eating another meal before the previous meal is digested; irregularity in eating habits; or eating unaccustomed foods, are additional causes. Impure food and water, food poisoning, parasites, changes in seasons, stomach flu or emotional disturbances like panic or grief can also bring it about.

TYPES OF DIARRHEA

Diarrhea is most commonly a Pitta condition, as Pitta has a damp and hot quality and the mildest tone of the colon. Yet it may be due to high Vata, high Kapha, high Ama (toxins) or psychological factors.
- Pitta diarrhea is usually yellow, foul smelling, and mixed with pus or blood. There may be a burning sensation at the

184

rectum. There may be thirst, dryness and possibly fever. This is what is usually seen in most acute cases of bacterial dysentery.

- Vata diarrhea involves pain, cramping, tenesmus, passing of gas and frequent motions without much stool being passed. Diarrhea and constipation may alternate, or a period of constipation or lack of bowel movements may precede the diarrhea.

- Kapha diarrhea is whitish in color, viscous and contains phlegm. There is a feeling of heaviness, torpor and lassitude. Motions are not frequent but tend to have more quantity.

In Chinese medicine, diarrhea is classified as either excess or deficient. Excess type is usually owing to the accumulation of damp-heat in the stomach and large intestine. It is very similar to the Pitta-type in Ayurveda and is often acute. Deficient type may be owing to chi (energy) or yang deficiency. Its treatment has similarities to the Vata and Kapha kinds but does not directly correspond.

General Treatment of Diarrhea

In the beginning astringents (stool-binding herbs such as alum, oak bark or raspberry) should not be used because they can cause the toxins to be held in the body. There should be fasting with herbs to burn up toxins (spices and bitters). An initial purgative—castor oil or rhubarb root—should be taken to flush the colon of toxins. Many anti-parasitical herbs may be helpful like wormwood, mugwort, pomegranate, and vidanga.

Foods for improving absorption in the small intestine should be taken first. Buttermilk is good, along with a bland whole grain diet, mung gruel or kicharee. An anti-Ama or detoxifying approach is best. Good spices for diarrhea include ginger, pippali, saffron, coriander and cardamom. The best common spice for stopping diarrhea is nutmeg. Take 1-2 teaspoons before meals with warm water.

Ayurvedic formula no. 9, Herbal Absorption, is excellent, as well as Nutmeg compound. A good general Western herbal formula is equal parts nutmeg, raspberry leaf, mullein leaf and marshmallow. Take such herbs every two to three hours until the condition improves.

Should severe or watery diarrhea persist for more than a few days, the use of astringents to bind the stool will be required, as well as the administration of tonic herbs like ashwagandha or ginseng to restore collapsed vitality.

PITTA TYPE DIARRHEA

An anti-Pitta diet is required. Hot spices should be avoided, particularly chilies and garlic. Do not take any form of alcohol. Oily, greasy and fried foods will also make the condition worse. No oil massage should be given. The abdomen should be kept cool. Yoga postures like shoulderstand can help reverse the downward movement of prana.

Herbal therapy involves primarily bitter herbs and secondarily astringents. Typical herbal bitters are good, such as barberry or goldenseal. Sometimes an initial bitter purgative like rhubarb root or senna leaves is necessary to cleanse the system of impurities. Good Ayurvedic herbs include bilva, kutaj, katuka, gentian, chiretta, cyperus, aloe and barberry. Formulas include Bilva compound, Cyperus wine and Kutaj wine.

Chinese bitters for diarrhea are coptis, scute and phellodendron. Other specific anti-dysentery herbs are purslane and anemone. Formulas for diarrhea include Coptis and Scute combination. Useful Western herbs include bitters —goldenseal, barberry, gentian and wormwood—and astringents—raspberry leaf, alumroot and potentilla. For blood in the stool astringent and demulcent herbs such as raspberry leaf, mullein leaf, and marshmallow are indicated. The general anti-diarrhea formula (listed above) can be given with barberry or goldenseal for added fire-clearing action.

VATA TYPE DIARRHEA

An anti-Vata diet is indicated along with carminative spices like ginger, cardamom, fennel, and asafoetida. Buttermilk is specific, particularly with a little nutmeg powder added. Castor oil can be given first to cleanse the colon.

Other important Ayurvedic herbs are haritaki (in small doses), kutaj and pomegranate rind. Ayurvedic formulas include Nutmeg compound, Asafoetida 8 and Cardamom compound. The Herbal Absorption formula is also useful or the general anti-diarrhea formula can be used with fresh ginger.

Kapha Type Diarrhea

Kapha diarrhea involves mucus in the stool. The treatment consists of an anti-Kapha diet. Dairy, fats, oils, sweets, pastries and breads should be avoided. Hot spices work well including cayenne, dry ginger and black pepper and others herbs to increase the digestive fire including nutmeg.

Useful herbs include expectorant and digestive stimulants such as calamus, bayberry, basil and sage. The Ayurvedic formula Trikatu or Clove combination can be taken.

Amoebic Dysentery

Amoebic dysentery is commonly picked up in travelling, particularly through third world countries where sanitation is not very good. The specific Ayurvedic compound for it is Vatsaka compound. Kutaj is the main Ayurvedic herb and its formulas.

Eating of garlic is a preventative, taking a quarter to half a clove every morning. Wormwood is very good (one ounce infused in a pint of water and taken daily for 3-7 days). The common summer weed purslane, particularly taken fresh, is good eaten or infused, one ounce three to four times a day. Amoebic dysentery easily becomes a chronic condition and may cause emaciation or wasting away of tissues. Then tonics like ashwagandha or ginseng are necessary to restore strength.

Bacillary Dysentery

Bacillary dysentery is much like Pitta diarrhea. It is initially an infectious disorder and much that is said there is relevant here.

The specific Ayurvedic compound is Kutaj wine or jelly. Kutaj tablet is also good. Many bitters such as chiretta, katuka, barberry, neem, goldenseal, wormwood, rhubarb root and coptis have an antibacterial and anti-inflammatory action on the digestive tract and are used in this condition. One ounce of any of these herbs can be infused in a pint of water and taken daily. If the condition becomes chronic, spices are required like ginger, garlic and asafoetida, or restorative tonics like ashwagandha or ginseng.

INFANTILE DIARRHEA

Infantile diarrhea and griping is usually caused by an inability to digest mother's milk or cow's milk. It is mainly a Kapha or Ama (toxic) condition.

Spices to help digest milk are excellent like fennel, dill, cardamom and calamus. These can be taken by the mother or by the infant in small, pinch-full dosages. Dill water, sold at most Indian markets, is very good. Nutmeg is also good for stopping the condition, particularly taken with a banana. Care is needed, however, as babies easily suffer from dehydration. In that case make sure to increase fluid intake or take moistening herbs like shatavari or marshmallow.

HEMORRHOIDS

Hemorrhoids are caused by varicosity of the veins around the anus. Initially they may only involve pain or difficult evacuation. Prolapse and bleeding can also occur. The causes of this condition include wrong diet, constipation, diarrhea, wrong posture, sedentary life-style, stress, irritability, excessive worry or excessive sexual activity.

Hemorrhoids can be due to any of the three doshas, but are most commonly Vata and Pitta types. For their treatment Agni, or the digestive fire, must first be improved with the right spices. Turmeric is a special spice for reducing swelling and inflammation of the muscle tissue and can be applied locally as a paste or in the form of various Turmeric cremes.

General Treatment of Hemorrhoids

Astringent herbs are indicated to tighten the tissues—haritaki, alum, pomegranate, red raspberry and mullein. Haritaki herbal wine is specific. These herbs are good applied topically as a wash, a paste or used as a suppository. Purgatives or laxatives will help to ease elimination when the cause is constipation, but should not be taken if the cause is diarrhea. Squatting and the use of cold water to clean the anus after defecation are helpful.

According to Chinese medicine such prolapse conditions are caused by sinking of the central chi (primary energy). They are treated by tonics—ginseng and astragalus—and special herbs to raise the yang—bupleurum and cimicifuga (black cohosh). The most typical formula used is Ginseng and Astragalus. This sinking of the central chi resembles low Ojas in Ayurvedic thought and requires a similar long-term tonification therapy.

Vata Type Hemorrhoids

Vata hemorrhoids involve pain not only in the rectum but also in the thighs, back, lower abdomen and urinary bladder. There is loss of appetite, nervousness and anxiety. The hemorrhoids are dry, rough, and irregular. There is seldom bleeding or swelling of the hemorrhoidal tissue.

Vata hemorrhoids are caused by constipation, dry stool, or straining at evacuation. They are more common in the elderly or the bedridden. Factors include too much cold, raw, dry, light or astringent food and a sedentary life-style with a lack of exercise. Emotional factors include worry, anxiety and fear.

The treatment consists of an anti-Vata diet, much like that for constipation, with an emphasis on warm, moist, oily food. Buttermilk with a little cumin and rock salt is very good. The colon must be lubricated properly. Warm sesame oil can be applied to the lower rectum or taken as an enema (1/2 cup in the evening).

When the digestion is weak and a pronounced tongue coating exists, spices to improve digestion and improve circulation in the colon should be taken. These include basil, dry ginger, black pepper, cayenne, and turmeric. Ayurvedic herbs include haritaki, amalaki, ashwagandha, shatavari, Triphala, Draksha or Asafoetida 8 formulas. Bulk laxatives like psyllium are also excellent. Application of heat and sitz baths are very helpful.

PITTA TYPE HEMORRHOIDS

Pitta type hemorrhoids involve redness, swelling, and bleeding or discharge of pus. There is often a burning sensation at the rectum or along with the passing of the stool. The stool is usually loose and yellow or greenish in color. Prolapse may occur after frequent or hot type diarrhea. There will be thirst, hunger, irritability and anger. The causes are too much spicy, sour or salty food, alcohol, and exposure to the sun or heat. Emotional factors are irritability, anger and aggression.

The treatment is similar to that of Pitta diarrhea. It requires an anti-Pitta diet with emphasis on salads and green vegetables. Nightshades—tomatoes, potatoes, eggplant and peppers—should be avoided, particularly where there is rectal bleeding. Pomegranate juice is great. Mainly bitter and astringent tastes are prescribed.

Good herbs are aloe gel, turmeric, cyperus, barberry, katuka and neem. A good simple formula is turmeric, cyperus and barberry in equal parts, which can be very effective. Formulas include Triphala with ghee, as well as the anti-diarrhea formulas.

Good demulcents and astringents for bleeding hemorrhoids include mullein leaf, raspberry leaf and marshmallow, or the Ayurvedic herb ashok. Aloe powder should not be used as a purgative because it aggravates rectal bleeding. But aloe gel can be applied to the anus to relieve inflammation.

KAPHA TYPE HEMORRHOIDS

Kapha type hemorrhoids are large, whitish or pale in color and slimy to touch. They are mainly an accumulation of phlegm or fat and may be associated with polyps or swollen glands in other parts of the body. There will be mucus in the stool, which will be pale in color. The urine may be milky in color. The patient frequently suffers from colds, cough, runny nose, excess salivation or sweet taste in the mouth.

The treatment is similar to Kapha constipation. Fasting or light anti-Kapha diet is indicated, strictly avoiding all mucus forming foods. Use strong cleansing and stimulating spices like cayenne, black pepper, dry ginger, bayberry, and calamus. Good formulas include Trikatu and Triphala taken together with honey.

PARASITES

Intestinal parasites are not as uncommon as we might think, though with the improved sanitation of Western countries they are not the major problem here that they once were. The main causes are impure food and water, travelling in unsanitary areas and weak digestion.

Parasites are more common in Kapha and Vata constitutions and are usually associated with Ama, undigested food. Long-term parasite infestation causes wasting away of tissues and aggravates Vata. Pitta types seldom suffer from parasites because their digestive fire is usually high. Even when contracted, the parasites are burned up in the process of digestion.

In Ayurveda, parasites are classified according to the medium in which they reside. Vata caused parasites reside in the stool, Kapha caused parasites reside in the mucus or mucus membranes, and those caused by Pitta reside in the blood.

General Treatment for Parasites

An initial fasting or anti-Ama (detoxifying) diet comes first. Sweets, meat and dairy products should particularly be avoided. Usually a purgative is given, then a course of 3-5 days of anti-parasitical herbs. Purgation is then given again and the stool examined to see if the parasites have been dispelled. This process works better in acute conditions. In chronic conditions, tonic and nutritive herbs are required to balance out the depleting effect of the parasites.

Parasite growth is encouraged by low Agni (weak digestive fire) and in turn causes low Agni. The use of hot spices to promote digestion—cayenne, black pepper and asafoetida—is a major part of anti-parasitical treatment.

Bitter taste is indicated in treating for parasites because of its powerful cleansing and reducing properties. Good bitters for worms include wormwood, tansy, goldenseal, rhubarb root, and aloe powder. The last two are excellent purgatives for parasites.

Other herbs have anti-parasitical actions through a special property (prabhava) and may not be unpleasant tasting. An example is pumpkin seeds, which can be eaten freely during a fast to help dispel worms. Some strong anti-parasitical herbs can be toxic, like pinkroot and male fern, and must be used with care (though they are less toxic than drugs for the same purpose).

The main Ayurvedic herb for parasites is vidanga, which is effective even for tapeworms. Pomegranate, particularly the root bark of the tree, is good for tape, round or pin worms. Other good herbs are holy basil, katuka, betel nuts and cyperus. Additional Western herbs are santonica (for all kinds of worms), wormseed (for round, hook or tapeworms), and rue.

Specific Treatment for Parasites

Vata type parasites are indicated by gas, constipation, abdominal pain and bloating, insomnia, anxiety and other high Vata symptoms. Additional treatment involves an anti-Vata diet with a limited intake of rich foods. Garlic and hot spices can be taken freely. Formulas include Vidanga compound, Garlic compound and Asafoetida 8. Castor oil can be used as a purgative. When malnutrition or low energy exist herbs such as ashwagandha, bala and ginseng may be necessary as supplements.

Pitta type indications are fever, burning sensation, diarrhea or loose stool and other high Pitta signs. Pain in the gall bladder and liver area is common. Additional treatment involves an anti-Pitta diet with a lot of raw food, vegetable juices and greens. Spices should be avoided, and digestive bitters taken instead, before meals. The bitter side of the general therapy is used. Formulas include Vidanga compound taken with aloe gel or juice. The best herbs are strong pure bitters—coptis, chiretta, katuka, gentian and goldenseal.

Kapha indications are phlegm, nausea, fatigue, feelings of dullness and heaviness, lack of appetite and poor digestion. Additional treatment involves an anti-Kapha diet with free use of spices, as hot as one can bear like cayenne and garlic in liberal amounts. All sugar and dairy must be avoided. Formulas include Vidanga compound, Trikatu or Asafoetida 8. Aloe powder or rhubarb root can be used as purgatives when necessary.

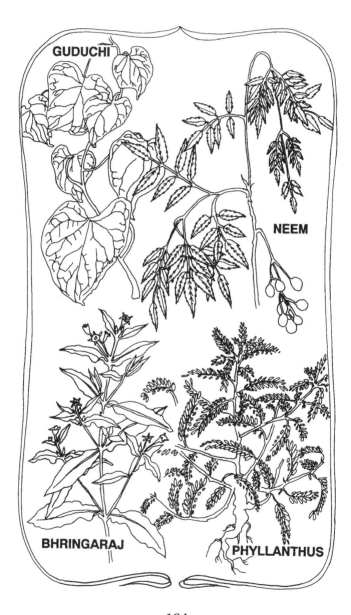

II.3
Disorders of the Respiratory System

The lungs and stomach are the primary sites of Kapha, the biological water humor. Phlegm is produced in the stomach, accumulates in the lungs, and then travels throughout the rest of the body producing Kapha diseases. Most respiratory disorders, therefore, are Kapha disorders. Kapha or water types are prone to colds, fluís, sore throat, swollen glands, bronchitis, asthma, pneumonia and other diseases of the respiratory system.

Yet we must consider the role of the other doshas as well. The lungs are an important site of air, Vata, where prana comes into the body. Respiratory disorders involving lack of strength, shortness of breath, wasting away of tissues, and dehydration, such as consumption or tuberculosis, are usually Vata diseases. On the other hand, most severe infectious conditions of the respiratory tract (as of all the systems) are Pitta conditions.

Whenever there is poor digestion there tends to be accumulation of mucus, regardless of the doshic condition involved. Mucus does not necessarily indicate high Kapha, it may simply indicate low Agni. Therefore, improving the digestive fire is also a major treatment for respiratory system disorders.

Causes of respiratory disorders include wrong diet, exposure to the elements, seasonal changes, poor posture, poor breathing practices, excess or deficient exercise, and breathing bad or stagnant air. Psychological factors include attachment, grief and fear. As the lungs are near the heart, emotional pain often weakens the lungs as well.

The treatment of respiratory disorders requires not only the right herbs and diet but also yoga practices including Pranayama (breathing exercises). Local applications of herbs are essential including gargles, herbal oils or decoctions through the nose (nasya), smoking herbs, and applying herbal oils or pastes to the head, back or chest.

195

A good lung tonic with commonly available herbs is 2 parts elecampane root, 2 parts comfrey root, and 1 part each cinnamon, ginger and licorice. For Kapha types, add 1 part each of cloves and calamus. For Pittas, use burdock root instead of elecampane. For Vata, add 2 parts ashwagandha or ginseng. Or the Lung Tonic (no. 3) can be taken, with a teaspoon of honey for Kapha; honey and ghee in proportions of two to one for Vata; or with honey and ghee in proportions of one to two for Pitta.

Emetic Therapy

The main Ayurvedic treatment for Kapha disorders is emesis or therapeutic vomiting (Vamana). It is one of the strongest herbal treatment methods and requires caution. It is preferable to go to a Pancha Karma clinic or be under the supervision of a qualified Ayurvedic practitioner to receive it. Once the art of vomiting is learned, however, it is possible to do it for oneself. Regular or daily therapeutic vomiting to cleanse the stomach and lungs is important for maintaining health and promoting longevity, particularly for Kapha types. The same effect can be achieved over longer periods of time with an anti-Kapha diet and expectorant (phlegm-dispelling) herbs.

Pranayama

Pranayama, yogic control of the breath, is a primary long-term treatment for lung disorders. Pranayama practices can correct most lung problems including long-term allergies and asthma. Breath control increases energy, gives strength and promotes circulation.

In the beginning keep inhalation and exhalation of the same length and lasting as long as it is comfortable for you to easily do. Eventually you can aim at making exhalation twice the length of inhalation and can also lengthen the breathing time. There should be no forceful attempt to hold the breath.

196

For Pranayama to be effective, right posture or asana must first be achieved. Otherwise the lungs will be contracted and proper breathing will be difficult. Pranayama should not be attempted in acute conditions of asthma without the help of an experienced teacher.

ALTERNATE NOSTRIL BREATHING

For most lung disorders, alternate nostril pranayama is excellent. In this form of pranayama one breathes in through one nostril while holding the other nostril closed and then breathes out the opposite nostril. Breathing in through the right nostril and out through the left is called *solar pranayama* and increases heat and fire in the body. Breathing in through the left nostril is called *lunar pranayama*. It increases cold and dampness in the body.

- For Kapha, or congestive conditions of the lungs, one should breathe in through the right nostril and out through the left or solar pranayama.
- For Pitta, or inflammatory conditions of the lungs, one should breathe in the left nostril and out through the right or lunar pranayama.
- For Vata conditions, or cold and dryness in the lungs, alternate the two types of breathing. However, when there is dryness in the lungs or dry cough with insomnia, lunar pranayama is better. When there is cold and congestion, solar pranayama is better.

Right Nostril	Solar	Pitta	Hot	Dry	Stimulating	Reducing
Left Nostril	Lunar	Kapha	Cold	Wet	Calming	Building

SOHAM PRANAYAMA

Soham pranayama consists of mentally chanting the mantras SO on inhalation and HAM (pronounced 'hum') on exhalation. Simply hold the sound inwardly along with the breath and let the breath naturally deepen of its own accord. Soham Pranayama is an excellent gentle and balanced pranayama. The sound SO naturally deepens inhalation and improves Prana. The sound HAM naturally increases exhalation and removes excess Apana, the downward moving air. Soham pranayama is good for all constitutions.

COMMON COLD/FLUS

The common cold is still our most common disease. It is the first stage of disease, indicating a breakdown in our bodily defenses from which further diseases can arise. Many different rhinoviruses are behind it. The cold usually starts in the head where, through the mouth and the senses, we have our greatest exposure to external pathogens.

Colds and flus are usually Kapha (phlegm) diseases and the symptoms are of that dosha. There is accumulation of mucus, runny nose, sore throat, congestion, cough, bodyache, headache and chills with mild fever. Causes include exposure to cold air or wind, cold, damp or mucus forming food, and seasonal changes as well as other Kapha-increasing factors.

General Treatment of Colds

An anti-Kapha and anti-Ama (detoxifying) diet is prescribed. The diet should be light, warm and simple: for example, whole grains and steamed vegetables in moderate quantities with spices. Avoid dairy products, especially cheese, yogurt and milk. Avoid heavy, oily and damp food like meat, nuts, breads, pastries, candies and sweet fruit juices. Fasting is helpful if the individual is not too weak.

Take lemon and ginger juice with warm water and a little honey. Fresh ginger or other spice teas like cinnamon, basil and cloves are excellent. Tonic herbs like ashwagandha, shatavari or ginseng should be avoided owing to their heavy nature.

Herbal treatment employs diaphoretic, expectorant and anti-cough herbs to promote sweating and relieve mucus. The peripheral circulation needs to be restored and the cold dispelled. After drinking a warm spice tea, the patient should go to bed under a warm blanket and brought to a mild sweat. Other sweating methods such as dry sauna or steam box also can be used. The patient should only be mildly sweated; profuse sweating should be avoided.

Typical Ayurvedic herbs include ginger, cinnamon, pippali, licorice, basil, cloves, and mint. The main formulas are Sitopaladi powder or Talisadi powder taken with honey or ghee. The Lung Tonic, (no. 3), can be taken in the same way.

In Chinese medicine a cold is called a 'surface wind-chill syndrome', and is treated with warm spicy surface-relieving herbs, like ginger and cinnamon. Formulas include Ma Huang decoction, a strong diaphoretic, and Cinnamon branch decoction, a mild diaphoretic. Additional good Western diaphoretics are sage, hyssop, thyme, osha and bayberry.

TYPES OF COLDS

Although colds are generally of a Kapha nature, they can be of a Vata or Pitta nature.

Vata type colds involve dry cough, insomnia, scanty phlegm, hoarseness or loss of voice. A few drops of sesame oil can be placed in the nose with an eyedropper. Herbs include not only the spices and warming diaphoretics mentioned above but also demulcents such as licorice, comfrey root, shatavari and ashwagandha. Sitopaladi powder can be taken with warm milk or along with Shatavari compound or Ashwagandha compound.

Pitta colds involve high fever, sore throat, red face, yellow or blood-streaked mucus. Treatment is with cooling diaphoretics such as mint, burdock, yarrow, elder flowers and chrysanthemum—what Chinese medicine calls 'spicy-cool surface-relieving agents.' The Chinese patent medicine Yin Qiao San is excellent for this and most other types of colds.

For colds with high fever (usually a Pitta condition) a good formula is equal parts basil, sandalwood and peppermint, 2-3 teaspoons of the herbs infused per cup of water, and taken every 2-3 hours.

COUGH

Cough is also usually a Kapha disorder. It is caused by accumulation of mucus, or by irritation to the mucus membranes of the respiratory tract. Treatment concentrates on bringing out the phlegm, not just suppression of the cough, which is what most allopathic anti-cough drugs and syrups do.

Cough may be due to the other doshas as well. Treatment is largely the same as for a cold. In addition specific cough-relieving herbs are used.

Ayurvedic herbs and spices for cough are cloves, cinnamon, ginger, sumac, pippali, bibhitaki, and calamus. Turmeric powder by itself is good. A good home remedy is equal parts honey and lemon juice in teaspoonful dosages. Vasa is a special Ayurvedic anti-cough remedy. It is often given as an herbal jelly or as an herbal wine.

Typical Ayurvedic formulas for cough include Clove combination, Sitopaladi powder or Talisadi powder, 1-6 grams 3-4 times a day. Draksha can be taken in tablespoon dosages. Catechu is a good astringent for cough and sore throat in Kapha and Pitta conditions. Other astringents like alumroot can be used the same way but they may aggravate Vata (dryness) conditions.

Types and Treatment of Cough

KAPHA COUGH

Kapha cough involves expectorating thick or slimy mucus, clear or white in color with an infrequent cough. Symptoms are distaste for food, a feeling of heaviness, and a sweet taste in the mouth with excess saliva or feeling of nausea. The patient will complain of cold and the lungs will be full of phlegm.

Treatment involves an anti-Kapha diet, avoiding dairy and other mucus-forming foods. Avoid ice, cold water and fruit juices. Hot spicy herbs, particularly pippali, dry ginger or chitrak as a milk decoction are helpful as is Trikatu compound taken with honey.

PITTA COUGH

Pitta type cough involves expectorating yellow phlegm, sometimes streaked with blood. There will be a burning sensation in the throat and chest, along with fever, thirst and dryness of the mouth. The mouth will taste bitter or pungent.

Treatment is much like that for Pitta type colds. Ghee can be used to soothe the throat. Powdered lotus seeds with honey is helpful. Licorice combination can be used, or take simple licorice tea with a little cinnamon. Western herbs are mullein, horehound and coltsfoot.

VATA COUGH

Vata type cough is usually a dry cough with little expectoration. Cough will be frequent, painful and with a particular sound. Pain in the chest and heart, or a headache, is typical. There will be dryness in the mouth, hoarseness and perhaps nervousness, anxiety or insomnia. (This is like 'yin-deficient' cough in Chinese medicine).

Treatment involves an anti-Vata diet. Make sure to have enough liquid in the diet, with soups and milk preparations. Anti-cough and demulcent herbs are indicated such as licorice, marshmallow, comfrey root, shatavari and ashwagandha, particularly as taken with honey. Formulas include Cardamom combination and Draksha, plus what is indicated under the common cold.

OTHER HERBS FOR COUGH

Chinese herbs for cough include apricot seeds, coltsfoot, loquat leaves, fritillary and pinellia. Loquat and fritillary cough syrups are particularly good for dry cough. Ophiopogon combination is specific for a dry, hacking night cough.

Western herbalism also has many cough-relieving herbs such as horehound, wild cherry, yerba santa, grindelia, thyme, spikenard, osha and mullein. Syrups or candies made from these are helpful (sugars soothe the throat).

Usually anti-cough herbs are used for their specific action.

They are not used energetically, so the energetics will depend upon the other herbs in combination. One or two anti-cough herbs can be added to formulas for treating various kinds of respiratory disorders, depending upon the condition.

SORE THROAT

This is usually a complication of the common cold and receives similar treatment. Sore throat with congestion and phlegm is a Kapha condition. It requires mainly diaphoretics, expectorants and astringents.

Sore throat with dryness, hoarseness and constipation is a Vata condition. Sesame oil or ghee, particularly made with calamus or licorice, should be applied to the throat. Licorice tea is also excellent.

Severe, swollen sore throat and strep infection is usually a Pitta condition. It requires the use of antibiotic, blood and lymph cleansing herbs such as katuka, goldenseal, yellow dock or isatis.

Gargling with astringent herbs is recommended, particularly for Kapha and Pitta types. Use alum, turmeric, sumac, sage or bayberry. A simple gargle of turmeric and salt in warm water done every hour is often sufficient. If there is dryness in the throat, demulcents like licorice or slippery elm are required. Other Ayurvedic herbs are cloves, haritaki, bibhitaki and turmeric. Formulas include Sitopaladi and Talisadi.

Typical Chinese herbs for severe sore throat include honeysuckle, forsythia, isatis and platycodon. Special Western herbs include echinacea and mullein. Echinacea tincture, 10-30 drops every few hours, is excellent for severe sore throat.

LARYNGITIS

Laryngitis is the loss of voice that accompanies many respiratory disorders. Sometimes it arises from too much speaking or other straining at the voice.

Kapha type laryngitis is characterized by phlegm blocking the throat and the larynx. Its treatment requires an anti-Kapha diet and expectorant herbs. Good spices include cloves, peppermint and calamus; useful herbs are bayberry, bibhitaki, and haritaki. These herbs can also be smoked in a pipe. Formulas include Clove compound.

Pitta type laryngitis is indicated by severe sore throat, yellow mucus and fever. Bitter herbs are used for it—katuka, turmeric, and barberry, prepared or taken with ghee.

A dry throat and low voice characterize Vata type. It is apt to be chronic. Treatment involves an anti-Vata diet and demulcent herbs like shatavari or marshmallow. Apply a little ghee or sesame oil to the throat. Simple licorice tea is good. For improving the voice and speaking ability, Calamus ghee is excellent, 1 teaspoon three times a day.

BRONCHITIS/PNEUMONIA

Bronchitis is an infection of the bronchi located in the respiratory passages. It is treated as a severe form of the common cold or cough. Though mainly a Kapha condition, like a cold, it can present varieties relative to the three doshas. Expectorants and diaphoretics like bayberry, cloves, ginger, calamus, nutmeg and licorice are still effective. Cooling anti-cough agents like vasa, gotu kola or mullein are good for the febrile stage, as is the Ayurvedic lung tonic vamsha rochana (bamboo manna).

Inhaling the steam of aromatic herbs is another excellent remedy. Essential oils of eucalyptus, camphor, mint or wintergreen are excellent in this regard. Place 10-30 drops of such oils in hot water. Put a towel over ones face above the pot of heated herbs and inhale for ten minutes. Alternatively, boil the leaves of such herbs in a pot, put a towel around ones head over the heated herbs, and inhale the steam. Other forms of steam therapy (swedana) are helpful, but avoid dehydration.

Pneumonia can be similarly differentiated relative to the doshas but is more dangerous because the infection tends to be at a deeper level and the fever is often higher. Deer horn ash

(Shringa bhasma) is specific for pneumonia. Gypsum ash (Godanti bhasma) is effective for the high fever stage of these lung diseases, as is the Chinese formula Gypsum combination.

In such acute conditions antibiotic herbs are useful—echinacea, goldenseal, katuka and isatis, taken every two to three hours in dosages of 3-5 grams of the powder or twice that in decoction. The Herbal Febrifuge (no. 7) is good, taken with honey. Antibiotic drugs may be necessary when the condition is severe.

In convalescence from weak lung conditions, including tuberculosis, Chyavan Prash is excellent, or other lung tonics like comfrey root, slippery elm, shatavari, ashwagandha or ginseng preferably taken as milk decoctions.

ASTHMA

Asthma is a chronic form of cough and lung condition that involves gasping, wheezing and difficult breathing. Causes include allergies, complications of other lung diseases and hereditary factors. It is mainly a Kapha syndrome and treatment is like other Kapha lung disorders, though it varies somewhat in different doshic types as well. Bronchial asthma can be from any of the three doshas but is most often Kapha in nature. Cardiac asthma is usually Pitta, and renal asthma is usually Kapha. But the doshic complications also vary with symptoms. For example, in the fall with wind and dryness as aggravating factors Vata may be more involved.

TYPES OF ASTHMA

- Vata type asthma is characterized by dry cough and wheezing. Additional symptoms are thirst, dry mouth, dry skin, constipation, anxiety and craving for warm drinks. Attacks occur predominantly at Vata time, dawn and dusk.
- Pitta type asthma is characterized by cough and wheezing with yellow phlegm. Other symptoms are fever, sweating, irritability and need for cool air. Attacks are at Pitta time, noon and midnight.
- Kapha type asthma is characterized by cough and wheezing

204

with abundant clear or white phlegm. The lungs will be full of water, producing a railing sound. Attacks are at Kapha time, morning and evening. Smoking of herbs is very helpful.

General Treatment of Asthma

Care must be taken to differentiate syndromes as the condition can change quickly. Acute wheezing is treated by bronchodialators such as ephedra, lobelia or vasa. Lung tonics like ashwagandha or ginseng may aggravate this condition as they consolidate or close the energy of the lungs. Acute asthmatic attacks can be dangerous and should be treated by a professional. In clinical situations in Ayurveda asthma is mainly treated with emetic therapy. Milder symptoms are treated with diet and herbs.

Long-term treatment requires tonification to rebuild the energy of the lungs. Tonics should be taken between acute attacks. In Ayurveda such herbs include ashwagandha, shatavari, bala, gotu kola and licorice. Formulas are Chyavan Prash, Ashwagandha compound and Shatavari compound.

In Chinese medicine, chronic conditions require such tonic formulas as Rehmannia 6 plus Ophiopogon and Schizandra. Human placenta can be used as a single herb.

Special Ayurvedic treatment involves smoking bronchodialating and antispasmodic herbs such as cloves, bayberry, ephedra, and tobacco. For allergic type asthma, turmeric power is helpful. It should be warmed in butter with raw sugar and taken frequently in teaspoonful doses during acute attacks.

Specific Treatment of Asthma

For Kapha types, treatment involves an anti-Kapha diet, avoiding all mucus-forming foods, as well as yogurt and sour fruit. Freely use hot spices such as cayenne, mustard, ginger and pepper. A milk decoction of pippali taken daily can correct chronic asthma. Mustard or ginger paste can be applied to the chest. Important Ayurvedic herbs are pippali, calamus, bayberry, and ephedra. Formulas include Trikatu, Sitopaladi, Talisadi compound and Clove compound.

Important Chinese herbs for this condition are ma huang and apricot seeds. A typical formula is Major Blue Dragon. Good Western herbs include mullein, bayberry, sage and thyme.

For Vata types, an anti-Vata diet is prescribed along with spices. Sour fruit juices are good, like lemon or lime, to hydrate the tissues. Ayurvedic herbs include those for Kapha along with tonics for the lungs like ashwagandha because Vata conditions always tend towards wasting of the tissues.

For Pitta types, an anti-Pitta diet is prescribed along with cooling herbs like coriander, gotu kola and burdock. Vasa is particularly good for asthma. Brahma Rasayana works well as a long-term restorative food.

HAY FEVER/ALLERGIC RHINITIS

Hay fever is another immune system derangement and relates to hypersensitivity of the nervous system. It is usually a Vata disorder because Vata types are the most sensitive, but Pitta and Kapha types exist. Pitta is involved in the more severe allergies with toxic blood and symptoms of fever, red eyes and rashes. Kaphas get allergies along with their general accumulation of dampness and mucus. Hay fever most often occurs in a weaker or debilitated constitution.

- Vata type allergies are caused by dust, wind and dryness and manifest more in the autumn. Vata symptoms are cough with a little phlegm, headache, insomnia, restlessness and anxiety.
- Pitta allergies are caused by heat and sunlight and manifest more in the summer. Pitta symptoms are burning eyes, thirst, fever, yellow nasal discharge, and skin rashes.
- Kapha allergies are caused by dampness and mold and manifest more in the spring. Kapha symptoms are abundant clear or white phlegm, dullness and heaviness.

206

In acute conditions the treatment for allergies is similar to that for the common cold, with a detoxifying diet. Dairy and other mucus-forming foods should be avoided. Between attacks, however, it is important to strengthen the immune system and the lungs, particularly for Vata constitution individuals, with a diet according to constitution. For this tonification therapy important Ayurvedic herbs are ashwagandha and bala; Chinese herbs are ginseng and astragalus; and Western is comfrey root. Chyavan Prash is a good general tonic to take or the Energy Tonic (no. 2). Brahma Rasayana is excellent for both expectorant and nervine action.

Treatment of Hay Fever

All kinds of hay fever require special herbs to clear the sinuses, open the head and dispel phlegm. Basil tea (particularly holy basil or Tulsi from India) is good, taken with honey. Coriander and cilantro (coriander leaf) are best for Pitta. For Kapha, the old standby Trikatu is good, or dry ginger powder as a snuff.

Ayurvedic herbs include calamus, gotu kola, ginger, cloves, camphor (in very small amounts), ephedra and bayberry. Calamus ghee applied in the nose is excellent. Gotu kola oil or ghee is similarly used for Pitta conditions.

Chinese herbs include magnolia flower, xanthium (cocklebur), mint, angelica, wild ginger and chrysanthemum. Additional Western herbs are peppermint, sage, eucalyptus, wintergreen, bay leaves and mullein flowers.

When Pitta is involved, bitters and blood cleansing herbs such as echinacea, barberry, dandelion and burdock must be added.

Essential oils like menthol, eucalyptus or camphor, or a paste of spicy herbs like ginger can be applied to the temple or root of the nose (avoiding the mucus membranes). Sandalwood oil on the forehead is good when there are hot or febrile sensations.

For red, itchy eyes, ghee, particularly that made with Triphala can be applied to the eyelids. Triphala ghee is best, and ghee by itself is helpful. Camomile, eyebright or chrysanthemum in luke-warm infusions can be used to wash the eyes.

A good formula for hay fever is gotu kola, calamus, angelica, wild ginger and licorice in equal parts of the powders. Vata and Kapha types can take this with honey, Pitta with aloe gel or with the addition of other bitter herbs. Also, the Lung Tonic (no. 3) can be taken with the Brain Tonic (no. 6).

NASYA THERAPY

Nasya, or nasal application of herbs and oils, is important not only for hay fever and sinusitis but also for all diseases of the head and sinuses. Go to an Ayurvedic practitioner for a special facial massage and nasya therapy for the sinuses. Alternatively, simply put a few drops of medicated oil into the nostrils with the help of an eyedropper. Vata types should take licorice in sesame oil (Anu Tail). Pitta types should take gotu kola in sesame oil or Brahmi oil, and Kapha types should take calamus, eucalyptus or camphor in sesame oil.

NETI POT

Yoga employs a small pot for pouring water into the nose as a yogic means of cleansing the nostrils. This is called a neti pot. A daily use of a neti pot or washing the nostrils with a saline solution works wonders in many allergy cases. Usually one takes about an 1/8 teaspoon or a pinch of salt in the neti pot. But you can also add a little sesame oil and a little of the power of ginger or calamus for a stronger action. This opens the head and sinuses and removes phlegm and congestion. However, in very congested conditions a snuff of herbal powders or an application of oils works better than the neti pot, which can cause water to get lodged in the head.

II.4
CIRCULATORY SYSTEM DISORDERS

HEART DISEASE

According to Oriental medicine, the heart, not the brain, is the seat of consciousness. It is the site of the Atman, the true or Divine Self. An old European adage states, 'As a man thinks in his heart, so is he.' This thought is also found in the *Upanishads*, the great ancient scriptures of India. How we feel in our hearts is the measure of who we really are. What we think in our heads is often no more than a superficial impression, passing momentarily through us via the senses. Hence, heart diseases reflect deep-seated issues of identity, feeling and consciousness. Heart disease is perhaps the main cause of death in this country. This is largely because the heart is denied in our culture which aims at personal achievement rather than communion with others. Many of us literally die of broken hearts or spiritual starvation, even those who may outwardly appear successful. We can be so driven by achievement that we deny our hearts, which then fail owing to our neglect of them.

The American diet that concentrates on sweet and salty food, animal fats and fried food makes us culturally prone to heart attacks. So do our life-styles which are sedentary and sluggish, lacking proper exercise or ventilation.

Heart diseases include heart attacks, stroke, angina, arteriosclerosis and hypertension. Heart attacks, the end result of most heart diseases, are preceded by palpitations, insomnia and numbness or severe pain in the chest or middle back that radiates down the arms. Other indications are cyanosis (blue color of lips and tongue), loss of consciousness, fever, cough, hiccup, shortness of breath and vomiting.

Causes of heart disease include wrong diet, physical or emotional trauma, congenital or hereditary factors, suppressed emotions or excess strain and anxiety. It may occur as the complication of other diseases (rheumatic diseases or liver disorders). As the heart is an organ of emotion, emotional causes should always be considered first. These include difficulties in work or relationships, usually indicating that on an inner level we are not in touch with our own hearts. They may show insensitivity to the hearts of others.

Most coronary heart disease is Kapha in nature, reflecting overweight and stagnation in the tissues and organs. Yet as Pitta relates to the blood, heart disease, particularly involving hypertension, is commonly a Pitta disorder. The red faced, angry, ambitious, hard driving executive who suddenly dies of a heart attack is typically a Pitta person who denies his true heart.

Vata type heart disease is more common in the elderly, where there is drying out of the tissues and hardening of the blood vessels. Kapha (water or phlegm) type occurs mainly from overeating and the accumulation of mucus, fat and cholesterol that obstruct heart functioning.

Importance of Meditation

The first treatment for heart disease involves an extended period of rest or reduced activity, both physical and mental. Strain and worry should be set aside. Patients must get back in touch with their real hearts and what they really want to do in life. Yogic asanas and pranayama are good with no forceful efforts at control of the breath. Heavy exercise and travelling should be avoided.

Probably the best thing is meditation to calm the mind, nerves and emotions. Take a meditation retreat in a lovely natural setting where one has contact with spiritual friends and teachers. Look into your true heart and try to discover your deeper wishes and values. Contact friends and family and honor the value of all relationships, particularly those that you have neglected. Give up anger, aggression and assertion. Calm rajas and develop sattva.

HERBS FOR THE HEART

Arjuna (Terminalia arjuna, a relative of the Triphala herbs) is a special powerful Ayurvedic herb for all kinds of heart diseases. As Ayurveda's heart medicine par excellence, it tonifies the heart and lungs, stimulates blood circulation, strengthens the heart muscles, stops bleeding and promotes the healing of tissues. Arjuna in the proper combinations is good for all three doshas. It is usually given with ghee or in the form of a medicated ghee. All people with heart weakness can benefit by this herb, regardless of the nature of their disease. Take 1-3 grams of arjuna powder daily. Vata types can take it with ashwagandha, Pitta types with gotu kola and Kaphas with elecampane for better results.

A good heart tonic for all three doshas is saffron, prepared in a milk decoction, $\frac{o}{}$ gram per cup of hot water. It is a special tonic and rejuvenative for Pitta and for the female reproductive system. Elecampane is another excellent herb for heart disease associated with Kapha and congestion in the lungs.

The Heart Tonic, (no. 11), can be taken with honey for Kapha, with ghee for Pitta and with milk and ghee for Vata. Arjuna combines well with ashwagandha and guggul as an all-around heart tonic. Another useful Ayurvedic and western herb for heart pain and high cholesterol is elecampane.

A special Chinese herb for heart disease is salvia (dan shen), a kind of sage. Salvia improves circulation, strengthens the heart and calms the emotions. It is excellent for angina pain, acting like a natural nitroglycerin (taken with a small amount of cardamom and sandalwood). It is helpful both before and after heart attacks and is good for thinning the blood. Salvia is particularly useful in Pitta and Kapha conditions, but can be used on Vata with warm spicy herbs like cinnamon.

The best Western heart tonic is hawthorn berries. It improves circulation, strengthens the heart muscle and helps dissolve cholesterol. Hawthorn is particularly good for Vata and Kapha and increases longevity. It works well as a tincture and makes an excellent herbal wine.

Myrrh is useful (like the Ayurvedic guggul) for cleansing the blood, clearing cholesterol, improving circulation and strength-

211

ening the deeper tissues. As a heart tonic, take ten to twenty drops of the tincture three times a day.

Many spices like ginger, cardamom and cinnamon possess circulatory stimulant properties and are great for the heart. They are particularly useful on Vata and Kapha conditions. They energize the heart, uplift the emotions and promote joy. Sandalwood is a specific herb and essential oil for calming and cooling the heart. Garlic is an important heart-stimulant and tonic with rejuvenative powers, particularly for Kapha and Vata types. Take one clove a day with honey for one month to restore weak heart function.

GEMS FOR THE HEART

The heart is like the sun for the body and the other organs work by its power, just like the planets reflect the light of the sun. Many gems and metals, either worn externally or taken internally as tinctures or specially prepared ashes (bhasmas), are great for the heart. They work on a subtle and long-term level to protect it and to fortify our longevity.

Gemstones for the sun like ruby, garnet and gold are heart stimulants and restoratives. Those for the moon like earl, moonstone, emerald, jade and silver calm the heart. Jupiter stones: yellow sapphire and yellow topaz tonify and strengthen the heart. Gold stimulates the heart and silver sedates it. Purifying drinking water by keeping it over night in a copper vessel will help prevent arteriosclerosis.

Types of Heart Disease

Vata type heart diseases appear as palpitations, tremor in the heart, numbness, tightness in the chest, and throbbing, breaking or bursting pain in the heart region. There will be insomnia, labored breathing, dry cough and constipation. Often there will be a dark discoloration around the eyes or dark patches on the skin. The individual becomes intolerant of noise and loud speech. Heart problems will follow stress, overwork or excessive exercise. Psychologically, there will be restlessness, fear, even fright, anxiety and sometimes fainting, after which the symptoms will worsen.

Pitta type heart disease symptoms are a burning sensation in the region of the heart, a feeling of smoldering heat, spontaneous sweating, fever and a general feeling of heat all over the body. The face will usually be flushed, with red or bloodshot eyes. There will be dizziness, sometimes fainting, and the eyes and skin will become pale and yellow. Vomiting of bile or sour fluids may occur, along with loose yellow stool. There may be nosebleeds, a tendency to bleed easily or slow healing of cuts and bruises. Emotionally, anger and irritability will prevail, with outbursts of temper which aggravate the symptoms.

Kapha type heart diseases are indicated by a feeling of heaviness and stiffness in the region of the heart. There will be congestion in the chest, accumulation of phlegm, cough, excess salivation, lack of appetite, nausea and perhaps vomiting. Fatigue and excessive sleeping are symptoms, and mentally the patient may feel dull and lack clarity. Emotionally, there will be greed and attachment and an unwillingness to let things go.

In short, most nervous heart conditions are Vata in nature; most inflammatory heart conditions such as myocarditis, endocarditis and pericarditis, relate to Pitta; most congestive heart conditions or cardiac edema are Kapha.

SPECIFIC TREATMENT OF HEART DISEASE

Vata Type Heart Disease

An anti-Vata diet should be followed, avoiding dry, light and artificial foods and irregular diet. Fish is good, as well as oily vitamins such as A, E, and D. Garlic can be used freely, particularly as a milk decoction. A small amount of red wine or the herbal wine Draksha can be taken with meals. The patient should rest, relax, be quiet, spend time in nature, meditate and do sitting yoga postures.

213

It is helpful to wear a ruby or garnet set in gold, on the ring finger of the right hand, to strengthen the heart. Sandalwood oil can be applied to the forehead or chest when palpitations or pain occur. The mantra SHAM is good to help calm the heart. The mantra RAM can be used to strengthen the heart.

Important herbs are ashwagandha, garlic, arjuna, cinnamon, cardamom, sandalwood, guggul, elecampane, and licorice. Take a milk decoction of ashwagandha, 3-6 grams of the herb and 1 teaspoon of ghee per cup, 2-3 times a day.

Formulas include Ashwagandha compound or specifically, Ashwagandha ghee or Ashwagandha herbal wine, as well as the Arjuna preparations. Garlic compound is excellent. Additional helpful Western herbs include comfrey root, Solomon's seal, hawthorn berries and myrrh. Additional Chinese herbs are dang gui, rehmannia, zizyphus, ginseng, astragalus and formulas like Ten Major Herbs.

Pitta Type Heart Disease

Treatment requires an anti-Pitta diet, avoiding particularly alcohol, hot spices, too much oil or greasy food, red meat and too much salt. Exposure to sun and strong exercise should be limited. Emotionally, strain, anger, hatred, resentment and violent urges should be set aside. One should cultivate peace, love and forgiveness.

An emerald set in silver, worn on the middle finger of the right hand, is helpful. Pearl and moonstone are also recommended. Sandalwood oil should be applied to the third eye and to the chest. The mantra 'Sham' is indicated for its cooling and calming action.

Good herbs are arjuna, saffron, sandalwood, shatavari and gotu kola as well as bitters such as aloe gel, katuka and barberry. Katuka or barberry can be given in equal parts with licorice and taken with ghee (dosage two grams taken after meals). Purgation is helpful in acute conditions. Important formulas include Arjuna preparations, Gotu Kola compound and Brahma Rasayana.

Additional Western herbs include motherwort, myrrh and goldenseal. Chinese herbs include salvia, coptis and formulas such as Coptis and Rhubarb combination, particularly for acute conditions.

Kapha Type Heart Disease

Kapha type heart disease is caused by the development of high cholesterol through a Kapha-increasing diet. An anti-kapha diet should be followed avoiding sugar, dairy, cheese, butter, eggs, fatty meats, lard and salt. Draksha herbal wine can be taken.

Similar to Vata, Kapha types benefit from wearing a ruby or garnet set in gold. Camphor, mustard or cinnamon oil can be applied to the chest. Chanting of OM is helpful for its clearing and opening action.

Expectorants (phlegm dispelling herbs) should be taken or a mild emetic therapy. Guggul, or myrrh as a substitute, are excellent (take the tincture 10-30 drops twice a day). Other good herbs include arjuna, calamus, cardamom and cinnamon. Equal parts elecampane and pippali (cayenne can be used as a substitute) taken with ghee are excellent for Kapha heart disease. Take one gram (two '00' capsules) after meals. Licorice should be avoided because it increases cardiac edema.

Formulas include Arjuna preparations and Trikatu, or the Digestive Stimulant (no. 1), taken with honey. Additional Western herbs include cayenne, myrrh, bayberry and motherwort.

Western herbalists have found cayenne to be good for reviving the heart after attacks. It is excellent for Kapha heart disease and useful in Vata conditions. It will aggravate Pitta, however, and should only be used for short-term heart revival in their case. According to Ayurvedic practice, cayenne would be better taken in ghee. Motherwort is another famous heart herb used in the West and in China. It has cooling and diuretic properties, making it good for Kapha and Pitta and for cardiac edema.

215

HYPERTENSION

Hypertension is high blood pressure. It is one of the main complications and causes of heart disease and is also often involved with liver problems. It is most commonly a Pitta condition, reflecting the driven nature of fiery types. But it can occur in the other doshas as well.

Most of its indications and treatment are similar to that of heart diseases, with the addition of specifically nervine herbs such as gotu kola, calamus, valerian, skullcap, and jatamamsi. The Heart Tonic (no. 11) can be combined with the Brain Tonic (no. 6) or the latter taken alone with honey or ghee as per the dosha.

Types and Treatment of Hypertension

Pitta hypertension is indicated by a flushed face, red eyes, violent headaches, sensitivity to light, nosebleeds, anger, irritability and burning sensations. The pulse will be wiry, taught and tight. It is often a complication of liver disorders and the accumulation of internal heat.

Use bitters like aloe gel, barberry and katuka. In strong types purgation is indicated with bitter herbs such as aloe, rhubarb root or senna. Gotu kola is specific for Pitta hypertension, calming the nerves and relieving heat and stress. Formulas include Gotu Kola preparations, Brahma Rasayana and Saraswat powder. Gotu kola and skullcap in equal proportions works very well.

Vata type hypertension is irregular in nature. The blood pressure may rise suddenly and fall suddenly with nervous tension. The pulse will be irregular or erratic both in rhythm and strength. An increase in blood pressure will follow worry, strain, overwork, anxiety or insomnia. It is frequently involved with nervous system disorders.

Treatment is mainly tonification therapy. Garlic is particularly good not only as a spice, but also eating an entire crushed clove (with honey) once or twice a week. Nutmeg in a warm milk decoction is good, as is Saraswat powder. Long-term tonification through Ashwagandha preparations is usually required. A good formula for Vata hypertension is—ashwagandha, valerian and

216

gotu kola in equal parts. Take 1-3 grams of the powdered herbs with warm water or with ghee.

Kapha hypertension is constant in nature, with the blood pressure remaining continually high. There is usually obesity, tiredness, edema and high cholesterol. Dairy, butter, eggs and high fat foods should be avoided. Good herbs are cayenne, myrrh, garlic, motherwort and hawthorn berries. Use hot spices freely in the diet, particularly mustard and onions. Licorice should be avoided. Formulas include Arjuna preparations and Trikatu.

ARTERIOSCLEROSIS

This is a condition of high cholesterol and clogging of the arteries. Both Kapha and Pitta types are due to fat accumulations. Vata type is owing to hardening of the arteries. Treatment is as for heart diseases generally and for hypertension, which usually follows from arteriosclerosis.

Guggul is a specific herb for lowering high cholesterol in all doshic types but particularly for Kapha. It improves circulation, reduces pain, removes accumulations and promotes healing. Take 1 gm. morning and evening for three months. The formula Triphala guggul is excellent and cleanses cholesterol from the blood.

Garlic is a good herb for high cholesterol in Kapha and Vata constitutions, particularly as taken with honey. Calamus and turmeric are excellent, as is elecampane. Aloe gel with turmeric or safflower, or the Ayurvedic katuka, are good for Pitta. Other good herbs are myrrh, saffron, motherwort, and hawthorn berries. The main Chinese herbs are he shou wu (fo ti) and salvia.

LOW BLOOD PRESSURE

Low blood pressure (hypotension) is not as problematic as high blood pressure but it is involved in many chronic conditions and often occurs along with debility, anemia and malnutrition. Low blood pressure is related to weakness of the digestive fire. It is most common in Vata types, who tend towards poor circulation. In Kapha it occurs because of congestion and stagnation, with phlegm clogging and reducing the blood flow. In Pitta it is mainly associated with anemia or damaged liver function.

To counter low blood pressure, circulatory stimulants are primary—turmeric, cinnamon, ginger, cayenne, garlic, black pepper or cardamom. For Vata types garlic or Garlic compound are good. Kapha types should take cayenne or Trikatu. Pittas should take saffron or turmeric in a base of aloe gel. When associated with anemia take also blood tonics like amalaki or turmeric ghee.

Wearing of ruby or garnet (not for Pitta constitution) is important because the condition is often chronic and requires long-term remedial measures. Such stones increase circulation. Pitta types should use red coral or pearl.

BLEEDING

Bleeding, or hemorrhage, is due to a variety of causes. It may occur because of injury. Disease factors that cause bleeding include fever, infection or doshic imbalance. Minor bleeding includes most nosebleeds and slight amounts of blood in the phlegm or stool. Internal bleeding suggests serious complications, like infection and tumors. One should have a medical examination as to its origin, even if we choose to treat it with natural methods.

Bleeding is mainly a Pitta disorder. It is called 'rakta-pitta' in Sanskrit, which we could translate as a condition of heat or bile in the blood. When the blood is overheated it flows easily, the veins and arteries become fragile and bleeding occurs.

Causes of bleeding are mainly those which aggravate Pitta, such as exposure to heat or sun, excessive exercise or travelling and overeating of spicy, sour or salty foods. Anger or a too aggressive life-style can bring it on.

In weaker Vata types, malnutrition and dehydration can cause bleeding. Moreover, long-term or chronic bleeding results in anemia and malnutrition. Fever can cause bleeding; and blood loss in turn can bring fever. Cold can cause bleeding in Kapha and Vata types as well but it is usually not severe.

Types of Bleeding

- Vata caused bleeding is dark red, frothy, thin or dry. It is usually from the lower orifices, the anus and urethra, and is difficult to treat.
- Pitta caused bleeding is dark, purple or black. It may be mixed with bile. It can be from either the upper or lower orifices.
- Kapha caused bleeding is thick, pale, oily and slimy and may be mixed with mucus. It originates mainly in the lungs and stomach. Kapha caused bleeding is usually from the upper orifices: the mouth, nose, eyes and ears. It is more easily curable.

General Treatment of Bleeding

Immediate treatment requires the use of astringent and hemostatic herbs to stop bleeding. Most spicy herbs should not be used as they promote the flow of blood. Local application of ice or cold water by its contracting action stops bleeding. A cool shower is often sufficient to stop bleeding from the nose.

A little alum powder (a mineral) applied to the site will stop most bleeding; or the powder of any herb with a large amount of tannin, such as white oak bark or alumroot. Common herbs and weeds such as self-heal, yarrow, plantain, chickweed or blessed thistle can be made into a paste and applied directly to the site. In Ayurvedic common usage, turmeric powder is applied locally, particularly for injuries. It is excellent for all soft tissue injuries. Turmeric root heals wounds naturally without scarring. Aloe gel can be used in the same way.

Good Ayurvedic astringents include aloe, manjishta, saffron, turmeric, arjuna, ashok and the Triphala formula. Good Chinese herbs are pseudoginseng, agrimony, cattail and mugwort. Pseudoginseng, a ginseng relative (and also rather expensive) is good for any kind of bleeding. Yunnan Bai Yao powder, a Chinese patent medicine made from it, can be used internally or externally. Additional Western astringents and hemostatics include arnica, yarrow, self-heal and mullein.

219

PITTA TYPE BLEEDING

Treatment requires keeping the patient cool. An anti-Pitta diet should be followed, avoiding hot, spicy food and sour and fermented food. Pomegranate juice is a good drink to take. Strong exercise or exposure to heat should not be allowed. Anger should be released as much as possible. Milk is good, particularly for bleeding from the lungs, and can be taken with a little turmeric. The general treatment applies here. Aloe gel is excellent, internally or externally.

VATA TYPE BLEEDING

Vata bleeding is caused by dryness of the mucus membranes or blood vessels. It may accompany dry cough or constipation. When large amounts of blood are involved, severe Vata disorders are indicated.

Treatment for mild conditions requires demulcent and tonic herbs to strengthen the mucus membranes—shatavari, licorice, ashwagandha, bala and their compounds. Hemostatics like turmeric can be added to these. Triphala is good for lower orifice bleeding, particularly taken with a hemostatic tea, like red raspberry or agrimony, as a vehicle.

KAPHA TYPE BLEEDING

For Kapha conditions, bleeding is due to blockage of the vessels by phlegm, which drives the blood the wrong way. Most hemostatics can be used, as above, along with hot spices such as cayenne, ginger and the Trikatu formula.

EPISTAXIS OR NOSEBLEED

Nosebleed requires a local application of herbs. Apply an infusion of astringent herbs like alumroot to the nose with an eyedropper. Daily nasya therapy, applying medicated sesame oil in the nose, often cures this problem which is mainly caused by dryness.

For a Vata (dryness caused) condition sesame oil should be applied to the nose nightly. Astringent tonic herbs like ashwagandha or haritaki are good. For a Pitta type (with red face and feeling of heat or fever) apply sandalwood oil to the forehead and ghee or coconut oil to the interior of the nose. Herbal teas such as coriander, vetivert, sandalwood or gotu kola are good, as is the treatment under Pitta liver disorders. Kaphas require additional expectorants like sage, hyssop, turmeric or elecampane.

ANEMIA

Anemia is called 'pallor disease' in Sanskrit (panduroga) because it makes the body turn pale. There is a deficiency of blood, in quantity or quality. Anemia is mainly a Pitta disorder because Pitta rules the blood. It is usually classified with such liver disorders as jaundice and hepatitis. Physiologically, it is caused by bile entering into and thinning the blood, which is the general movement of Pitta in its disease development.

High Vata or high Kapha can also cause anemia. For Vata types, anemia is usually part of a pattern of general deficiency and malnourishment that affects all the tissues and organs. For Kapha it is part of a pattern of obesity, edema and congestion. Excess fat or phlegm prevents proper nutrition to the blood.

Symptoms of anemia are a pale and lifeless appearance, lack of energy, low-grade fever or burning sensation, irregular elimination, yellowish and scanty urine, indigestion, vertigo, fainting and fatigue. For women, there is scanty or pale menstrual flow or absence of flow altogether.

The causes of anemia are wrong diet, eating of too much pungent, sour and salty food (tastes that aggravate both Pitta and the blood), alcohol or malnutrition. Anemia may follow traumatic injury, pregnancy, excessive menstruation or other conditions of excessive bleeding. It may be brought about by febrile diseases, the heat damaging the quality of the blood, or by liver disorders, which impair the liver's ability to build up the blood. Excess sexual indulgence, which depletes Ojas and weakens the bodily fluids, can result in anemia as well.

221

Women are prone to anemia owing to their monthly blood loss during menstruation. The majority of women can benefit from diet and herbs to improve the blood, particularly right after the menstrual cycle is over.

TYPES OF ANEMIA
- Pitta caused anemia is due to bile thinning the blood. There will be a burning sensation, fever and thirst. The skin and nails will be pale with a yellowish tinge, and bodily discharges will turn yellow.
- Kapha caused anemia is due to excess mucus blocking proper digestion and thinning the blood. The face, eyes, skin and urine will be white, with excess phlegm and salivation. There will be edema, often overweight, excess sleeping and heaviness of the limbs.
- Vata type involves dry skin with a darkish tinge, anxiety, tremors, insomnia, constipation and possible dehydration.

GENERAL TREATMENT FOR ANEMIA
A nutritive diet is indicated with foods, herbs and supplements to build the blood. Good foods include red meat, bone soups, dairy products, mung beans, almonds and sesame seeds (black). Some fruit is good for building the blood, particularly the juice of pomegranate or black grapes. Sugars are helpful, especially jaggary and molasses.

Iron supplements are indicated, as well as vitamins A and E. However, as iron preparations weaken the digestion, they should be taken with herbs to improve digestion such as ginger or cinnamon. The Ayurvedic tonic jelly Chyavan Prash is excellent—2-3 teaspoons twice a day with warm milk. Turmeric ghee is good or, as an alternative, ghee to which turmeric powder is added (the basis of most Indian cooking).

The bowels should be regulated with laxatives as in liver disorders (laxatives help stimulate liver function by draining out excess bile through the large intestine). But use mild laxatives such as aloe gel, Triphala or cascara sagrada.

Important Ayurvedic herbs are aloe gel, amalaki, haritaki, saffron, shatavari, manjishta, and punarnava. Or simply take 1/4 gram of saffron in warm milk daily with ghee. Special Ayurvedic iron preparations are excellent: humanized, non-toxic iron oxides that are prepared by repeated incineration of iron, as well as cooking it in various herbal substances. Most common are Iron ash and Navayas compound. Good formulas without iron are Shatavari compound, the Energy Tonic (no. 2) and the Woman's Tonic (no. 4).

Red coral, garnet and ruby are good gems for improving the blood, particularly for Vata and Kapha constitutions. Pearl or moonstone is good for Pitta and Vata types.

Chinese treatment involves special blood tonic herbs such as dang gui, rehmannia, fo ti, and lycium. Formulas include the Four Materials for simple blood deficiency and Woman's Precious Pill for combined blood deficiency and weak digestion (evidenced by loose stool, lack of strength and shortness of breath). The latter is commonly available as a patent medicine in Chinese and other herb stores.

The favorite Western herb is yellow dock, which contains large amounts of iron in its root. Prepared with blackstrap molasses, it becomes a good blood tonic, particularly for Pitta and Kapha type conditions. Its blood cooling, bile moving and laxative properties are also helpful.

SPECIFIC TREATMENT FOR ANEMIA

The general treatment is similar in all three doshas. Diet and spices, however, vary considerably.

For Pitta type raw salads, green vegetables, sprouts and common green herbs such as nettles, dandelion leaf, and red raspberry leaf are good. Chlorophyll helps cleanse bile from the blood, improving its quality, particularly in Pitta conditions. Milk and ghee are good. Bitters like aloe gel, barberry and katuka are helpful for controlling liver function.

Vatas should take rich food including dairy and oils, like ghee or sesame. They should avoid raw food and raw vegetables, except taking some cilantro or parsley. Ghee made with Triphala is good taken along with raw sugar. Herbal wines like Draksha are excellent.

Kaphas should concentrate on improving their digestion and getting rid of phlegm. Spices with circulatory stimulant properties should be used—cayenne, cinnamon, saffron, turmeric or the Trikatu formula taken with honey. Exercise and deep breathing is also helpful.

TRAUMATIC INJURIES

Herbs are part of nature's medicines for treating traumatic injuries. But as allopathic medicine became more effective in this area, herbal remedies are seldom used today, except when allopathic treatment is not available. Common astringents—nature's first aid chest—grow almost everywhere. Yarrow, self-heal, mullein, aloe, comfrey, chickweed and plantain are commonly available in forests, fields and gardens. These herbs were once very important medicinals, highly regarded in the materia medica of earlier times for wounds and injuries of all types.

Such herbs work well if picked fresh, crushed and applied as a poultice to the injured part. They not only stop bleeding but aid in the healing of tissues. Herbal ointments can be made from them or purchased and used as part of an herbal first aid kit, or the herbs can be mixed with a little honey and applied. The same herbs can be taken internally for internal injuries in the initial phase.

Bitter antiseptic herbs such as goldenseal, echinacea, aloe and myrrh are useful to counter infection. They are effective both externally and internally. Once the wound is closed and any fever or infection reduced, use herbs to promote blood circulation to stimulate healing like cinnamon, ginger, cayenne, sassafras, and saffron. If healing is slow or if tissue damage and blood loss have been extensive, tonics should be taken, like ashwagandha, ginseng or comfrey root.

Aloe gel is nature's best natural topical herb for cuts, wounds, sores and burns. Fresh chickweed has similar properties. Many

224

green and leafy herbs, especially plantain and comfrey leaf, are great as poultices.

Turmeric is a major herb for soft tissue and muscle injury. In India, fresh turmeric root is applied directly to cuts and wounds and they are found to heal without a scar. Treat strained muscles and joints with turmeric as well; it is great for sports injuries. Ayurvedic turmeric creams are helpful not only for nourishing the skin or removing acne and blemishes but also for promoting healing of injured tissue.

Ashwagandha is a good tonic for broken bones. Use 5 grams per cup in milk decoctions along with a small amount of turmeric or cinnamon. Other useful herbs in this condition are comfrey root and Solomon's seal, which provide nutrition to the bone tissue to promote healing.

Myrrh is an important herb for removing stagnant blood and preventing necrosis. Its Ayurvedic relative, guggul, is used similarly. The formula Triphala guggul is a natural antiseptic and antibiotic that promotes the healing of the deeper tissues in the body. Take 3 pills 3 times a day up to one week for severe injuries. Or take 2 pills twice a day for up to a month for milder injuries or for injuries that are slow to heal.

Other plant resins, those of various pines, liquidamber, or the sap of various tropical Indian fig trees, have important astringent, antiseptic and healing properties. Such resins can be dissolved in rubbing alcohol and combined with a little camphor for treatment of bruises and sprains.

Castor oil packs are effective for reducing swelling and promoting healing of bruised or damaged tissue. They can be applied with good results for abdominal pain and tumors. Castor oil can be applied on cotton and wrapped or taped around the affected part.

In Chinese medicine, salvia is used to promote healing of damaged tissue and to prevent scarring and adhesions. Siberian ginseng (often mislabeled as 'ginseng'), Eleuthrococcus senticosus, is used for sports injuries and also helps improve performance by strengthening the muscles, tendons, ligaments and bones.

Heart tonics like pseudoginseng or arjuna are useful in the same way.

Traumatic injury is an external factor so it is not treated according to the doshas. Generally, any severe injury over the long-term will derange the life-force, Prana, and aggravate Vata. Initially, Pitta may be aggravated with fever and infection.

POST-SURGERY

Surgery, like traumatic injury, disturbs the prana and deranges homeostasis. Anesthetics and antibiotics complicate this condition. Many people suffer from poor healing after surgery. Scars and adhesions, particularly in the abdominal area, cause various digestive system disorders such as gas and constipation, as well as lingering pains. This is partly because Western medicine does not consider post-surgical care beyond clearing up infections with antibiotics.

Turmeric is important both externally and internally and helps prevent scars and adhesions from forming. Take 1-3 grams of the powder three times a day with honey. Another excellent but expensive herb is saffron; safflower or calendula can be used as a substitute.

Aloe gel is good for healing any damage to the female reproductive organs, as well as for the liver and spleen. Myrrh is helpful for the female reproductive system, and after bone or joint surgery (for which the gugguls, particularly Triphala guggul, are specific). The Triphala formula itself is excellent after colon surgery. Gotu kola, particularly in the form of Brahma Rasayana, aids in the healing of nerve tissue. It also helps remove any emotional trauma that may be involved. Calamus works to restore nerve and sensory function and is particularly good for clearing out the effects of anesthetics. Arjuna is helpful after heart surgery.

Chyavan Prash is a good herbal food to take when recovering from surgery; it nourishes the blood and the deeper tissue. Ashwagandha in milk decoction helps calm the mind and fortify Ojas. It is good for rebuilding the bones and nerves. Shatavari helps calm and nourish the heart and restore sensitivity of feeling.

Both Ashwagandha and Shatavari compounds can be used or the Rejuvenative Tonic formula (no. 2).

Fennel is a common spice that promotes healing of hernias. You can also use it for treating lower abdominal pain and post-surgical digestive disorders. Castor oil packs are excellent for healing and reducing swelling, or occasional massage with castor oil in milder conditions.

II.5
DISEASES OF THE URINARY TRACT AND WATER METABOLISM DISORDERS

The kidneys are a very important organ in the body. Their action is closely related to the nervous system and to the reproductive organs. They are as important to the water metabolism as the colon is to food (metabolism of the earth element). Just as wrong eating habits damage the stomach and the G.I. tract, improper intake of liquids damages the kidneys and the urinary tract.

The kidneys are weakened by drinking either too much or too little water, by excessive sexual activity, by alcohol, by taking diuretic drugs, by antibiotics, and by not heeding the urge to urinate. Excess consumption of calcium or of foods like spinach which contain oxalic acid are additional factors. Too much travelling or excessive thinking weakens kidney function. Fear and fright damage the kidneys on a psychological level. The kidneys weaken with old age. They are delicate in sensitive or traumatized children, or in anyone who has suffered stress to the adrenals. They are often weak after childbirth.

Care of the Kidneys: Kidney Flush

Toxins accumulate and lodge themselves in the kidneys and urinary tract, particularly when the kidneys are not filtering the blood properly. Symptoms include lower back pain, sciatic pain, difficult or painful urination, urinary tract infections, swollen prostate or kidney stones. An occasional kidney flush is a great preventative measure, much like an occasional flushing of the colon. It should mainly be done during the warm season.

KIDNEY FLUSH PROCEDURE
Fast for one full day, then drink a quart or two of water the following morning. Add to it a small amount of mild diuretic herbs like coriander, parsley, lemon grass, horsetail or corn silk, or the Kidney Tonic (no. 10). This will increase the urination.

Over-use of diuretics, however, can weaken the kidneys. Diuretics aggravate Vata by overstimulating the kidneys and drying out the system. Too much water, particularly cold or ice water, will weaken the kidneys and usually increase Kapha.

It should be remembered that the human body is composed not primarily of water but of plasma, an oily solution. Drinking too much water, particularly distilled water, can drain essential substances from the plasma and leave the body depleted.

Water not only brings fluid into our body, it also brings Prana, the life-force. Hence, water devitalized by chlorination or distillation will not energize the life-force properly and this can contribute to many health disorders. Fresh spring water is preferable. The quality of our water can be improved by putting it in a copper vessel overnight. Aeration of water gives it Prana, such as pouring it back and forth between two cups before we drink it.

SHILAJIT

The best Ayurvedic herb for tonifying and strengthening the kidneys is shilajit, a special mineral pitch exuded by various rocks in India. It improves kidney and bladder function, increases sexual vitality, strengthens the nervous system, reduces tumors, and is antiseptic and helps dissolve stones. Shilajit is good for all three doshas and is an important rejuvenative (rasayana). It is useful for urinary tract disorders, whether cleansing or building actions are needed. The purified mineral can be taken in dosages of 1/2 - 1 gram twice a day or Shilajit compound can be used. It can be used for any of the conditions below and is excellent for diabetes.

DIFFICULT URINATION (DYSURIA)

Most kidney disorders reveal themselves through some abnormality or difficulty in urinary function. Difficult or painful urination can be caused by any of the three doshas. We use the symptom to diagnose and treat underlying poor kidney function.

- Vata caused dysuria is indicated by severe pain in the lower back, rectum and urinary channel. Urination will be frequent but scanty, with sharp or colicky pain. Constipation, insomnia and other high Vata conditions will prevail.
- Pitta dysuria involves dark yellow or red urine. Urination is frequent, often profuse, with a burning sensation. There will be feverishness, irritability and other high Pitta signs.
- Kapha dysuria involves pale or milky urine, passed with mucus. There will be a feeling of heaviness in the lower abdomen and a dull pain in the kidney region.

General Treatment for Dysuria

Diuretic food and herbs must be taken. The best general diuretic for all three doshas is gokshura (Tribulis terrestris), the common goatshead or puncture vine whose little stickers are a nuisance in our lawns and fields. Its action is sure but mild, and it has tonic properties for the kidneys that prevent it from aggravating Vata. Gokshura is best taken 1 teaspoon of the powder per cup of hot water.

The best general diuretic herb from Chinese Medicine is the mushroom hoelen (fu ling). It is mild and has tonifying action, particularly for the spleen and heart. Many good Western herbal diuretics can be found as well, like common cleavers and plantain as the diuretic property is very common in the herbal kingdom. Sarsaparilla is one of the best diuretics with tonic properties.

Specific Treatment for Dysuria

For Kapha type dysuria, an anti-Kapha diet is indicated, avoiding cold drinks, fruit juice, dairy, cheese, oils and fats. Hot spices and diuretics are indicated, like cubebs, cinnamon, and juniper berries along with parsley, uva ursi or cleavers. Formulas include Trikatu and Sandalwood compound or the Kidney tonic (no. 10) with warm water.

Treatment for Pitta is much the same as for urinary infections, avoiding spices, oils, and sour fruit. Cooling diuretics are indicated —

231

gokshura, punarnava, uva ursi, pipsissewa, horsetail, burdock or plantain. Formulas include Sandalwood compound or the Kidney tonic (no. 10) with cool water.

For Vata demulcent-diuretic herbs should be used, which soothe the mucus membranes and aid in urination. These include gokshura, bala, marshmallow, licorice and sarsaparilla. Formulas include Gokshura guggul or the Kidney tonic (no. 10) with milk.

EDEMA

Edema is a classic symptom of high Kapha, excess water in the system, but can occur in the other doshas as well. Kapha types tend towards edema, particularly as they get older. They easily accumulate water in the lower abdomen and thighs.

- Kapha type edema has a pronounced swelling, with moist and white skin. When pressed, the tissue holds the shape of the imprint for a short time.
- Vata type edema is indicated by dry skin and visible veins. The tissue is spongy and comes right back up when pressed.
- Pitta type edema is associated with swelling, redness and burning sensation.

Treatment for Edema

As edema is usually a long-standing condition, dietary therapy is particularly helpful. Good diuretic foods include grains like corn, barley and rye, vegetables like celery, carrot, parsley and cilantro, and fruit like cranberries and pomegranate. Most beans are diuretic, particularly aduki beans.

One cannot relieve edema merely by taking large amounts of diuretic herbs or drugs. These can weaken the kidneys by over-stimulating them. Mild diuretics are best—gokshura, corn silk, hoelen, lemon grass, and coriander and formulas such as Gokshura guggul or the Kidney tonic (no. 10). Vata types can take such herbs with milk or warm water, Pittas with aloe gel or cool water, and Kaphas with honey. Shilajit is important for edema, particularly in weak types, 1-2 grams twice a day with water or milk. Vatas do well with a combination of ashwagandha and gokshura for strengthening the kidneys.

URINARY TRACT INFECTIONS

Urinary tract infections involve difficult, frequent or burning urination, with pain, bleeding or discharge of pus in the urine. Acute infections are usually due to high Pitta. To treat them effectively the diet should be strongly anti-Pitta, avoiding alcohol, spices (except coriander) and nightshades, particularly tomatoes. Cranberry, coconut or pomegranate juices are good. Sexual activity should be curtailed for the duration of the infection.

General Treatment for Urinary Tract Infections

Typical Ayurvedic herbs for burning urination are sandalwood (a natural urinary antiseptic), coriander, punarnava, lemon grass and fennel. For urinary pain gotu kola is excellent. Formulas include Sandalwood compound and Gokshura guggul or the Kidney Tonic (no. 10) taken with aloe gel.

Typical Chinese formulas are Dianthus combination (strong diuretic action), Polyporus combination (moderate) and Anemarrhena, Phellodendron and Rehmannia (weak, with tonic action).

Western herbs are uva ursi (strong), pipsissewa (moderate), horsetail, plantain and spearmint. A good formula is pipsissewa, plantain, marshmallow, coriander, lemon grass and gotu kola in equal parts. Take 1-2 teaspoons of the cut and sifted herbs per cup of hot water every few hours until the condition improves.

Specific Treatment for Urinary Tract Infections

Vata urinary tract infections will be chronic, low-grade and irregular in onset and development. Herbs are necessary to tonify the kidneys—ashwagandha, bala and shatavari—along with mild diuretics like gokshura and marshmallow. Ashwagandha compound can be taken with Gokshura guggul or the Rejuvenative tonic (no. 2) can be taken with the Kidney tonic (no. 10). Sarsaparilla and corn silk are other good Western herbs for this condition.

Kapha type infections are due to mucus in the kidneys. All dairy products and fats should be avoided and spices should be freely used. Good herbs include cinnamon, cubebs, juniper berries and parsley. Standard anti-Kapha formulas like Trikatu are excellent, along with shilajit for its diuretic properties.

STONES IN THE URINARY TRACT

Urinary tract stones can be caused by any of the doshas. The main factors are Kapha (phlegm) which accumulates in the urinary tract and Vata (wind) which dries it out, creating the stone. They are related primarily to wrong diet but other factors come into play as well.

Strong diuretics and stone-dissolving (lithotriptic) herbs are specifically indicated. These include corn silk, gravel root, Ayurvedic pashana bheda and shilajit, and Chinese lygodium and desmodian. Take them as teas along with demulcents such as marshmallow or licorice to deal with burning or pain. Guggul, myrrh and gotu kola are also helpful for pain relief. Take large amounts of water, sweet or astringent (not sour) fruit juices and herb teas to help flush out the stones.

Purgation is helpful, particularly when the pain is acute. Castor oil or rhubarb root can be used in the usual, or in high, dosages. Constipating food like beans and cabbage family plants should be avoided. Two ounces of corn silk infused in a pint of water taken daily is helpful for most urinary tract stones. Take it with a small amount of lemon grass to improve its taste and effect.

Types of Kidney Stones

- Kapha stones are mainly composed of calcium. They are soft, smooth and white, and passed without severe pain. The urine will be pale or white and in large quantity.
- Pitta stones are yellow or red in color and composed mainly of oxalates. They are sharp and painful. There will be dark yellow, red or burning urine, mixed with blood or pus.
- Vata stones are brown or black in color and composed mainly of phosphates. They are rough, dry and irregular and cause severe pain throughout the lower abdomen and thighs. Urination will be difficult, scanty and irregular and may be associated with extreme pain.

Specific Treatment for Kidney Stones

Pitta types should avoid the nightshades tomatoes, eggplant, peppers and potatoes, along with spinach, chard, onions and other foods that increase oxalic acid. Cilantro juice is good. Purgation with bitter herbs like rhubarb root is often helpful. In addition, take strong cooling diuretics such as uva ursi, corn silk, gravel root, tribulis or pashana bheda.

Vatas should avoid food that is too light or dry, including dry grains like corn. Tonic and demulcent diuretics like sarsaparilla, sandalwood, marshmallow and ashwagandha are good as well as the milder diuretics like corn silk and tribulis. Purgatives such as castor oil or Triphala can be used.

Kapha should avoid dairy, cheese, fats and oils. Strong bitter and pungent diuretics can be used—uva ursi, juniper berries, cubebs and gravel root. Purgation can be helpful as well.

DIABETES

Diabetes is a disease of profuse urination in Ayurveda. It is described mainly as a dysfunction of the water system (Ambhuvaha srotas) or a water metabolism imbalance. Ayurveda lists twenty such diseases according to the three doshas that cause them, but diabetes, as we commonly know it, relates mainly to two types, diabetes insipidus and diabetes mellitus.

Diabetes is a severe disease, difficult to treat and with many complications. Natural remedies cannot often cure it, particularly that of juvenile onset, but they can alleviate many of its side effects and improve the quality of life and energy. For juvenile onset, and once the pancreas function is totally lost, the condition is generally not reversible.

Types of Diabetes

Diabetes manifests itself as excess thirst and excess urination. Initially, in adult onset type diabetes, it is primarily a Kapha disease caused by obesity and excess consumption of sweet, Kaphogenic foods. Kapha increases in the stomach due to low pancreas function, then enters the other tissues, causing frequency or turbidity of urination.

Long-term and juvenile onset diabetes involves thirst and wasting away of tissues, and is or becomes primarily a Vata disease. This is true in diabetes mellitus, the most common type of diabetes. Vata accumulates in the large intestine and travels to the pancreas, deranging pancreas function.

Pitta can also cause diabetes, including the juvenile type. It accumulates in the small intestine, then travels to the liver and pancreas upsetting their functions. Pittas have a high Agni that can burn out the pancreas.

Wrong diet is a main causative factor in diabetes, with excessive consumption of sugar, sweets, dairy products, alcohol, fat and breads. It can be caused by obesity, excessive sex, sleep in the day time, lack of exercise, worry, stress and anxiety or it may be hereditary. Psychologically, diabetes is a disease of desire, thirst and lack of contentment in life.

General Treatment for Diabetes

The best general herb and common spice for regulating pancreas and liver function, particularly useful in the initial stage of diabetes, is turmeric. Take it as a powder, 1-3 grams two to three times a day, with a little aloe gel or aloe juice.

The main Ayurvedic herb in severe or long-term conditions is shilajit, usually taken in the form of Shilajit compound. Another important Ayurvedic herb is gurmar (Gymnema sylvestre). It is the subject of modern scientific research throughout the world for its anti-diabetic properties. Sushrut, one of the greatest ancient Ayurvedic doctors, gave it the property of destroying the taste of sugar (gur-mar means sugar-destroying). It is able to reduce excess sugar in the body as well as countering sugar cravings. It is usually taken along with shilajit and is part of Shilajit compound.

Most bitters help control sugar metabolism, especially gentian. Spices like ginger and cardamom also aid in the digestion of sweets. Guggul and myrrh are useful for the obesity that is often behind the problem and also have sugar-regulating properties. Vasanta Kusumakara, a special mineral preparation, is great in severe cases. Though sugar should be generally avoided, pure, unheated honey can be used.

In gem therapy, Jupiter stones like yellow sapphire or yellow topaz are used for improving sugar metabolism and for protecting the life. These are usually set in gold and worn on the index finger of the right hand.

Specific Treatment for Diabetes

For Kapha types, a long-term anti-Kapha diet is the main treatment. Bitter taste is indicated because it helps control sugar and fat metabolism and liver and pancreas function. Bitter melon (karela) is an excellent food. Good bitter herbs for diabetes are aloe, gentian, katuka, neem, barberry, turmeric, goldenseal, and myrrh. Black pepper, cayenne and ginger and other pungent herbs are helpful for weight reduction that is a necessary part of treatment. Useful Ayurvedic formulas include Chandraprabha and Shilajit, as well as Trikatu.

Vata type diabetes involves emaciation, thirst, dehydration, extreme hunger, insomnia, low energy and burning sensation in the hands and feet, as well as the usual high blood sugar and profuse urination. An anti-Vata diet is indicated, avoiding sugar and sweet juices. Complex carbohydrates, nuts and dairy should be taken instead. Ghee is very helpful taken 1-2 teaspoons 2-3 times a day, particularly calamus or ashwagandha ghee. Oil treatment is essential; particularly the application of warm sesame oil to the head or forehead in a series of drops (shirodhara) at least two nights a week. (This is also good for Kapha types).

Herbal treatment aims at tonification using herbs such as shilajit, ashwagandha, bala and shatavari and their formulas, as well as Chyavan Prash. Important Chinese herbs for tonification therapy in diabetes are ginseng, astragalus, dioscorea, schizandra, trichosanthes root, rehmannia, and lycium and the formulas Rehmannia 6 and Rehmannia 8. Good Western herbs include comfrey root, Solomon's seal and American ginseng in strong decoctions.

Pitta type or Pitta stage diabetes involves fever, acidity, bleeding, ulcerative sores, red, yellow or bluish urine, irritability and hypertension. Treatment is anti-Pitta. Bitter herbs are indicated as under Kapha, along with cooling demulcent tonics such as shatavari, aloe gel or marshmallow for weaker types. Gotu kola ghee is excellent. The Liver Tonic (no. 8) is helpful. Chinese formulas include Major Bupleurum for liver excess type and Gypsum combination for lung and stomach heat type.

II.6
REPRODUCTIVE SYSTEM DISORDERS
Gynecological Disorders, Male Reproductive System Problems, Venereal Diseases

THE AYURVEDIC VIEW OF SEX

Ayurveda stresses maintaining the health and vitality of the reproductive system. This is not simply to allow for a better sex life. It is also to afford greater vitality for the body as a whole and for the nervous system specifically. Sexual energy can become creative energy and facilitate mental or spiritual work. Many yogis use herbs for the reproductive system for this general energizing effect. Such herbs enhance Ojas, our underlying vital essence; they do not irritate the sexual nerves or promote unwanted sexual activity.

Most diseases involve some wrong use of sexual energy because sexual energy is the primary energy of both body and mind. Most psychological disorders are based upon an inability to form right relationships and are largely sexual in origin. Therefore, the right use of sexual energy is a key to physical and mental health.

Our highly sexually oriented culture is suspicious of any weakening of the sexual drive. Lack of interest in sex, however, is not always a sign of disease. It can be a sign of the development of higher consciousness, with the awakening of detachment. It may be a sign of good health. Toxins in the system irritate the nerves, creating a sexual drive not easy to satisfy. In a body free of toxins the sexual drive is mild and easy to satisfy.

It is natural for interest in sex to decline with age. Constant preoccupation with sex is not necessary; nor is it the highest human good. This does not mean there is anything wrong about sex; it has its place in nature. Guilt and shame about sex causes more problems than it solves.

On the other hand, increased sex drive is not necessarily a sign of poor health or lack of spiritual development. The awakening of the subtle energies of the mind, stimulating the lower chakras, can increase both the sexual drive and mental creativity.

239

This, however, can cause health disorders if not managed properly; or if not transmuted it can be difficult to deal with.

Moreover, abstinence from sex can be a causative factor in disease. If the energy is merely repressed, vitality can stagnate and weaken. For this reason, sexual abstinence usually requires some use of asana, pranayama and meditation to turn it into a positive force. Sex is a creative force that must be used, and that if turned inwardly can transform our consciousness.

Excessive sexual activity causes Vata and Pitta disorders because it depletes the essence of water from the body. It weakens the immune system and makes us susceptible to infectious diseases. Toxins transmitted through sexual secretions can circumvent our defenses and directly lodge in our deepest tissues. Sex without love depletes the vitality and deranges the emotions, causing many human problems.

According to Ayurveda, masturbation can cause diseases because it does not provide the emotional and energy exchange to maintain balance in the system. Disrupting balance, it aggravates Vata. Overstimulating the imagination, it can make us vulnerable to negative psychic or astral forces. Ayurveda also sees homosexual activity as more likely to cause disease than heterosexual activity. It does not create a natural balancing of the system because the two physical and emotional bodies are of the same polarity.

Vata constitutions have the greatest interest in sex but the lowest vitality for it. They are most easily fatigued by sex. They are also more likely to have different or deviant sexual patterns. Kapha types have the best sexual vitality with continuous but moderate interest. For them the family life as a whole is important and sexual activity is seldom exhausting. Pitta falls between with the drama and passion of sex the main things for them.

Vatas need partners who are calming and nourishing to them and help ground them. Love makes them flower and feel secure. Generally Vata people need a Kapha influence in the people around them to keep them in balance. Pittas require partners whom they can work together with to achieve a common cause. They benefit from some Kapha around them to cool them down and counter their anger. Kaphas need partners who help stimulate them and get them going. For this they need Pitta or Vata energy to balance their heaviness and inertia. However, relationship as a whole is a way of increasing Kapha which is love, caring and attachment.

Seasonally, sexual activity is best in the winter and spring when Kapha predominates. At this time reproductive secretions are higher. Sexual activity is more depleting in the summer and fall, in Pitta and Vata seasons, when reproductive secretions are low. It is better done at night than during the day when the body's energies are internalized. Sexual energy is also higher when the moon is waxing than when it is waning. Sex is not advisable during a woman's menstrual period, in which Apana Vayu is active and pushes the life-force downward.

Sexual Abstinence (Brahmacharya Chikitsa)

Abstinence from sex is an important therapy for treating many diseases. It is helpful whenever there is debility, emaciation or underweight, or in convalescence. It is a major part of tonification therapy. Abstinence is valuable in treating mental and nervous system disorders because the extra sexual fluid can lubricate and nourish the nerve tissue.

Abstinence from sex naturally occurs in acute disease conditions like fevers. Disease lowers our interest in sex and causes us to preserve our vitality. Increased sexual activity, on the other hand, is used to treat Kapha diseases such as obesity and has its therapeutic value as well. However, one must discriminate between abstinence as a temporary treatment measure and forced abstinence that can lead to emotional unhappiness. As a therapeutic measure it is only necessary for the term of treatment.

Sexual activity easily increases rajas and tamas, disturbance and dullness in the mind, and reduces sattva, the mental clarity. Therefore, the system of Yoga emphasizes 'brahmacharya', control of one's creative energy through transmutation of the sexual force, as one of the main factors for spiritual development. Such a long-term abstinence is not necessary for ordinary health. It is a special practice for those who want to transcend the ordinary human condition.

GYNECOLOGICAL DISORDERS

Ayurveda has a special branch of gynecological medicine for the treatment of diseases of the female reproductive system. These diseases are primarily reflected in menstrual disorders. They often result from hormonal imbalances that derange the menstrual cycle. In this chapter we also discuss pregnancy and fertility.

The menstrual cycle is a good key to the health of a female. It can also be used to determine the Ayurvedic constitution, with Vata, Pitta and Kapha having their unique menstrual patterns. Regular menstruation, absence of pain or tension, smooth flow, and balanced emotions are signs of good health. However, most women suffer some difficulties with menstruation at one time of life or another, as part of the normal changes that life brings us.

Menstruation and Constitution

- Vata constitution women generally have a scanty menstrual flow. The blood is darkish-red or brownish and it is usually a little dry or old. Menstrual cramping may be severe with lower back pain or headache. Feelings of depression and nervous sensitivity may increase, with fear and anxiety, difficult sleep or insomnia. There will be lessening of vitality and resistance may be lowered. The vaginal wall will be dry. Constipation, gas or abdominal distention may occur. Periods are short, irregular and variable, lasting only 2-4 days.

- Pitta type women usually have an excess menstrual flow because of Pitta's association with the blood. The blood color is dark, red or purple, while the flow is profuse and warm, with possible clotting. There may be fever or burning sensation, along with flushed face or red eyes. Skin rashes or acne are possible. Emotional states include anger, irritability and short temper. Diarrhea or loose stool of predominately yellow color may occur. Periods are typically of medium duration, 4-6 days.

• Kapha women exhibit a moderate flow but the period will last longer, a week or more. The blood will be pale or light red with possible mucus and the flow will be continuous. There will be feelings of heaviness and tiredness with a desire to sleep. Some nausea or possible vomiting with mucus and saliva is possible. The breasts tend to swell and there may be edema, particularly in the lower legs. Sentimentality and nostalgia dominate the psychology.

Dual types will show a combination of the symptoms of the doshas. The menstrual flow can be disturbed by many factors. These include poor diet, stress, and overwork. Excessive physical exercise, particularly too much aerobic exercise, can interfere with the period. Our modern cultural emphasis on thin bodies is a factor. Without adequate fat the body cannot produce enough blood for easy menstruation. A premenstrual regimen of quiet and rest should be followed, avoiding any strong exercise (mild yoga asanas are good, however).

Treatment of Menstrual Disorders

Mild menstrual difficulties are treated with the same therapies as those for balancing the woman's predominant dosha. Most gynecological disorders involve a delay or difficulty in menstruation. Therapies to promote and regulate menstruation are usually indicated with the use of emmenagogue (menstruation-promoting) herbs like turmeric and saffron in Ayurvedic medicine or pennyroyal and motherwort in Western herbalism. Antispasmodics (for relieving muscle spasms) and nervines (to relieve cramping pain and calm the mind) are helpful, such as fennel, asafoetida, jatamamsi or valerian. Special tonics for the reproductive system are important when there is debility.

HERBAL TONICS FOR WOMEN

As blood loss frequently involves a weakening of vitality, herbal tonics are important supplements for the majority of women. They can be used like vitamin or mineral supplements. Typical preparations are Shatavari preparations, the Female Reproductive Tonic (no.4), the Ayurvedic herbal jelly Chyavan Prash or the Chinese patent medicine Women's Precious Pill.

Shatavari is the main Ayurvedic female reproductive tonic. It is highly nourishing, soothing, and moistening and calms the heart. Amalaki is also excellent, building all the tissues and calming Pitta as well. Aloe gel is very helpful and balanced in its action, cleansing as well as nourishing the female organs. Dan gui is the main Chinese tonic. It combines menstruation-promoting, blood-building and antispasmodic properties.

It should be noted that excess use of strong emmenagogue herbs like pennyroyal, tansy or rue can derange menstruation or cause excessive menstrual bleeding. This type of herb is usually contraindicated during pregnancy. They are sometimes used to help promote abortions but seldom work and can cause many side effects.

One of the main therapeutic actions of spicy or pungent taste is to move stagnation and increase the circulation of blood. Many common spices promote menstruation and have antispasmodic properties as well. Turmeric is the best general spice but many others are good—cinnamon, ginger, cayenne, black pepper, basil, dill, fennel, cardamom and asafoetida. Take 1/4-1/2 teaspoon of these spices in 1-2 teaspoons of aloe vera gel twice a day for mild menstrual difficulties.

The Female Reproductive Tonic (no. 4) can also help. Take 2-3 tablets, three times a day, a week or two before menstruation, with warm milk or warm water for Vata, with aloe gel or cool water for Pitta and with honey for Kapha.

PMS

PMS (premenstrual syndrome) has come to signify many of the difficulties associated with menstruation such as absence or

244

delay of menstruation, early menstruation, premenstrual head-aches, menstrual cramping, and swollen breasts. Specifically, it indicates the emotional or nervous problems associated with menstruation including irritability, rapid shifts of moods, depression and anxiety, along with their complications.

As a psychological condition, yoga therapies are excellent, combined with herbs and foods to promote sattva (harmony of mind). Gemstones, which have a special action to calm the mind, help in the long run. Pearl or moonstone, gemstones for the moon, are good for PMS because they calm the mind and heart and strengthen the female reproductive system. Pearl is generally the woman's gemstone and strengthens the feminine nature physically and psychologically.

PMS can be caused by any of the three doshas, as an indication of general imbalance. As a psychological or nervous condition, it is mainly a Vata disorder. Emotional or mental agitation upsets the normal secretion of hormones regulating menstruation. Provoking factors include poor nutrition, stress, overwork, travelling, difficulties in relationships and suppressed emotions. The general treatment is like that for the female reproductive system, as above.

Types of PMS

Vata type PMS is characterized by anxiety, depression, insomnia, constipation, headache and severe cramping pain. There will be nervousness, agitation, feeling spaced out, dizziness, fainting or vertigo with ringing in the ears. Moods may shift rapidly; the person will be very hard to please. Anxiety and feelings of abandonment may occur. The individual will complain of feeling cold, with thirst and dry skin. She may even feel like she is dying or have suicidal feelings, however, once the period starts to flow freely most of the symptoms will disappear. The period may be delayed or irregular. The flow is usually scanty, brown or black and the period lasts only a few days, the usual Vata menstrual pattern. Pain is worse at sunrise or sunset (Vata time).

245

Pitta PMS is distinguished by anger, irritability, and proneness to argument, with temper and possible violent outbursts. There may be diarrhea, thirst, sweating or fever and the individual will feel hot, particularly in the upper half of the body. There will be acne or possible skin rashes. The blood flow is usually abundant or excessive and may contain clots. The period will tend to come early and there may be spotting between periods. Symptoms are worse at noon and midnight (Pitta time).

Kapha type PMS is indicated by tiredness, heavy feeling, crying, feeling sentimental or needing to be loved. Emotional changes will not be as severe. Susceptibility to colds or flu and mucus discharges will increase. There will be lack of appetite and some nausea. There will be swelling of the breasts or edema. The period will tend to be late. Menstrual flow will be whitish or pale, thick, mixed with clots or mucus. Symptoms will be worse in early morning or early evening (Kapha time).

Specific Treatment for PMS

Vata Type PMS

For Vata type PMS, an anti-Vata diet is necessary, with tonic food like garlic and cooked onions. Spices to promote menstruation such as turmeric and ginger, combined with antispasmodic spices such as nutmeg, can be taken in warm milk before sleep. Warm sesame oil should be applied to the head and lower abdomen. It can also be applied to the vagina or a douche can be made with demulcents like shatavari. All stimulants like coffee and tea, tobacco, alcohol and drugs should be strictly avoided. Red gemstones are indicated—red coral, garnet, ruby or bloodstone build the blood and white stones like pearl or moonstone increase body fluids.

Herbal treatment consists of sweet and spicy tastes with herbs like aloe gel, shatavari, ashwagandha, licorice, turmeric, cyperus, dill, fennel, valerian, jatamamsi and asafoetida. Formulas include Shatavari compound, Ashwagandha compound, Asafoetida 8 or the Female Reproductive Tonic (no. 4). A good simple formula is

246

3 parts shatavari along with 1 part each of turmeric, cinnamon, valerian and licorice. Take 2-5 grams of the mixture before meals with honey.

Chinese herbs are dang gui, rehmannia, white peony, and ligusticum. Important formulas include the Four Materials and Bupleurum and Tang Kuei. The latter is the basic PMS formula in Chinese medicine, sold as Bupleurum Sedative Pill. It is also good for Pitta. Western herbs include emmenagogues, nervines and tonics such as pennyroyal, rosemary, camomile, valerian, false unicorn, and comfrey root.

PITTA TYPE PMS

For Pitta type PMS an anti-Pitta diet should be combined with menstruation-promoting spices such as turmeric, coriander, fennel, saffron and safflower, but hot spices should be avoided. Good gemstones are pearl, moonstone and red coral. The use of fragrances and incense—jasmine, rose, sandalwood and gardenia—is also excellent, or a simple gift of flowers.

Ayurvedic herbs include aloe gel, shatavari, turmeric, cyperus, saffron, manjishta, lodhra, gotu kola and bhringaraj. Important formulas include Shatavari and its various preparations, and Aloe wine. A simple formula is 3 parts shatavari and 1 part each of turmeric, cyperus and gotu kola. Take 2-5 grams of the powder before meals with warm water and a natural sugar.

Chinese herbs are salvia, motherwort, peach seeds, safflower, bupleurum, cyperus, and mint. Formulas include Bupleurum and Peony. Western herbs are nettles, yarrow, red raspberry, black cohosh, skullcap, and betony. Simple dandelion tea is often effective.

KAPHA TYPE PMS

For Kapha type PMS the anti-Kapha diet should be followed. Heavy or oily foods should be avoided: spices and light vegetables can be used freely, including all hot spices. Short-term fasting or skipping the evening meal can be helpful. More activity, deep breathing and going outdoors are important life-style recommendations.

Ayurvedic herbs include aloe gel, turmeric, cyperus, cinnamon, black pepper, pippali, ginger and calamus. Formulas include Trikatu or Clove compound. Or simply take one tablespoon of aloe gel with 1/4 teaspoon of dry ginger before meals.

Chinese herbs are ligusticum, safflower, hoelen, alisma, and the Tang Kuei and Peony formula. Western herbs include pennyroyal, rosemary, myrrh, cayenne, cinnamon and most typical emmenagogues.

AMENORRHEA

Amenorrhea is delay or absence of menstruation. As a premenstrual difficulty, much that is listed under PMS is applicable here. As a long-term or frequent condition it is mainly a deficiency disease due to Vata. But the other doshas can cause it as well. Lack of body fat and too much exercise can bring it about, which is why athletic women often fail to get their period.

Causes are exposure to cold, poor nutrition, anemia, emaciation, and dehydration. Displacement of the uterus, hormonal imbalance, emotional trauma and other factors may be involved. It may result from severe or wasting diseases such as diabetes. Amenorrhea may occur along with constipation or caused by the same factors that produce it. In severe cases it is related to blood or liver disorders, which should be the primary focus of the treatment.

Treatment for Amenorrhea

Herbs to promote menstruation are indicated, generally along with tonics to rebuild the reproductive system. Myrrh by itself is good for amenorrhea and the resultant pain, particularly taken as a tincture 10-30 drops every 3-4 hours.

An anti-Vata or tonifying diet is primarily indicated using dairy, nuts, oils, whole grains and other nourishing foods. Iron supplements or Ayurvedic iron ash preparations are important. Warm sesame oil can be applied to the lower abdomen or used as a douche. A mild laxative can be taken such as Triphala, aloe gel or castor oil in low dosages.

248

For amenorrhea due to cold, spicy herbs such as ginger, black pepper, cinnamon, rosemary, or the formula Trikatu are best. Fresh ginger and pennyroyal in equal parts, one ounce per pint of water, taken 1 cup three times a day, is a good herbal treatment for this condition, which is usually easy to treat.

Ayurvedic herbs for Vata-type delayed menstruation include asafoetida, cyperus, myrrh, ashwagandha, shatavari, and black and white musali. Formulas are Shatavari compound and Ashwagandha compound, taken with fresh ginger tea. Chyavan Prash is also helpful as a tonic.

A good simple formula is shatavari and ashwagandha, 2 parts each, and turmeric and ginger, 1 part each. Use 1 teaspoon of the powder per cup of warm water. Or the Woman's Tonic (no.4) can be taken along with the Energy Tonic (no. 2).

Chinese medicine relates absence of menstruation to blood stagnation, which may be allied to blood deficiency. Chinese herbs are ligusticum, salvia, dang gui and motherwort. Formulas include Persica and Rhubarb (strong constitution) and the Four Materials (weak constitution). Additional Western herbs are emmenagogues such as wild ginger, tansy, rue and squaw vine. These work better with a demulcent and nutritive like comfrey root, marshmallow or American ginseng if there is debility.

Kapha type delayed menstruation is due to congestion and sluggishness in the system. It can also be treated by strong warming spices—ginger, cinnamon, cayenne, black pepper or Trikatu or Clove combination formulas. Most typical emmenagogues are also good, such as pennyroyal. Motherwort is a good Chinese and Western herb for this condition, good for Pitta types as well.

Pitta type delayed menstruation is usually mild and can be treated by common herbs like turmeric or saffron in warm milk. Good herbs are rose, cyperus, dandelion, and other cooling emmenagogues.

DYSMENORRHEA

Dysmenorrhea is difficult menstruation, usually with cramping pain. Much that is said under the previous categories is relevant here. Dysmenorrhea is more common in Vata types due to dryness in the uterus, lack of proper secretions, or spasms of the smooth muscles of the uterus. It is often associated with bloating, gas or constipation.

In Pitta and Kapha types dysmenorrhea is a congestive disorder caused by stagnant blood and congested lymphatics. In Pitta types it is associated with a burning sensation and loose stool or diarrhea. In Kapha it appears with edema, leucorrhea or mucus discharges.

Treatment for Dysmenorrhea

Antispasmodic, muscle relaxing, and pain relieving herbs are used along with emmenagogues. Cyperus is a special Ayurvedic and Chinese herb for menstrual cramping pain and can be used for all types. Myrrh or guggul are also useful, as is ashoka.

Vata type involves severe colicky pain, constipation, dry skin, headache, anxiety, palpitations, abdominal distention and gas. Treatment consists of an anti-Vata diet with moist and oily foods. Heat or warm sesame oil should be applied to the lower abdomen. Sesame oil or shatavari can be used as a douche.

Herbs are turmeric, nutmeg, asafoetida, ginger, valerian and jatamamsi. They function better with demulcents such as shatavari or licorice, which possess a soothing and cortisone-like effect. Formulas include Asafoetida 8, as well as Shatavari formulas.

Good Chinese herbs are corydalis, salvia, and ligusticum. Dang gui and white peony specifically relieve spasms of the smooth muscles of the uterus. Good Western herbs are camomile, lady's slipper and evening primrose.

For Pitta and Kapha types note the sections on PMS and on amenorrhea. Pitta dysmenorrhea requires cooling nervines like gotu kola, jatamamsi, skullcap, passion flower, and hops. Kapha needs spicy nervines and antispasmodics—ginger, calamus, myrrh, guggul, cinnamon and nutmeg.

MENORRHAGIA

Menorrhagia is excess menstrual bleeding. The menstrual period may be prolonged and bleeding or spotting may occur between periods as well. It is usually due to high Pitta that heats up the blood. It may be involved with other bleeding disorders, such as blood in the stool.

Causes include overeating of hot, spicy, sour or salty food, smoking or drinking (alcohol), unresolved anger, resentment or hostility. This condition may be caused by abortions, by incomplete miscarriages, by cervical erosion, endometriosis, polyps and tumors. IUD contraceptives can bring it about, as well as birth control pills. It can indicate infection or cancer and should be examined carefully.

General Treatment for Menorrhagia

An anti-Pitta diet is required with avoidance of all hot and oily food. The patient should be kept cool and should avoid exercise and exposure to heat and sun. During bleeding an ice pack can be applied to the lower abdomen.

Astringent and hemostatic herbs should be given, such as red raspberry or manjishta. If the condition has persisted for some time, tonics should be given as well. Once the bleeding is over take tonic herbs like amla, shatavari and dan gui as per the treatment of anemia.

Important Ayurvedic herbs include ashok, lodhra, ashwagandha, arjuna, shatavari, aloe, amalaki and bhringaraj. Shatavari and manjishta are excellent in equal proportions. Ashok herbal wine is indicated. Formulas include the Heart Tonic (no.11).

Chinese herbs include mugwort, gelatin, and pseudoginseng, with formulas like Tang Kuei and Gelatin. Additional Western herbs are agrimony, nettles, yarrow, self-heal and mullein.

LEUCORRHEA

Leucorrhea is an abnormal discharge from the vagina. The vagina has a natural acid environment that protects it from unfa-

251

vorable pathogens. If this acidity is not maintained, various bacteria, fungi or protozoa can proliferate. Douches of sour taste substances such as vinegar, yogurt or herbs with acidophilus supplements are effective for this reason.

In Ayurveda, leucorrhea is most commonly a Kapha or excess mucus condition, but can be caused by the other doshas. Treat the dosha rather than the specific pathogen.

- Vata type leucorrhea will be brown, sticky and dry, with severe pain.
- Pitta type is yellow, foul smelling, perhaps purulent or mixed with blood, with a burning sensation.
- Kapha type is white, mucoid, thick or profuse, with feelings of dullness and heaviness.

Causes are mainly those that increase Kapha; eating too much sweet, sour, salty, heavy and greasy foods such as dairy, sugars and starches. Lack of cleanliness, excessive sex, excessive use of antibiotics, infections or venereal diseases contribute to the problem.

Treatment for Leucorrhea

The most specific form of treatment is a douche. Otherwise treatment is according to the dosha. Ayurvedic herbs for douching are alum, turmeric, aloe gel, and licorice.

For Vata type leucorrhea use yogurt as a douche or demulcent herbs such as shatavari and licorice. Take ashwagandha, shatavari and their preparations as herbal teas.

For Pitta type leucorrhea use bitter herbs as a douche—aloe powder, katuka, alum, coptis, goldenseal and gentian. For internal use, aloe gel, turmeric and barberry are indicated or the Herbal Febrifuge and Blood Purifier (no.7).

For Kapha type leucorrhea bitter, astringent and pungent herbs are combined for douching like aloe powder, alum, calamus, prickly ash and ginger. For internal use, Trikatu can be taken with honey.

Good Western herbs include wormwood, tansy, rue, alumroot, oak bark, usnea, goldenseal and echinacea. Two ounces of a combination of any of these herbs can be decocted in a pint of water for twenty minutes, then strained and applied as a douche morning and evening. Goldenseal, sarsaparilla and prickly ash in combination with a small amount of alum are excellent for acute conditions.

MENOPAUSE

Menopause, the change of life in women, can be a time of health disturbances with the shifting of hormones. Treatment requires special herbs for strengthening and rejuvenating the female reproductive system along with herbs to regulate the hormones and calm the emotions. As menopause is associated with the movement into old age, the Vata stage of life, symptoms are primarily of high Vata with increased nervousness, anxiety, insomnia and depression. But Pitta is usually involved as well, owing to the decreasing Kapha or secretions in the body.

The general treatment is anti-Vata. Herbs that tonify the female reproductive system are crucial, including aloe gel, shatavari, saffron, kapikacchu, and ashwagandha, taken in milk decoctions or in different preparations like Shatavari compound. Chinese tonic herbs such as dang gui, rehmannia, white peony, lycium and Woman's Precious Pill are great.

Aloe gel is specific for maintaining the youthfulness of the female reproductive organs. It is particularly effective for night sweats and sensitivity to heat. Chyavan Prash is important for its general rejuvenative effect. Shatavari maintains nourishment to the female organs and moistens the mucus membranes and skin. Sandalwood oil applied to the forehead helps with the night sweats as well.

Pitta type menopause appears as anger, irritability, and short temper, with frequent or pronounced hot flashes. Treatment is anti-Pitta including aloe gel and shatavari, a saffron milk decoction or Shatavari compound.

Kapha type involves feelings of heaviness, sleepiness, lack of motivation, weight gain or holding of water. Treatment is anti-Kapha. Hot spices are used like the Trikatu formula along with aloe gel. Myrrh is also excellent, as is saffron.

HYSTERECTOMY

The uterus has functions other than reproduction; it is also an organ of emotion and creativity. When it is removed, feelings of emotional imbalance and insecurity can arise. Along with hormonal imbalance, the system will tend to become devitalized. The metabolism may be deranged and excess weight can be put on.

These factors primarily serve to increase Vata. Depression, ungroundedness and anxiety may increase. The other doshas can increase as well, usually according to what is predominant in the general constitution. Pitta types will experience anger, irritability and heat sensations. Kapha will accumulate water and phlegm, and feel more tired or sentimental.

The general treatment consists of tonics to the reproductive system—shatavari, aloe gel, saffron and their preparations or Chyavan Prash. Shatavari by itself, 2-5 grams morning and evening in warm milk, is excellent. Chinese tonic herbs such as dang gui, rehmannia and white peony, again, are important. Herbs that balance the mind and calm the emotions are helpful— gotu kola, calamus, bhringaraj, jatamamsi or Brahma Rasayana. Chinese mind-calming herbs, zizyphus and biota, are good as well as Western nervines, skullcap, valerian and lady's slipper. Immediately after surgery herbs are used to promote healing: turmeric and arjuna are best.

BREAST OR UTERINE CYSTS AND BENIGN TUMORS

Cysts in the breast or uterus are not uncommon occurrences. A significant percentage of women will get them. They are more common in women who do not have children and in women after forty. Most cysts are benign but malignancy does develop in some cases. Malignant tumors are hard to the touch and possess definite boundaries. Simple cysts are softer and more watery in nature. Cysts and tumors can be due to any of the three doshas but are most common in Kapha types, who tend to create excess tissues.

- Kapha type cysts consist of subcutaneous fat or mucus accumulations. They involve swelling, dampness and congestion. If large, they can be safely removed through surgery, if necessary. As the breast is a fatty organ it easily gets such cysts or tumors.
- Vata type cysts are characterized by pain. They are dry, variable in size and location. Vata individuals are prone to fear and are more likely to imagine that any swelling or cyst is cancer.
- Pitta cysts are distinguished by inflammation, infection, swelling and a hot sensation.

General Treatment of Cysts and Benign Tumors

An anti-Kapha regimen is indicated for most benign tumors. Fat-reducing herbs are used, combining pungent and bitter tastes. Good herbs are black pepper, cayenne, turmeric, calamus, katuka, goldenseal and barberry. A good formula is Trikatu taken with honey. Honey itself has a fat and tumor reducing property. Triphala or other laxatives are helpful as well.

Special herbs for reducing breast tumors include turmeric, saffron, safflower, dandelion, violet and cyperus. A saffron milk decoction is excellent; use a high dosage of saffron, 1-2 grams per day, for short periods of time. Alternatively, take 1-3 grams of turmeric after meals.

For the other doshas, the treatment is similar to that for dysmenorrhea. See also the section on Cancer for other anti-tumor approaches. Milder forms of these same treatments can be used for swollen breasts, such as occurs either premenstrual or during breast-feeding.

PID, ENDOMETRITIS AND ENDOMETRIOSIS

In their acute forms, PID (pelvic inflammatory disease), endometritis and similar conditions are Pitta disorders showing accumulation of heat and stagnant blood, with infection and inflammation. Often the liver has to be treated and the blood cleansed.

Treatment requires an anti-Pitta diet and regimen, avoiding all spices but turmeric, coriander and saffron, also refraining from salt, alcohol and refined sugar, and all oils but coconut and sunflower. Good herbs include shatavari, aloe gel, sarsaparilla, gotu kola, dandelion, myrrh and echinacea. Strong bitters like katuka, goldenseal, gentian or uva ursi can be added to these. Shatavari and manjishta in equal proportions works well. Other treatment follows menstrual symptoms (usually Pitta type menstruation). The Woman's Tonic (no. 4) is good taken with aloe gel or the Herbal Febrifuge (no. 7). In chronic conditions take shatavari with aloe gel, 1 teaspoon of the powder per 1 tablespoon of the gel twice a day on an empty stomach.

Endometriosis is more Kapha in nature with the excess growth of the uterine membrane. This is particularly the case when there is little infection. An anti-Kapha, anti-tumor and general detoxifying and reducing approach is useful with typical herbs like guggul, myrrh, turmeric and dandelion. Black pepper and katuka or goldenseal can be taken with honey.

DURING PREGNANCY

During pregnancy a mild nutritive therapy is the main thing. Avoid taking herbs that are strong or extreme in their action like emmenagogues, purgatives and toxic herbs. Very hot and spicy herbs like cinnamon, ginger and cayenne should be used carefully, as should very cold and bitter herbs like goldenseal or gentian.

Use herbs for building the reproductive tissue like shatavari, ashwagandha, bala, white musali and kapikacchu. Tonic formulas such as Shatavari compound, Ashwagandha compound and Chyavan Prash are indicated or the Energy Tonic (no. 2), preferably taken with milk and ghee.

Underweight Vata women in particular should follow a nutritive diet with tonic herbs. If their body fat level is too low, miscarriage, difficult birth, or poor health after delivery are possible. Pitta women should stay cool with an anti-Pitta diet and mild anti-Pitta herbs like shatavari. Kapha women do well with mild spices like cardamom, fennel and basil to keep their energy circulating.

POST-PARTUM

Immediately after delivery herbs should be used to cleanse the uterus and promote uterine circulation. These include emmenagogues like turmeric, saffron, safflower, myrrh and pennyroyal, but taken only for a few days up to a week in most conditions.

Then follow a mild nutritive therapy throughout the period of breast-feeding using whole grains like rice, wheat and barley. Use dairy products like milk and yogurt, particularly for Vata and Pitta constitutions. Herbs to increase the breast milk include shatavari, marshmallow and licorice, prepared in milk decoctions. Chinese herbs such as dang gui and rehmannia are excellent.

Herbs to facilitate the flow of the breast milk include fennel, dandelion and nettles. Sage is good for stopping the flow of milk when it is excessive or when breast feeding time is over or a paste of mung bean flour can be applied to the breast.

MISCARRIAGE/HABITUAL ABORTION

Miscarriage, or habitual abortion, has several causes. More commonly it is a Pitta condition of excessive movement of the downward moving air (apana). Kapha types are usually fertile but may have a false or ectopic pregnancy. Vata types are more likely to be unable to conceive in the first place, but when underweight or nervous can lose the fetus from lack of strength.

The general treatment for miscarriage involves an anti-Pitta diet, with avoidance of spicy and oily foods. Dairy products are helpful, particularly milk and ghee. The patient needs adequate rest and relaxation, avoiding travel and exercise. Exposure to sun and heat should be limited.

After a miscarriage, care must be taken first to move out all stagnant blood and heal the uterus with emmenagogue herbs such as aloe gel, myrrh, turmeric and manjishta. After a week or two follow this therapy with tonification therapy.

Herbal therapy aims at tonification and calming the emotions. Ayurvedic herbs are shatavari, amalaki, ashwagandha, aloe gel and gotu kola. Formulas include Shatavari compound, Ashwagandha compound, and Chyavan Prash. Good Chinese herbs are mugwort, eucommia and loranthus, with formulas like Tang Kuei and Gelatin combination.

INFERTILITY

Infertility is usually associated with poor nutrition or lack of proper development of the reproductive organs. Accumulation of fluids or stagnation of blood can also cause it. Generally, Kapha types are the most fertile and Vata types the least fertile. Pitta types fall in between, losing their fertility when their system gets overheated.

An astrologer can be consulted for the best times for conception. This is usually when the moon is waxing and in fertile signs or nakshatras. The woman's overall fertility can also be determined astrologically.

Treatment of Infertility

Tonification therapy is generally best with an anti-Vata, pro-Kapha diet using nourishing and strengthening foods: dairy products, particularly milk, nuts and oils such as ghee or sesame. Treatment requires mainly the tonic herbs for strengthening the female reproductive system.

Typical Ayurvedic female tonics such as shatavari, ashwagandha, aloe gel, saffron, and licorice are good. Formulas include Shatavari compound, Dashamula, and Phalaghrita.

The best Chinese herbs are dang gui and rehmannia. Formulas include Woman's Precious Pill and Four Materials. Additional Western herbs are comfrey root, marshmallow, saw palmetto and false unicorn.

Where it is a congestive disorder or due to sluggish function, as in those overweight (Kapha types), energy moving and circulation promoting herbs must be employed. Cinnamon, saffron, ginger and myrrh and formulas such as Trikatu and Triphala together with honey are useful. Pittas can use saffron, aloe gel and shatavari.

DISEASES OF THE MALE REPRODUCTIVE SYSTEM

Reproductive system disorders are given less emphasis in men but should not be overlooked. Men should consider treatment of their reproductive systems and sexual habits as a primary factor for health.

MALE SEXUAL DEBILITY

Sexual debility is lack of sexual vitality or inability to perform adequately sexually. Symptoms include low energy, fatigue, tiredness, lack of sexual motivation and impotence. Nervousness, palpitations, spermatorrhea, nocturnal emissions and premature ejaculation may occur. Sometimes weak kidney indications, frequent urination or lower back pain will happen.

Sexual debility can be caused by overwork, too much exercise, stress or trauma. It may be a complication of underweight and malnourishment where there is insufficient energy. Or it can be caused by overweight that slows down and dulls the reflexes. Emotional factors are fear, difficulties in relationships and feelings of rejection. For a strong sex drive the male ego has to have some confidence; failure or lack of success in life can cause it to weaken. According to Ayurveda, sexual debility is frequently caused by excessive sex, the product of sexual exhaustion.

In Ayurvedic terms it is mainly a Vata condition. Abstinence from sex is an important initial treatment. Rest and relaxation are helpful.

Treatment for Sexual Debility

Tonification therapy is generally required, with anti-Vata diet and foods to increase the semen. These are dairy products, ghee, nuts, lotus seeds, garlic, onions, okra and Jerusalem artichokes. Shellfish and red meat are also good but tamasic in nature.

Special tonic herbs for the male reproductive system are indicated such as ashwagandha, shatavari, bala, cuscuta and licorice. Kapikacchu (Mucuna pruriens) is one of the best Ayurvedic herbs in this respect. Important formulas are Ashwagandha compound and Chyavan Prash, as well as the Energy tonic (no. 2). These can be taken with milk and ghee. See also Male Sexual Vitality formula (no. 17).

Additional Chinese herbs are he shou wu (fo ti), lycium, astragalus seeds and formulas such as Rehmannia 6. Good Western herbs include saw palmetto, comfrey root and marshmallow.

Sexual debility can also be a Pitta condition, where Pitta burns out the semen. Treatment is also tonification. Aloe gel is good, as is shatavari or Shatavari compound taken with milk, sugar and ghee.

Kapha type sexual debility is characterized by lack of interest in sex, obesity, congestion and sluggishness in the system. Sugar is often used as a sex substitute. It is treated by aphrodisiac stimulants such as pippali, garlic, cloves, damiana and yohimbe. Formulas include Trikatu and Clove combination taken with honey. Guggul and shilajit are also useful here (and can be helpful for the other doshas).

MALE STERILITY

Inability to produce the right quantity or quality of sperm to bring about conception results in male sterility. Sexual function may otherwise be normal.

Following a tonification therapy similar to that for sexual debility can improve sperm count, as above. Key foods are dairy products, ghee, sesame oil, garlic and onions. Good herbs are ashwagandha, kapikacchu, bala and pippali. Indian clinical studies show that ashwagandha is quite effective in raising the sperm count. It works well in a milk decoction. Pungent, bitter and astringent tastes should be reduced as they cause depletion of sperm. Excessive sour articles can do this as well.

ENLARGED PROSTATE

Prostate enlargement is common in old age with weakening of sexual function. It can happen in younger men through excessive sexual practices or from undue suppression of ejaculation. Modern medical treatment generally regards it as an infection and uses antibiotics.

The best general Ayurvedic herb is gokshura, particularly when combined with ashwagandha. Shilajit is useful. The western herb saw palmetto is effective, particularly for Vata types.

Most commonly enlarged prostate is a Vata condition and comes in the Vata stage of life (old age). Symptoms include low back pain, low energy, and constipation. The treatment involves a standard anti-Vata diet with more oily and nutritive food. Good herbs are bala, kapikacchu, guggul and marshmallow. Formulas include Ashwagandha compound, Gokshura guggul and the Kidney tonic (no. 10).

Pitta type enlarged prostate involves infection, swelling and possible fever. The urine will be dark yellow or red. The treatment is similar to that for urinary tract infections, with cooling and diuretic herbs like uva ursi, echinacea or punarnava, added to tonic herbs like ashwagandha and gokshura or formulas such as Chyavan Prash. Lemon grass tea can be taken regularly.

Kapha type is due to water retention and excess phlegm. Treatment is similar to that for edema. Hot spicy diuretics are excellent—cinnamon, ginger, cloves, cubebs and juniper berries. Shilajit and guggul are important as long term remedies.

VENEREAL DISEASES

In the sexual act we bring together the deepest tissue levels of our bodies. This allows reproduction to occur; but it can also allow toxins to be transmitted directly into the most interior tissues. We can be invaded by pathogens, potentially devastating in their effects, which could otherwise be easily fought off. The greater the variety of our sexual partners and practices, the more likely we are to become vulnerable. Venereal diseases can become epidemics and threaten the health of a whole culture, which is what we are seeing in our world today.

GENITAL HERPES

Like any highly infectious condition this is largely a Pitta disorder, particularly during the acute phase. But it can involve the other doshas, particularly when there is debility or toxins (Ama) in the system. Genital herpes involves heat in the liver that is transmitted downwards along the liver meridian through the urino-genital region. The blood is usually impure, and excess bile may clog the system. In addition there will be accumulated stress, anger or anxiety.

Pitta type herpes is indicated by fever, thirst, irritability and other Pitta signs. The lesions will be red, swollen, painful or infected.

Vata type herpes involves dry skin, constipation, lack of energy, insomnia, anxiety and other Vata symptoms. The lesions will be painful and hard but not very red or inflamed.

Kapha type herpes involves general Kapha signs of mucus accumulation and lymphatic clogging. It involves weeping or oozing lesions with little redness or pain, but notable discharges.

Sarsaparilla is a good herb for venereal disease in any of the three doshas; it has good anti-viral properties. Gotu kola helps to calm the mental unrest of the condition and has excellent cleansing properties for the urino-genital system. Turmeric is excellent for its blood and liver cleansing properties.

TREATMENT FOR PITTA TYPE HERPES

Follow an anti-Pitta and blood-cleansing diet. Avoid hot spices, alcohol, sour food, and too much salt and sugar. Raw vegetables, salads and vegetable juices, including various green or chlorophyll drinks, should be taken fresh. Coriander is the best spice to use, and cilantro or parsley are also good. A mung bean or kicharee fast helps during acute attacks.

Stress should be reduced, with adequate rest and relaxation. Sexual activity should be avoided. During acute attacks sandalwood oil should be applied to the head and coconut oil to the body. Pancha karma treatment can be followed, with emphasis on purgation. Wash or douche the sores with cooling herbs like gentian, goldenseal, sarsaparilla and alum. Coconut oil or ghee can be applied to the sores as well.

Herbal treatment aims at cleansing the liver and blood. Diuretics and purgatives are helpful for their cleansing action. Mainly bitter taste is indicated. Good Ayurvedic herbs are aloe gel, gotu kola, barberry, gentian, sarsaparilla, sandalwood, gokshura, punarnava, shatavari, manjishta and katuka.

A typical Ayurvedic formula for acute conditions is 3 parts manjishta, 2 parts shatavari, and 1 part each of gotu kola, katuka, gokshura, sarsaparilla and lemon grass. Add 1 or 2 parts rhubarb root if constipation exists. Typical Ayurvedic patent medicines are Sarsaparilla compound or Sandalwood compound, taken with aloe gel. Tikta and the Liver Tonic (no. 8) are also good. In chronic conditions or between attacks one can take Chyavan Prash, Brahma Rasayana or gotu kola tea. Shatavari is excellent for women suffering from the condition.

Chinese treatment consists of heat-clearing therapy with Gentian combination, usually with the addition of special antiviral herbs such as isatis or honeysuckle during acute attacks. Between attacks, tonification is given with Rehmannia 6 or Anemarrhena, Phellodendron and Rehmannia formula. Excellent Western herbs for acute attacks are echinacea, goldenseal, plantain, uva ursi, and pipsissewa, along with marshmallow as a soothing demulcent. A tincture of 10-20 drops of echinacea can be taken every three or four hours when symptoms are strong.

Treatment for Vata Herpes

Cleansing herbs such as sarsaparilla, aloe gel, turmeric, barberry, sandalwood and gotu kola are required, with typical tonics like ashwagandha, bala, shatavari and licorice. Combination blood cleansing and tonification therapy is indicated. The diet should be anti-Vata, avoiding hot spices.

Formulas include Sarsaparilla combination with milk or ghee and Ashwagandha compound when severe weakness exists.

TREATMENT FOR KAPHA HERPES

Use liver cleansing herbs like aloe, barberry, turmeric and gentian along with hot spices, cayenne, dry ginger, pippali and cloves. Formulas include Sarsaparilla combination with Trikatu. A simple but effective treatment is regular taking of turmeric and cinnamon.

OTHER VENEREAL DISEASES

Other infectious venereal diseases like syphilis and gonorrhea can be treated like herpes, with a similar differentiation of doshic syndromes. Sarsaparilla compound is especially good for syphilis. For women, cleansing emmenagogues such as aloe gel, myrrh, saffron, safflower and other menstruation-regulating therapies are good, as per symptoms.

AIDS

According to Ayurveda AIDS is primarily a disease of low Ojas, the vital sap of the body, the essence of the reproductive system that maintains the immune system. The AIDS virus can only affect us if our Ojas is already low. Factors that deplete Ojas include excessive sexual activity, poor diet, junk food, use of drugs, too much thinking or worrying and lack of sleep. Some people have weak constitutions that make them vulnerable to such diseases as well.

As Ojas is the essence of Kapha, symptoms of low Ojas usually involve both high Pitta and high Vata. There will be anxiety, restlessness, irritability, vertigo, insomnia, palpitations, and chronic fever with low energy and poor endurance.

Ojas relates to sattva, so a sattvic life-style should be followed. Sattvic herbs for the mind like gotu kola, calamus and sandalwood are helpful. Tonics like ashwagandha, shatavari and amala-ki are excellent. Yogic postures and breathing exercises, particu-larly lunar pranayama (breathing in through the left nostril and out through the right), are important.

Treatment for AIDS

Both anti-Pitta (anti-fire) and anti-Vata (anti-air) regimens should be combined. Spicy, sour, bitter and astringent tastes should be reduced. Take food to strengthen Ojas that is sattvic in nature: sesame seeds and oil, almonds, chickpeas, milk, yogurt and ghee (clarified butter). Apply sesame externally, with sandal-wood or Brahmi oil applied to the head.

It is important to abstain from sexual activity or at least reduce it as much as possible. Anal sex, above all, should be avoided as it drains Ojas from the system. (It overly-stimulates apana, the downward moving air, and drains away prana, posi-tive vitality.) Masturbation should also be avoided; it is very reducing to Ojas. (The lack of emotional interchange drains ener-gy from the nervous system.)

Typical Ayurvedic herbs for building Ojas include most strong tonics and tonics to the reproductive system such as ashwagand-ha, shatavari, gokshura, bala and kapikacchu. Shilajit is excellent. Take 1-3 grams twice a day with milk and ghee. Formulas include Ashwagandha compound, Shatavari compound, Chyavan Prash or the Energy Tonic (no. 2).

The Ayurvedic special preparation, diamond ash (hira bhas-ma) is important. A Mercury compound, Makaradhwaj, is also good for restoring vitality but should not be taken in acute infec-tions.

Mantras for increasing Ojas include OM, SHUM and SHRIM. Gems to wear include Jupiter stones (yellow sapphire, yellow topaz, citrine) and Venus stones (diamond, clear zircon).

Ojas-increasing herbs should be combined with diuretics, gokshura or sarsaparilla, for cleansing the urino-genital tract and with gugguls or myrrh for cleansing the deeper tissues. Triphala guggul is good. Guduchi is excellent for clearing deep-seated fevers and strengthening the immune system. Much of the treatment for other venereal diseases is useful here as per symptoms.

Brahma rasayana, gotu kola herbal jelly, has cleansing and clearing effects. Saffron, in a milk decoction, is an excellent herb for most AIDS conditions.

A typical Ayurvedic AIDS formula is—gotu kola, sarsaparilla, ashwagandha, shatavari, gokshura, sandalwood and coriander in equal parts. Guduchi, guggul and shilajit can be added if available.

According to Chinese medicine AIDS is largely one of kidney essence deficiency. Usually it is more a yin than yang deficiency, but can be both. In addition the immune system or chi is weak, along with an internal accumulation of dampness and heat. Typical Chinese formulas for AIDS include Rehmannia 6 or Rehmannia 8 plus Astragalus. Other heat-clearing and blood-moving herbs may be added including salvia, red peony and isatis.

Good Western herbal tonics for AIDS include American ginseng, marshmallow, Solomon's seal and saw palmetto. A good AIDS formula with commonly available Western herbs is gotu kola, sarsaparilla, American ginseng, marshmallow, plantain, sandalwood and coriander in equal proportions.

II.7
MISCELLANEOUS CONDITIONS
Febrile Diseases, Skin Diseases, Arthritis and Gout, Cancer

FEBRILE DISEASES

Ayurvedic medicine has treated all types of febrile and infectious diseases, including collective plagues and epidemics. For this it employs powerful herbs, special foods, and sweating therapies. As antibiotic drugs begin to fail today, these natural methods are again becoming important. While they may not be as strong or as immediately effective in acute conditions as drugs, they are more useful in chronic conditions. Moreover, their side effects are much less. Natural therapies are less likely to weaken or suppress the immune system. In fact, after treatment our resistance will be stronger. We are not rendered vulnerable to new pathogens as happens with drugs. Antibiotic herbs do not breed new resistant strains of bacteria. When used at an early stage and with support therapies of right diet and life-style, herbs can be as effective as antibiotic drugs.

Of course we should be careful trying to treat high fevers or infections ourselves merely using common herbs. We should not take such conditions lightly and should always seek the proper help. But even if we are compelled to take antibiotics, such herbal methods can aid in the process of healing.

The main indication of all febrile diseases is a rise in body temperature. This is generally accompanied by a rapid pulse, bodyache, absence of sweating, restlessness, insomnia, delirium and lack of appetite. Depending on the type of disease there may be sensitivity to temperature changes, thirst or debility.

Febrile diseases usually relate to high Pitta, since excess Pitta causes fever and infection. However, fever can be created by any of the three doshas or by any combination of them. In addition, fever can arise from external causes such as injuries. Vata type fevers arise indirectly from an accumulation of gas or dryness in the body fluids. Kapha type fevers are the result of congestion and stagnation of fluids.

Ayurveda classifies many different types and degrees of fevers. As most of these relate to acute conditions that require medical supervision, we will deal only with the more common conditions here. We have already examined specific febrile conditions relative to different organ dysfunctions. Here we will take an overview of the subject.

Types of Fevers

- Pitta fevers are characterized by high body temperature, burning sensation, thirst, red tongue with yellow coating, red eyes, perspiration, yellow or burning urine, yellow stool or diarrhea and possible bleeding. There will be irritability, restlessness and disturbed sleep.
- Vata fevers show irregularity and changeability in symptoms, along with more severe pain. Their onset is variable: the temperature rise changes and does not remain the same. Additional symptoms of high Vata occur such as anxiety, restlessness, constipation, insomnia, pain and stiffness in the body, and ringing in the ears.
- Kapha fevers are usually low-grade with only a mild increase in body temperature. There will be loss of appetite, loss of taste, sweet taste in the mouth and excess salivation. The body will feel heavy, tired and cold and there may be cough and discharge of mucus.

It is important with fever to discriminate Ama and Nirama conditions—whether or not the undigested food mass (Ama) exists. When there is a pronounced tongue coating, Ama is indicated and herbs to promote digestion are needed, such as common spices like ginger and cinnamon or the Trikatu formula.

GENERAL TREATMENT OF FEVERS

Bitter herbs are indicated, especially for severe fevers. Many bitters contain antibacterial and antiviral properties. Some have been proven to possess antibiotic action in vitro against specific bacteria or viruses. Bitters will first target the pathogen, which is separated out from the tissues in which it is lodged. In excess, however, the herbs will have a reducing effect on the body itself, (to a lesser degree than antibiotic drugs,) therefore they should be used with discretion.

Each herbal tradition in the world has its particular panacea bitter febrifuge and anti-inflammatory herbs. Western herbalism has goldenseal or barberry. The Chinese have coptis or gold thread. Ayurveda has chiretta or katuka and the formula Tikta.

In addition, diaphoretic herbs are used to help sweat out a fever. A rise in body temperature works to kill many pathogens. Simple, fresh ginger tea is great for this purpose. Even better is basil tea, particularly the Indian tulsi or holy basil, which is good for all kinds of fevers. Take one cup of the infused herb every two or three hours until the fever breaks.

In Ayurvedic medicine, a smaller amount of hot pungent herbs such as Trikatu is added to bitters to help burn up the fever. Dry ginger by itself is good, with honey for Kapha, butter for Pitta and ghee for Vata. The usual dose is 1/4 teaspoon of dry ginger per teaspoon of honey every two or three hours.

Generally, diaphoretics work better in the initial stage of a fever, when there is Ama. They are also more effective in Vata and Kapha fevers. Bitters are better for Pitta and Kapha fevers. Diuretic herbs can be employed to drain the fever downwards (as fire is relieved by downward action). Purgatives can be used in the same way, but they are contraindicated in initial or new fevers, which require a more diaphoretic or sweating approach.

In both Ayurvedic and Chinese medicine the mineral gypsum is employed for lowering dangerously high fevers. The Chinese use the strained decoction of the crude mineral. Ayurveda makes a special incinerated ash called Godanti Bhasma.

Avoid eating during high fevers, particularly heavy or oily foods. If you are very hungry take whole grains, particularly barley, mung, rice or Kicharee. Mung water or mung bean soup is excellent for all types of fevers, infections and toxic blood conditions. Adequate liquids should be taken, preferably herbal teas or hydrating juices like coconut or pear. In initial fevers, do not drink cold water because it tends to drive the fever deeper into the body. A cold water sponge bath can be applied to the head and limbs if you need to cool down the body. Rose water sprinkled over the head and sandalwood oil applied to the forehead are cooling; also try henna and vetivert if you have access to these herbs. In the beginning or acute stage the patient should rest.

The initial treatment of fevers, as for the common cold, consists of hot spicy herbs for stimulant and diaphoretic action. Pippali or dry ginger can be used, taken with honey, or Trikatu formula with warm water. Other good herbs include bayberry, cinnamon, ginger, cloves and cayenne.

Old or mature fevers, which are fevers that have lasted several days or longer, are treated with typical bitter herbs like goldenseal or katuka. At this stage purgatives become helpful if there is also constipation or tense pain in the lower abdomen. Use rhubarb root or aloe powder for Pitta and Kapha, Triphala or castor oil for Vata.

Chronic low-grade fevers usually require tonification. Good herbs for high Vata or chronic Pitta conditions include aloe gel, shatavari, barberry, amalaki, bala and marshmallow. Shatavari has a special moistening and hydrating effect on fevers that have caused dryness, dehydration or depletion of the body fluids. Guduchi is a special Ayurvedic herb for long-term or low-grade fevers. Its extract or starch, guduchi sattva, has proven effective for many types of difficult lingering fevers. It also restores the immune function and brings back the appetite. Guduchi is perhaps the best herb in such conditions. Take 2-4 grams of the powder or about 1/2 teaspoon every three or four hours in warm water.

Formulas for low-grade fevers include Shatavari compound. The Ayurvedic herbal jelly Chyavan Prash is excellent: 2 teaspoons twice a day taken with warm milk. Sometimes this condition requires herbs to strengthen the immune system such as ashwagandha, bala, ginseng or astragalus.

SPECIFIC TREATMENT FOR FEVERS

Pitta fevers require primarily bitter herbs. Important Ayurvedic herbs are katuka, chiretta, neem, vetivert, lemon grass and sandalwood. Formulas include Sudarshan and Mahasudarshan powders as well as the Herbal Febrifuge and Blood Purifier (no. 7). After the fever, a bitter purgative like rhubarb root may be good to clear out residual toxins. Good Chinese formulas are Coptis and Scute (for septic fever) and Gypsum combination for high fever with thirst and delirium.

Vata fevers need bitter and pungent herbs such as black pepper, galangal, ginger, garlic and barberry. Formulas include Sudarshan powder or the Herbal Febrifuge with Trikatu, 1-2 grams of each twice a day with warm water.

Kapha fevers require primarily hot pungent herbs, though bitters can still be used. Black pepper or pippali can be taken mixed with honey. Formulas include Trikatu or Clove compound taken with honey.

INFECTIONS

For infections, bitter natural antibiotics and alteratives (blood-cleansers) are used. In Ayurveda, the most common is katuka. Chiretta, gentian, barberry, and isatis are also useful. In Chinese medicine, coptis is the main bitter. Other herbs are lonicera, forsythia, isatis, scute, phellodendron and rhubarb root. The usual Western herb is goldenseal. Also used are barberry, gentian, echinacea, sarsaparilla and usnea. Many herbs possess cooling energy and can be used in this way. A tincture of goldenseal and echinacea, 10-30 drops every 2-3 hours, is good for most infections.

Myrrh or guggul are also excellent, particularly for deeper-seated or long lasting infections. The formula Triphala guggul will remove infections from the blood. The rest of treatment for infections is like that for fevers. The condition is mainly high Pitta. Below we will examine one form of general infection, boils and carbuncles.

BOILS AND CARBUNCLES

Boils and carbuncles are local infections of the skin and hair follicles by staph and other bacteria. A toxic blood condition, they are characterized by swelling, pain, fever and discharge of pus. They occur more commonly on the back, legs and arms but can erupt anywhere on the surface of the body. Acne is a much milder condition, which can be treated by the same line of therapies.

In Western medicine boils are related from external factors. In Ayurveda internal impurity is considered to be the main cause and indicates the need for internal cleansing. Boils are an Ama (toxic) condition resulting from poor diet but can also come about from other impure conditions. The liver is the main organ involved, therefore a toxic liver will be prone to them.

Types of Boils

Pitta type boils are characterized by redness, swelling, thirst and fever. Kapha type boils are indicated by large amounts of pus, dullness, heaviness and lassitude. Vata boils are hard, dry and painful. They are slow to come to a head and may migrate to other points in the body.

Boils generally result from impure food and water, or overeating of spicy, hot, sour and salty foods (Pitta-causing foods). Intake of excess sweet, oily or greasy foods can cause them. Sweet taste in excess, which leads to poor digestion and fermentation, will acidify the blood. Exposure to sun or heat, too many saunas or hot baths, and other such Pitta-aggravating elements may also contribute to the infection. Anger, irritability, stress or suppressed emotions are psychological factors that can bring it about. The condition may be brought on by travel to a hotter climate with a higher bacterial count.

Western medical treatment is largely with antibiotics. The main danger is that the infection will become septic, spreading through the body and infecting the internal organs. It can even cause death.

272

General Treatment of Boils

In acute conditions, a detoxifying and anti-Pitta diet and therapy is essential. Salads, sprouts and vegetable juices, preferably fresh, should be taken. Dairy products, breads, sweets, oils, meat, fish and mushrooms should be avoided. All stale, recooked and canned food, junk food or otherwise devitalized food such as white sugar and white flour should be strictly avoided. No spices should be used except turmeric and coriander. No oil should be applied to the body, but the essential oil of sandalwood or gardenia can be applied to the forehead. Strong or aerobic exercise should be avoided.

Herbal bitters are indicated, with some use of astringents. Alterative (blood-cleansing) teas are great including alfalfa, plantain, red clover, burdock and dandelion. Specific herbal therapy involves the use of natural antibiotic herbs and special herbs to help dissolve pus (suppuratives).

Treatment is both external and internal, applying herbal packs or poultices to the sore. Important Ayurvedic herbs are manjishta, katuka, neem, isatis, turmeric and barberry. Aloe gel can be taken in 2 teaspoon dosages, 3 times a day with a little turmeric. Formulas are the Herbal Febrifuge and Blood Purifier (no. 7) and the Herbal Laxative (no. 5). Ghee can be helpful externally, the older the better (even if it smells).

Chinese herbs include honeysuckle, forsythia, isatis, coptis, scute and phellodendron. Formulas are Honeysuckle and Forsythia combination for milder conditions and Coptis and Scute combination for severe cases. Western herbs are burdock, sarsaparilla, sassafras and red clover for mild infections, with myrrh, chickweed, dandelion, barberry and goldenseal for severe conditions.

Specific Treatment of Boils

Vata boils are caused by exposure to the wind, by dryness in the blood and by distention and constipation. Laxatives such as Triphala help clear toxins from the large intestine. Triphala guggul or myrrh tincture are excellent. Sarsaparilla is a good single herb, and garlic often works well, particularly to bring boils to a head.

Kapha boils relate to impurities in the lymph system and may accompany phlegm diseases. They require the use of expectorants (pus can be a kind of subcutaneous phlegm) and spicy taste substances. Good herbs include cinnamon, angelica, turmeric, sassafras and calamus. Most of the Pitta herbs can also be used, along with Trikatu or dry ginger.

SKIN DISEASES

The skin is the largest organ in the body and the one most exposed to the external world. The skin either protects us from external forces of heat and cold, wind and dryness or allows them to enter into our body and cause various diseases. Therefore, the skin is closely connected to the immune system. A good, lustrous and slightly oily skin indicates a good immune system and a good resistance to disease. Skin that is discolored, too dry or too oily, or inflamed indicates poor resistance to disease and possible impending health problems.

The skin reflects the plasma (rasa dhatu), which is the first tissue produced from the food that we have digested, and mirrors overall bodily health and nutrition. Right care of the skin, therefore, is essential for good health. Many diseases manifest through the skin or show up as various skin problems.

Regular oil massage protects the skin and strengthens the immune system, particularly heavier oils like sesame and almond that coat and protect the skin. Steam, sweating and sauna therapies cleanse the skin. These two procedures are the basis of Ayurvedic snehana and svedana, oleation and sweating therapies that are the basis of Pancha Karma therapy. They are also essential to any healthy life-style as regular health maintenance procedures. We should all take good care of our skin, not simply out of cosmetic purposes but to protect our health as a whole and for disease prevention. If we use cosmetics we should choose natural remedies that protect the skin and stimulate its proper growth.

There are many types of skin diseases such as psoriasis, eczema, skin rashes and contact dermatitis. In Ayurveda, these are classified succinctly according to the three doshas. Those caused by external toxins, like poison oak or poison ivy, can usually be treated like the Pitta type.

Skin diseases are more common in Pitta types because Pitta can overheat the blood and irritate the skin. Skin diseases that involve loss of skin pigmentation, such as leucoderma, are usually Pitta disorders, as Pitta governs complexion.

Factors causing skin diseases include too much use of sour, salty or pungent tastes, too heavy, sweet or oily food, drinking of alcohol, exposure to the elements and overuse of cosmetics. They are similar to boils, carbuncles and other toxic blood conditions in their origin and treatment.

The skin relates to the plasma, to the outer disease pathway and to the blood. Skin diseases, therefore, relate to the lungs and the liver. The use of expectorants and diaphoretics to cleanse the lungs, and alteratives and bitter tonics to cleanse the liver, are important in the treatment of skin diseases.

General Treatment of Skin Diseases

There are many good herbs for cleansing and healing the skin. Among the best are common blood-cleansing herbs like dandelion, burdock, red clover, plantain, yarrow and self-heal. Ayurvedic herbs include turmeric, barberry, sandalwood and guggul. Chinese herbs are honeysuckle, forsythia, isatis and bupleurum. Such herbs are mainly for acute cases. In chronic cases, demulcents and tonics such as marshmallow, licorice, shatavari and gokshura are required.

Psoralia, Sanskrit bakuchi, is an important Ayurvedic herb for leucoderma, for restoring normal skin pigmentation and a rejuvenative to the skin, nails and hair. Take 5 grams of the powder twice a day before meals with a little coriander and honey to mask its bitter taste. It can also be taken as a medicated oil.

275

Herbs for skin diseases should be applied externally as well as internally. Externally, herbal decoctions can function as washes for the skin, herbal plasters or poultices can be applied to skin inflammations, or herbal oils used for massage.

Ghee is excellent externally for inflammatory skin diseases, rashes and burns. It is best prepared by placing it in a copper vessel along with about half the amount of water. It should be kept for a month, stirring it occasionally with a copper spoon if possible. The ghee will become whitish in color and take on a pleasant coconut-like smell. (This preparation, done over a shorter period of time by rapid stirring of water and ghee in a copper vessel is called Shatodhara ghrita and is sold in India). Such ghee is more absorbable to the skin. It is excellent for all manner of skin rashes and burns.

Aloe gel is another helpful topical preparation for almost any kind of skin rash. Cilantro juice is good for most allergic skin conditions. Ayurvedic Turmeric cream can be useful, particularly for acne or for improving complexion (but some Ayurvedic Turmeric creams contain essential oils like sandalwood that in excess can irritate the skin).

Saffron is a special herb for nourishing the skin, taken as a milk decoction (1 gram per cup). Pearl ash (moti bhasma) or pearl powder is also excellent. Shatavari cools the skin and relieves inflammation. It also hydrates the skin and improves the complexion.

It should be noted that skin rashes sometimes get worse before they get better, as the heat and toxins are being dispelled from the body. One should not terminate a treatment too quickly if the diagnosis appears sound.

Types of Skin Diseases

- Pitta skin diseases are characterized by redness, swelling, fever, infection and irritability. Heat and exposure to the sun increase them. Application of most oils will make them worse.

276

• Vata types show up as dry or scaly skin, itching, distention or constipation. They are aggravated by wind and dryness and alleviated by the application of heavy oils, especially sesame.

• Kapha types involve oozing or weeping sores, with congestion, edema and itch. Dampness and cold aggravate them. Oils also tend to aggravate them.

Specific Treatment of Skin Diseases

For Pitta type skin diseases one should follow an anti-Pitta diet avoiding possible allergen foods like nightshades, tomatoes, peaches and strawberries as well as sour dairy products. Drink coconut, pomegranate or sweet pineapple juice to clear the system. Exposure to sun and heat should be avoided. The best oils for external application are coconut or sunflower and Ghee is also excellent. Aloe gel or cilantro juice is excellent externally. Brahmi or Bhringaraj oil, or the herbs in decoction, are good for rashes on the head, neck and face. Most typical alteratives, like burdock or red clover, are good. Bitter laxatives, rhubarb root or aloe, are helpful. Formulas include the Herbal Febrifuge and Blood Purifier (no. 7) taken with aloe gel or dandelion tea.

Vatas should follow an anti-Vata diet. Soothing oils such as sesame should be applied to the skin on a regular basis. Laxatives and enema therapy are helpful. Triphala should be taken on a regular basis, 5-10 grams before sleep. Triphala guggul or myrrh tincture is good. Avoid exposure to wind, cold and sudden temperature changes.

Kaphas should implement an anti-Kapha diet avoiding all heavy, greasy and oily food, particularly cheese and yogurt. No oils should be used externally or internally. Dry powders on the skin are often helpful, using such anti-Kapha herbs as calamus, ginger or mustard. Diuretic herbs are helpful like plantain, burdock seeds or pipsissewa. Formulas include Gokshura guggul or Triphala guggul, as well as the Herbal Febrifuge and Blood Purifier (no. 7) with warm water or ginger tea.

ARTHRITIS

Arthritis is one of the most common chronic and degenerative diseases. Yet, modern medicine has little more to offer for treating it than aspirin. In Ayurveda, arthritis is called 'Amavata', a toxic air condition. Arthritis is mainly a Vata disease. It involves pain and weakening of the bones, the main Vata tissue in the body. It can also be divided into types or stages according to the three doshas.

Causes for the disease include both internal and external factors. Arthritis is more common in windy, damp and stormy climates. It is related to low Agni and poor digestion that causes the accumulation of Ama (toxins). Poor colon function allows the toxins to be transported to the joints. Arthritis may also be caused by injury. Arthritis is another immune system disorder where the body attacks itself, therefore much of what has been said under allergies is applicable here.

General Treatment of Arthritis

In Ayurvedic thought the state of the bones is reflected in the state of the colon, where nutrients are absorbed for the bones. Vata (waste-gases) absorbed in the colon go to the bones and cause arthritis. So in treating arthritis consider treating the colon as well. If there is constipation or malabsorption in the colon, take 2-5 grams of Triphala regularly before sleep. Cleansing enemas are helpful, particularly made with Dashamula decoction. To tonify the bones take sesame oil enemas containing a cup of oil and a cup of warm water, holding for twenty minutes twice a week. Oil massage to the colon can be as helpful as massage to the bones and joints.

MEDICATED SESAME OILS

Externally, medicated oils loosen stiff joints, clear toxins, nourish tissues and relieve pain. The special medicated sesame oils of Ayurveda are excellent in this regard.

278

- Mahanarayan Oil, whose main ingredient is shatavari, is excellent for improving flexibility, relieving stiffness and stopping pain. It is good for muscular fatigue, treats varicose veins and nourishes the skin. This makes it good for dancers or athletes as well.
- Narayan Oil, whose main ingredient is ashwagandha, is effective for muscular and joint pain. It improves circulation in the lower extremities and helps counter the effects of the aging process.
- Sahachardi Oil, whose main ingredient is sahacharda, is specific to rheumatoid arthritis and is effective where there is muscular atrophy or degeneration of the nerves. These oils should be applied daily with a gentle massage.
- Chandanabalalakshadi Oil, whose main ingredient is sandalwood, is cooling and good for Pitta type arthritis.

When these oils are not available warm sesame oil itself can be used. Castor oil is also excellent for arthritic pain. It is particularly good for swelling and also improves the healing of the tissue. Apply castor oil to the affected joints and keep it on overnight for the best results. We can make our own medicated oils by cooking specific herbs in sesame oil (for more information see *Yoga of Herbs* pps. 82-4).

Sweating therapy with saunas or steam boxes is excellent. A hose is connected to the top of a pressure cooker where special herbs are cooking (typically Dashamula compound). Apply the steam to local areas for a more direct treatment (nadi sveda). Diaphoretic or sweat-inducing herbs add to the therapeutic power of the steam—ephedra, angelica, nirgundi, bay leaves or eucalyptus leaves.

Herbal essential oils like camphor, mint and wintergreen are good for external application, particularly for pain and swelling. They can be dissolved in rubbing alcohol or combined with tonic herbs like ashwagandha in medicated sesame oil preparations. Wintergreen contains methyl salicylate and can be used in place of aspirin for pain relief.

As arthritis is a toxic, or ama, condition it is necessary to burn up the toxins by reviving the digestive fire. Short fasting or hot spicy herbs can be helpful such as cayenne, cinnamon, dry ginger and galangal. Hot gemstones such as ruby or garnet set in gold can be used as well. Care must be taken with these hot remedies, however, when there is fever or inflammation. Avoid damp, heavy, Ama-forming foods and irregular eating habits.

Important Ayurvedic anti-rheumatic herbs are guggul, castor root, turmeric, cyperus, galangal, nirgundi and prasarini. These relieve pain in the joints and promote flexibility. Guggul is specific for cleansing the bone tissue, and for strengthening the bones and improving flexibility. It is also good for sports injuries that often lead to arthritis. Cyperus, an herb also used in Chinese medicine, is used in Ayurvedic medicine for stopping arthritic pain and contractions. Prasarini and nirgundi possess good analgesic properties for rheumatic pain. Prasarini can be used for abdominal pain as well, while nirgundi is a good anti-inflammatory agent found in most anti-arthritis formulas.

The most effective Ayurvedic formulas are Triphala Guggul, Yogaraj Guggul and Mahayogaraj Guggul (the latter two contain special minerals). Yogaraj Guggul is usually the best of the three. Yet recent clinical studies in India show that the simple guggul itself is as effective as these complex formulas if taken in higher dosages, such as 6 grams a day. The Antirheumatic formula (no. 13), a modern and purely herbal guggul combination, is excellent.

A good formula with Western herbs is angelica, wild ginger, cinnamon and licorice in equal parts. The herbs can be infused or taken as a powder in one teaspoonful doses with honey (as honey possesses a better cleansing action than sugar, milk or ghee). This formula will work quite well in initial arthritis and is better for Vata or Kapha types. Where more Pitta or inflammation is involved, one or two bitter herbs such as katuka, barberry or goldenseal should be added.

Chinese herbs include du huo, qiang huo, ligusticum, Gentiana macrophylla and Siberian ginseng. Ligusticum is the preferable analgesic. Siberian ginseng is excellent for chronic and degenerative arthritis, particularly in the elderly, for which condition it combines well with ashwagandha. Additional Western herbs are myrrh, chaparral and yucca. Kava kava is also excellent for joint pain and for improving flexibility.

Types of Arthritis

- Vata type arthritis involves severe pain that is variable, migrating, throbbing and cutting. It is relieved by the application of heat and aggravated by the application of cold. The skin is dry or scaly, the joints become stiff and crack, and movement is difficult. Deformation of the bones is likely to occur. There may be constipation, gas or abdominal distention and lower back pain. Nervousness, anxiety, fear and insomnia are common.
- Pitta type involves inflammation, swelling, fever or burning sensation. Pain is relieved by cold but aggravated by heat. Symptoms include sweating, loose bowel movements and irritability.
- Kapha type involves swelling and edema around the joints. Pain will be localized, dull, heavy and aching. It will be relieved by heat and aggravated by cold and by damp weather. The skin will be oily; there may be congestion in the chest or mucus in the stool.

Specific Treatment of Arthritis

Treatment for Vata type arthritis is similar to the general treatment with an anti-Vata, anti-Ama, detoxifying diet. Gugguls and medicated sesame oils are the foundations. Galangal is a special herb for this condition. When there is degeneration and atrophy of the bones, tonics such as ashwagandha and vidari are required. Take care, however, that tonics do not increase toxicity (the undigested food mass) by their heavy nature. The colon should be kept clean with castor oil or Triphala. Perform regular oil massage of the body, including the colon. Hot baths in mineral salts, like Epsom salt, can soothe the joints and help draw out toxins.

For Pitta type arthritis, additional bitter herbs along with an anti-Pitta diet are indicated. Sandalwood oil or paste, coconut oil or Brahmi oil can be applied to the joints. Cold fomentations or ice packs are helpful. Good herbs are guggul, shallaki, sandalwood, guduchi, aloe, neem, turmeric, saffron and other bitter tasting antirheumatic herbs. The Anti-rheumatic formula (no. 13) should be taken with aloe gel.

For Kapha hot spicy herbs are specifically indicated such as cinnamon, ginger, mustard, cayenne, turmeric or the formula Trikatu. Hot herbs like mustard, cayenne, or ginger can be used in pastes, plasters or in rubbing alcohol. Calamus powder is excellent as a dry massage to the affected area. Mustard oil can be used externally with a little cayenne. Sugar, dairy and oily food must be strictly avoided.

GOUT

Gout is a metabolic disorder in which uric acid is deposited in the cartilage of the joints. In the Ayurvedic view it is a condition similar to arthritis and many of the remedial measures are the same. The big toe is characteristically involved, becoming swollen and very painful. Gout is called 'Vata-rakta' in Sanskrit, meaning Vata in the blood. Treatment is to reduce Vata and cleanse the blood.

Causes include eating food that makes the blood toxic: too much salty, sour and spicy food, too rich, too oily, too hot or improperly prepared food. Avoid meat, sugar, jellies, pastries, beans, mushrooms, yogurt, pickles, acid fruits and alcohol. Fresh vegetables may be taken freely; also fresh fruit, rice, wheat, potatoes and milk.

Alterative herbs are used such as manjishta, guduchi, guggul, myrrh, neem, sandalwood and vetivert. Aloe gel, preferably with turmeric, is a good home remedy, or the Herbal Febrifuge and Blood Purifier (no. 7). Pinda oil or castor oil can be applied externally. Western herbs are dandelion, red clover, burdock and barberry.

DENTAL PROBLEMS/BLEEDING GUMS

The condition of the gums and teeth reflects the health of the bones in the body. Those with bad teeth tend to other Vata or bone diseases like arthritis. Those with good teeth are generally blessed with good longevity as well.

Many Ayurvedic toothpastes and toothpowders are sold in India, composed with extracts of various herbs. Several of them are already imported into this country. Ayurvedic toothpastes contain special herbs of spicy and astringent tastes to stimulate and tighten the gums. The same types of herbs are used in Ayurvedic toothpowders.

Actually, Ayurveda prefers toothpowders to toothpastes. These toothpowders, rubbed into the gums on a daily basis, can prevent or eliminate most gum problems. Rubbing the gums with oils like sesame or coconut is also good for maintaining the tone of the gums, particularly for Vata types or those with receding gums. Gum massage is essential for health and longevity of teeth and gums.

For bad breath or a bad taste in the mouth many spicy herbs are good, taken as teas, such as thyme, peppermint, cinnamon and cloves. Cloves, wild ginger and prickly ash are good analgesics for toothache. Several drops of the tincture should be applied directly to the site. Sucking cloves after meals is another good breath freshener.

Swollen or bleeding gums is usually a Pitta (fire or infectious) condition but may be only a local problem of poor hygiene. Vata types suffer more from receding gums. Kapha types generally have good gums but swelling and excess eating of sugar can cause them to deteriorate.

Treat swollen gums by applying astringent herbs to the site. These include alum, alumroot, turmeric, catechu, myrrh or Triphala powder. Simple Triphala powder is great. Bitters, such as goldenseal or katuka, help by their anti-inflammatory action. Unfortunately most of these herbs taste bad, so spices like peppermint, spearmint or licorice can be used along with them and aid in their efficacy by helping them penetrate deeper into the gums.

283

However, should there be receding gums use astringents with care.

If the problem is not just local, usually high Pitta will be the cause and hyperacidity or heat in the liver or stomach will be the provoking factor. This should be treated directly.

CANCER

In Ayurveda cancer is a disease that often involves all three doshas, though it typically starts with a predominance of one. The digestive fire and other Agnis are low, allowing a build-up of toxic substances. The cancer represents a negative life-energy, something like a parasite, which has become established in the body. Negative life-energy usually comes from an excess of Apana, the downward moving air. Hence, Apana disorders such as distention, constipation and diarrhea may be the basis of this condition. Cancer cells, lacking oxygen (prana), represent a growth in the body outside the rule of prana.

Cancer has many causes including our toxic environment, devitalized foods, sedentary life-style, and lack of spiritual purpose or effort in life. Its basis often is suppressed emotion or emotional stagnation, which causes accumulation of toxic material, and excess doshas. In older Western medicine, it was seen as a disease of melancholy or black bile, which also translates as suppressed emotions. Hence, physical remedial measures are usually not enough to restore health.

In the Vedic system cancer is viewed as a psychic disorder, a disruption in the aura allowing the entrance of a negative astral force. Emotional cleansing, mantra and meditation are important to counter this.

Spiritual Therapies for Cancer

Gem therapy helps guard against Cancer. Gems are able to balance the aura and protect the life. Blue sapphire set in gold is the best gem for antitumor properties. It helps ward off the negative force invading the body, but should be used with other stones that increase the positive life-force. Diamond is most important for sustaining life and longevity. Diamond, yellow sapphire, and yellow topaz are the best stones for increasing Ojas, the energy of the immune system. Ruby, garnet or red coral can aid in reestablishing proper circulation, which removes the stagnation behind the tumor. Emerald and peridot help increase prana and relieve pain and disharmony.

Special Ayurvedic diamond preparations (hira bhasma) are particularly useful. Mantra therapy is excellent for cancer. Simple chanting of OM is excellent for opening up the aura and clearing the psychic air. The mantra, RAM, is best to give protection and bring down the Divine healing force. HUM is effective for casting out negative life-energies.

Pranayama is important to increase Prana, the positive life-force, regular solar Pranayama for Kapha, lunar pranayama for Pitta, and alternating breath for Vata. Practice of Pranayama is an important cancer preventative.

Types of Cancer

- Vata type cancer involves emotional factors such as fear, anxiety, depression and insomnia. The tumors are dry, hard and variable in appearance. The skin will turn gray, brown or dusky in color. There will be distention, constipation and other high Vata symptoms. Colon cancer is often a Vata type.
- In Pitta types there is anger, irritability, resentment or hatred. The tumors will be inflamed, infected and associated with a burning sensation or bleeding. Most forms of skin, eye and liver cancer are of Pitta type.
- Kapha type cancer involves tiredness, excess sleeping, congestion and salivation. Usually benign tumors appear first and over time become malignant. Surgery is an effective treatment if the cancer is found early enough. Lung or breast cancer is often a Kapha type.

285

Herbal Treatment for Cancer

The herbal therapies for reducing cancer can be put into several categories. A typical anti-cancer formula combines aspects of all these approaches, varied according to conditions.

1. POWERFUL ALTERNATIVE OR BLOOD-CLEANSING HERBS

These herbs destroy toxins, counter poisons and reduce infections. The most famous anti-cancer herbs are found in this category and some eastern herbs such as red clover, dandelion, self-heal, stillingia, burdock, sarsaparilla, Indian sarsaparilla and Chinese oldenlandia. Such herbs are better if used fresh, and they go well with a radical detoxifying diet like wheat grass juice. Dosages of one to three ounces daily of decoctions of fresh herbs may be required. They are good for lymphatic or skin cancer, and are better for Pitta and Kapha varieties.

2. STRONG CIRCULATORY STIMULANTS OR BLOOD-MOVING HERBS

These herbs promote circulation, break stagnation, reduce masses and aid in the healing of tissues. Herbs used in this way include turmeric and its relative zedoaria, saffron, safflower, myrrh, madder and guggul. Additional Chinese herbs are salvia and spargania. Good for breast or uterine cancer, liver or pancreas cancer, many of these herbs work on all three doshas. Dosages of these herbs need not be as high as the blood purifiers.

3. IMMUNE STRENGTHENING TONICS

These include famous Chinese herbs such as ginseng, astragalus, dang shen, white atractylodes, schizandra and ligustrum; and the Ayurvedic herbs ashwagandha, shatavari, guduchi, bala, shilajit, kapikacchu and black and white musali. Both Chinese and Ayurvedic herbs of this type have proven their immune strengthening effects in modern clinical studies. Western herbs like American ginseng, comfrey root and Solomon's seal have a similar effect. These tonics are better in debility conditions, which are usually Vata in nature, and to protect the strength of the patient undergoing stronger therapies, whether herbal, dietary, surgical or chemotherapy. Dosages again must be high, for example an ounce or more per herb per day.

4. SPECIAL EXPECTORANT OR PHLEGM-DISPELLING HERBS
These include kelp, seaweed, Irish moss and the Ayurvedic bhallatak and Chinese herb fritillary. They are better for thyroid, neck or lymphatic cancer but can be useful in other types as well. Ayurvedically, they are more for Vata and Kapha cancers.

5. STRONG BITTER OR PUNGENT HERBS WITH FAT-REDUCING AND TOXIN-DESTROYING PROPERTIES
Such herbs include goldenseal, coptis, aloe and katuka (bitter) and cayenne, black pepper, calamus and prickly ash (spicy). These herbs increase Agni and reduce the tissues, an action that is useful on cancer cells as well.

Based on these principles a good general anti-cancer formula is equal parts turmeric, safflower (or saffron in 1/4 part), manjishta, dandelion, self-heal, sarsaparilla and ashwagandha. Take in a strong decoction, 2 teaspoons of the powdered herbs per cup of hot water, or 3-6 grams of the powder 3 times a day. Take the powder with honey and black pepper for Kapha, with aloe gel for Pitta and with fresh ginger tea for Vata.

Such herbs may reduce tumors, whether malignant or benign, if the tumors are not large, have not metastasized and the patient is still strong.

However, tumor reduction is not always a sign of cure. Improvement of energy, immune function and other vitals is equally important. Only time will tell the real result of treatment. However, such natural therapies generally improve the patient's condition and make their life more tolerable, even if they fall short of a cure.

If the patient is already weak or debilitated, add more tonic herbs to protect the energy and immune system. Above all, the appropriate Pancha Karma treatment (see section) should be sought for all doshas, unless the patient is too weak to handle it. Herbs for cancer in the different doshas are:

- For Vata—calamus, haritaki, myrrh or guggul and the Triphala formula or Triphala guggul. The colon must be kept clean. Asafoetida 8 is also useful.

287

- For Pitta—saffron, manjishta, dandelion, gotu kola and turmeric. Usually, very strong blood-cleansing therapies and raw vegetable and juice diets can be applied to Pitta types. The Herbal Febrifuge and Blood Purifier (no. 7) is helpful, or liver-cleansing therapies and formulas.
- For Kapha—cayenne, black pepper, pippali, bhallatak, dry ginger, guggul, myrrh, turmeric and the Trikatu formula. Strong expectorant approaches are indicated.

Dietary Treatment for Cancer

Anti-cancer herbs generally work best with a strong anti-Ama or detoxifying diet. Strictly avoid meat and dairy products, as well as too much protein (the cancer cell itself is pure protein). However, some proteins should be taken to insure the secretion of enzymes to help digest it. In this regard mung beans are probably the best protein source. Cancer is often a disease of too much animal products.

The diet should emphasize raw vegetables and juices such as wheat grass, barley grass, celery, and dandelion which are your typical green drinks. Raw green juices are full of prana and help clear out any negative life-energy. Sprouts like alfalfa, sunflower and mung are also excellent, containing special enzymes that help digest unwanted tissue. However, such cooling foods can weaken the digestive fire. Balance them with spices like ginger, cayenne and garlic to protect the digestive fire.

If the patient is too weak for such a detoxifying diet, put them on a kicharee diet, with equal parts mung beans and basmati rice. To the kicharee add spices like turmeric, ginger and garlic, but use oil sparingly, only a small amount of ghee. Add root vegetables to the mixture if the patient can handle them. Such a diet should be followed for as long as necessary, extending up to a period of months.

288

II.8
CARE OF CHILDREN AND THE ELDERLY

THE FOUR STAGES OF LIFE

The ancient seers of India divided human life into four stages of twenty-five years each called ashramas. Each stage of life has its appropriate behavior and activity (dharma) that is the same for everyone.

The Four Stages of Life

1. Birth—25 years	Brahmacharya	Student	Kapha	Kama
2. 25—50 years	Grihastha	Householder	Pitta	Artha
3. 50—75 years	Vanaprastha	Hermitage	Pitta/Vata	Dharma
4. 75—100 years	Sannyasa	Renunciation	Vata	Moksha

The first phase of life, childhood and adolescence to early adulthood, is the learning or formative stage of life, what we can call the *student phase*. It is the time of Brahmacharya, which means learning and the discipline that goes with it. Children should be taught to focus on meaningful learning, which is learning to understand themselves and the universe around them, and to avoid distractions. This is the period of life dominated by Kapha, the formative or watery force. At this time we are seeking *kama* or enjoyment, gaining experience about the world around us.

The second phase of life, the prime adult phase from twenty-five to fifty, is the main period for earning a livelihood and raising a family. It is characterized as the *householder* phase. Meeting one's material and family needs are the primary obligations. This is the period of life dominated by Pitta, the fiery force. At this time we are seeking *artha* or wealth, gaining the necessities of life for ourselves and for those under our care. For this we are willing to sacrifice our own pleasure and enjoyment.

The third phase of life, the late adult phase, is meant as a withdrawal from the family duties of the householder phase while taking on the greater duties of social responsibility and spiritual practice. At this time people become grandparents or elders guiding society. It is called the *hermitage phase* because in ancient times people left their homes and took up a small hermitage just outside the village, from which point they could live in retirement but still be close enough to provide help and advice as needed. Sometimes a couple would simply retire to a smaller room at the back of the house and let their children take charge of the main household duties. This stage marks the transition between Pitta and Vata. At this time we are seeking *dharma*, meaning honor and truth, and the need for wealth gradually subsides.

The fourth phase of life, the *renunciation phase*, consists of preparing for death and the next life, or seeking to be liberated from the cycle of birth and death altogether. This stage is strongly under the domination of Vata, which brings about decay and death. At this time we are seeking moksha or liberation. We naturally lose interest in the outer affairs of life. We are like a traveler getting ready to move on to a new destination.

The time limits on these four phases are general. Some advanced souls can go directly in the Sannyasa phase. Other immature souls never get beyond the values and needs of adolescence. The beauty of the Vedic system of life-stages, which Ayurveda also follows, is that each stage has its appropriate behavior and life-style.

The problem with modern culture is that we don't understand the hermitage and renunciation phases. We try to keep people in the realm of pleasure and wealth for their entire lives. This not only stifles the soul but can imbalance the psychology. We also don't prepare people to use their wealth for higher dharmic and spiritual goals. Successes of the householder phase are used not to develop great spiritual successes in the latter phases of life but become a blockage to any higher development. The result is that we have a society that is immature and does not understand the deeper and later phases of human life and consciousness.

The four ashramas, or stages of life, provide a good model of social health that we should learn to follow in order to heal our culture. In terms of health there are special health concerns for the first or childhood phase, particularly up to the age of fifteen, and for the third and fourth or retirement phases, particularly after the age of sixty.

THE CARE OF CHILDREN

Ayurveda considers that the proper care of children is the foundation of health both for a person and for a culture. The best way to judge a person's health is to see how they grew up as a child—the diet, exercise and way of life that they followed. The best way to judge the health of a culture is to see the health of its children and how it raises children. By this standard modern culture is in trouble. Our children are raised on artificial food, mass media impressions that are often distorted, and have much time spent alone or without proper parental supervision.

One of classical Ayurveda's eight main branches is pediatrics. Disease propensity in life is created by the lack of understanding and care for the unique constitution of the child. An ancient Vedic verse states, "The One God has entered into the mind, born at first, he plays within the child." This Divine Child is worshipped in India as the infant Krishna. All parents were to consider their child as Krishna. This was a way of bringing out both care and understanding in the parents. Krishna, though a Divine incarnation, was portrayed as a young boy stealing butter so that parents would recognize the divinity even behind childhood pranks and treat children with the proper care.

It is important to determine the Ayurvedic constitution of your child. An Ayurvedic diet and life-style should be prescribed accordingly. The same diet is not good for all children, anymore than the same education is. Without understanding the unique nature of the individual—and that of the child may be different from that of the parent—we are likely to impose a restrictive or inappropriate pattern upon them. This makes it difficult for them

291

to discover who they really are and what their real needs may be. We can also examine childhood as a whole from the Ayurvedic perspective.

The Stage of Childhood

The stages or seasons of human life have their own particular nature and needs. The age of childhood, being the formative age, is the most important. It is more uniform in different people, races and cultures, as children are children wherever we find them.

Childhood is the stage of life in which Kapha, the biological water humor, predominates. Water is the formative element, the origin of life and is responsible for growth and development. As children are producing new tissues, new water as it were, they will also produce more mucus as a by-product. More mucus indicates poor digestion, which allows phlegm to accumulate rather than new tissue to be built up. For this reason children mainly have diseases of excess mucus and suffer most from disorders involving the lungs, ranging from the common cold to bronchitis and pneumonia. These are Kapha diseases in Ayurveda. Though children may be individually of any of the three doshas, the state of childhood will keep Kapha at a higher concentration. Therefore, with all children, we must be careful to keep the level of mucus in the system from becoming too high.

DIETARY CONSIDERATIONS FOR CHILDREN

Generally, children should have an even diet, avoiding too many sweets, strong spices, overly sour food or too much salt. A diet of whole grains and complex carbohydrates promotes a calm and harmonious child. It is easy to pervert the tastes of a child and such a condition can take years to correct, if ever. Tasty foods, used as a substitute for parental love and care, warp the child's sense of affection.

Yet, children need foods that are building and most of these increase Kapha. We cannot simply treat children by putting them on a water-decreasing or mucus-reducing diet because this will not afford them adequate nutrition for growth. In this regard dairy products and sugar are good for children if taken in the right way. According to the sages of ancient India, milk is an ideal food for children when taken properly and balanced with the right spices.

Dairy Products and Children

For proper growth in children, strongly nourishing foods are needed, including adequate amounts of protein. After mother's milk, the natural food of infants is cow's milk, which can be taken as the major food of most young children. The main exceptions are those whose culture has not used dairy; they may not genetically possess the enzymes to digest it.

For vegetarians it is helpful to add dairy products to the diet for improving nutrition. Dairy products are good meat substitutes and are equally as strengthening as meat without the negative effects and bad karma of taking an animal's life.

However, dairy products are mucus forming. This is true not only of milk, but also of cheese and yogurt to an even greater degree. Though good foods for children's growth, they are apt to aggravate children's diseases. To counter potential side effects, they should be prepared properly and taken in the right food combinations.

Most dairy products, particularly milk, do not combine well with other foods. Milk combines poorly with bread, sour fruit, beans, nuts, fish or meat. It is usually best taken alone or as a meal in itself. It does combine well with whole grains, however, and sweet fruit like bananas. Yogurt does not combine well with milk, sour fruit or nuts, though it combines better with vegetables and can be taken with meals.

Pasteurized milk is a kind of precooked food. It is devitalized and therefore more mucus forming. The best way to take milk is to use raw milk, heat it to the boiling point, which renders it more digestible, and then add mucus-decreasing spices. Such are cardamom, cinnamon, ginger and cloves. Cardamom is perhaps the best. A pinch to a 1/4 teaspoon of such spices per cup of warm milk, along with a little honey or raw sugar, not only tastes good but also makes the milk more digestible. To take cold pasteurized milk along with a meal of breads or meats makes a toxic combination.

Warm milk is a mild sedative to promote sleep. Its calming effect is increased by preparing it with a little nutmeg, about 1/4 teaspoon per cup. Milk is a mild laxative and good for constipation in children. However, it should be avoided in conditions of diarrhea or loose stool.

The mucus forming properties of cheese can be reduced by taking it with spices like cumin, mustard or cayenne pepper. Cheese is the most mucus-forming of dairy products and should not be used in excess.

Yogurt, according to the tradition of Indian use for thousands of years, is best taken with meals, mixed with fresh cucumber and spices like cumin, coriander, cilantro or cayenne pepper. It is heavy, hard to digest and somewhat constipating (making it good for treating diarrhea in children). Taken properly, yogurt adds good bacteria to the system and also promotes weight gain (according to Ayurveda, yogurt is not a good food for weight reduction, as is advertised).

Buttermilk is the least mucus forming of dairy products. The natural forms of buttermilk, to which little salt has been added, are preferable.

Dairy products should be supplemented with whole grains, like wheat or brown rice, with nourishing fruit, like bananas or papayas, and with complex carbohydrates like potatoes, to afford adequate nutrients for growth.

Sugar and Children

We need a certain amount of sugar for adequate growth because sugars serve to build the body. White sugar, however, is not good, as it is a refined, a dead or tamasic food, and leaches the minerals out of the body. Jaggary (Gur) is the best form of cane sugar. It is made from the crude syrup and is rich in vitamins and minerals. Other raw or natural sugars are good, like maple syrup, molasses, rice or barley malt and unrefined sugar.

Honey is a very concentrated sugar. It is best used in small amounts as a sweetener or as a medicine. It is excellent with herbs, particularly tonics or expectorants, because it is a good flavoring agent and enhances their effects. But as a food and in cooking (except when the baking temperature is not high), it is harder to digest than sugar and similarly can overstimulate the pancreas.

Sugar, even in the form of fruit or fruit juices, does not combine well with most foods and causes gas and fermentation. Whenever gas or indigestion exists it is better to avoid sugar in any form until the problem is taken care of.

Ayurveda recommends a certain amount of raw sugars for children, particularly with whole grains or milk. Many such Ayurvedic herbal confections exist using sugar, honey, ghee, nuts and tonic herbs. These are good for the debilitated also.

Oils and Children

Proper oils in the diet, like ghee, sesame or olive, are important, as are nuts like almond, walnut and pecan for nourishing the brain and nerves. But as oily foods cause mucus, make sure not to give them if the child is suffering from congestion. According to Ayurveda, the best oils for the diet are ghee (clarified butter) and sesame oil. Ghee can be taken as a cooking oil or used like butter. It is easier to digest than butter and less mucus forming.

Oils are also useful in massage (though this is a topic in itself). Giving a warm sesame oil massage to a child calms the nervous system, helps promote sleep and nourishes the skin. Above all, it increases the child's feeling of being nurtured and cared for.

Spices and Children

Many spices are good for children and help regulate their metabolism. Hot spices, however, such as cayenne, hot chilies and black pepper should be used with care. They are drying and can irritate the stomach. The stomach must gradually learn to produce more mucus secretions to deal with them. Warm, mildly sweet spices are preferable such as ginger, cinnamon, cardamom, coriander and fennel. Other mild but not sweet spices are turmeric, cumin and basil.

For keeping the system clear of mucus and for improving mental function and sensory acuity, herbs and spices such as basil, thyme, sage, hyssop and mint are good. Spices for relieving colic, gas and distention are fennel, cardamom, cumin and dill. These help stop griping, ease the flow of energy and regulate peristalsis in the colon.

Herbs for Children

Children can benefit from various herbal supplements. In Ayurveda, special tonics for children are prepared and different companies have their own proprietary medicines. These not only have good nutritive properties but also help regulate growth hormones. Equivalent-type remedies can be made with herbs available here. For improving growth of bone, teeth and hair, use comfrey root, Solomon's seal, marshmallow, American ginseng, licorice and sesame seeds. They are best taken in warm milk, with approximately a teaspoon of the powder of the herb.

Good Ayurvedic tonic herbs for children include ashwagandha, shatavari, amalaki and bala. Formulas include Ashwagandha compound and the Energy Tonic (no. 2). For improving intelligence in children, calamus is excellent taken in small amounts (1/4 teaspoon) in milk with honey. Gotu kola improves the mind, cleanses the blood, and calms the emotions. Gotu kola is particularly good for children who are hyperactive from excess sugar consumption and poor liver function. The medicated ghees of these two herbs are excellent.

296

Ayurvedic herbal jellies such as Chyavan Prash or Brahma Rasayana are excellent growth foods for children. As such jellies are tasty it is easy to get children to take them. In Chinese medicine the famous kidney tonic formula Rehmannia 6, now used mainly for the elderly, was originally devised for children.

The general treatment rule for children is that no strong therapies should be used. For example, cayenne, a very hot herb, and goldenseal, a very cold herb, should not be used frequently or in large quantities. Herbs that are very reducing, like purgatives such as rhubarb root, or very tonifying like ginseng, should be used with discretion. Dosage of herbs is less for children. Infants do well with small amounts, a pinch to a quarter teaspoon of herbs in teas or milk. Children ages five to ten can take a quarter to half the adult dosage.

Spiritual Therapies for Children

It is also important to teach yoga to children at an early age. Their bodies are suppler and postures learned while young can be easily retained throughout life. While meditation is difficult for children, we should at least encourage them to sit silently or to participate in chanting and rituals. We should open them to the world of nature with walks, hikes or retreats that meditation can be worked into. Myths, stories and animal forms of the Divine, such as Hanuman, the monkey god in the *Ramayana*, are important for communicating to the subconscious mind of the child. The natural creative imaginative power of the child should be allowed to flower and be attuned to the symbols of the cosmic mind.

OLD AGE

Ayurveda means literally 'the science of longevity'. Its concern is not merely curing disease but maximizing the life span and providing for optimal living. This is not just to give us more time to enjoy the things of this life. It is to sustain a longer incarnation for spiritual growth, which requires time and patience to develop.

In India the later years are considered to be the appropriate season of life for spiritual growth, the time when worldly obligations to work and family are completed and when the soul naturally begins to long for the transcendent. The body matures around the age of twenty-one, but the mind does not mature until about the age of thirty. The soul, however, does not mature until the age of fifty, when the higher aspect of our lives truly begins. For this reason the time after the age of fifty is the most important for spiritual growth.

Much of the disease or imbalance of our culture comes in our failure to recognize the value of the final stage of life and our inability to offer the elderly the appropriate tools for developing the higher consciousness that is naturally awakening within them. Instead we try to force them into the values and activities of younger people and their physical and material goals, which they neither have the interest or the capacity to enjoy. This makes them feel depressed when they fail to fit in with the society around them. We eventually dump them off into rest homes in which they are turned into little more than children and deprived of their dignity. In this way people of our culture end up in a miserable old age and do not experience the real and joyous fruits of a well-lived and conscious human life.

Because of their spiritual basis, the tools of yoga and Ayurveda are of special importance to the elderly, providing them the tools for the spiritual climax of our lives. Spiritual study, devotion, yoga and meditation are precisely what the elderly naturally seek as their soul unfolds.

Our elders represent the fruit of our culture and in them we can see the final outcome of our cultural values for good or ill. How we have really lived is reflected in how we age and how we die. Our culture as a whole is adolescent-oriented. We deprive the elderly of their intrinsic value, placing them under a false standard of youth. It is only natural for us to lose interest in the things of the world as we age—things like sex, money, fame and work—

and to develop wisdom, detachment and discrimination. This is not a sign of decline but of appropriate growth, as the brilliant color of the autumn foliage or the ripening of fruit. We do not insist that leaves remain green. Yet we have little appreciation for the beauty and wisdom of our own season of old age.

It is important that we endeavor to develop spiritual awareness in our later years, as our last stage of life is what determines the nature of our next incarnation. Even if our bad habits like smoking or drinking do not kill us, they create a propensity towards such wrong actions in future lives.

Old age is the stage of life dominated by Vata, the biological air humor, and its attributes of coldness, dryness, decay and disintegration. At the same time, as our body weakens and our connection with it grows less, there is space for the development of an awareness beyond it. Typical diseases of old age are Vata disorders: dry and wrinkling skin, constipation, hair or teeth falling out, weakness of the bones, cracking of the joints, arthritis, poor memory and failure of hearing and of vision.

Herbs for the Elderly

Whatever ones constitution by birth, in old age we must consider anti-Vata (anti-air) treatment and anti-Vata diet. Oil therapy becomes important with oil enemas, massage, and external application of oils such as sesame and its medicated forms. Ghee helps maintain mental clarity and nourishes the nerve tissue and senses. Tonification rather than reduction therapies become the primary focus along with tonic herbal foods. Rejuvenation becomes important, with special herbs to rebuild the body organs and tissues.

Chyavan Prash is the best all-around tonic for maintaining health and youth of tissues. It was originally devised for making the old feel young again and for helping yogis live and practice longer. Brahma Rasayana is excellent for retaining memory and revitalizing the brain cells. When it is not available, gotu kola or gotu kola ghee can be taken. Gotu kola is also perhaps the best herb for improving hearing. For promoting visual acuity, calamus is the preferable herb.

Ashwagandha is the main herb for retaining strength of the bones and joints. It is also good for impotence, premature ejaculation, leucorrhea or urinary incontinence. It strengthens ojas and the immune system. Ashwagandha is an excellent tonic for the elderly in all respects.

Guggul is the best herb for arthritic pain, as well as swelling and cracking of the hands, feet and joints. It normalizes the function of Vata and guards against arthritis. If it is not available, myrrh tincture can be used. Shilajit is important for maintaining kidney and reproductive system function. For constipation in the elderly, Triphala is best and helps rejuvenate the colon. A healthy colon insures good longevity.

A good tonic for the bones and joints with commonly available herbs is comfrey root 2 parts, turmeric 1 part, licorice 1 part and cinnamon 1/2 part. Take 1-3 grams of the powder twice a day with warm water. This improves circulation and nourishes the bones.

For women, the use of aloe gel on a regular basis preserves vitality and renews the reproductive system. Shatavari is excellent. Take 1 teaspoon of the powder daily with warm milk. Also good is adding small amounts of saffron to the tonic herbs or to milk decoctions.

In Chinese medicine Rehmannia formulas are given to the elderly: Rehmannia 6 for old age debility plus internal heat (Pitta type), and Rehmannia 8 for additional internal cold (Vata and Kapha type).

Spiritual Therapies for the Elderly

Gems are important tools for protecting and extending the life. Yellow sapphire and yellow topaz (Jupiter stones) are good for maintaining endocrine function and improving longevity, for wisdom and giving one the power to guide others (a position that naturally belongs to the elderly).

Yoga postures are important for maintaining flexibility of the joints and for preventing arthritis. They should be practiced regularly at least one half hour a day. Pranayama is helpful in maintaining strength and vitality and strengthening the lungs. Meditation is essential for dealing with the aging process and discovering its spiritual potentials. Old age is the prime time for such spiritual practices, as well as for deeper study and contemplation of the meaning of life.

Premature Balding or Greying of the Hair

Balding and graying of the hair are a common part of the aging process. They occur earlier in Pitta (fiery) constitutions, sometimes in the late twenties and often in the thirties. They do not necessarily indicate old age or ill health, but can occur as a sign of disease, particularly in women. Balding and graying may be caused by stress, emotional trauma, too much thinking and worrying, sudden blood loss, or excess sexual activity. Drugs or smoking can also bring it about.

Pitta constitutions have delicate hair that grays at an early age. Pitta type alopecia (balding) often follows blood loss or high fever. The treatment is anti-Pitta. An anti-Pitta diet is indicated with food that promotes hair growth including milk, ghee and sunflower. Herbs for hair growth, as below, for Pitta types include amalaki, shatavari, gotu kola and bhringaraj.

Vata type hair loss involves dry skin, anxiety, insomnia, constipation and irregular digestion. It follows fright or occurs after a severe illness. Its treatment involves a nutritive anti-Vata diet and herbs. Good foods include onion, garlic, sesame, almonds, dairy products and eggs. Good herbs are ashwagandha, bala, amalaki and other tonics.

Warm sesame and other medicated oils should be applied to the head on a regular basis. Nasya (nasal application) of medicated oils should also be given. Herbs for improving the hair include gotu kola, bhringaraj, amalaki, bakuchi, sandalwood and licorice. These can also be taken in medicated oils (sesame or

301

coconut base). Formulas include Bhringaraj Oil and Brahmi Oil. Chyavan Prash also nourishes the hair.

Chinese herbs include he shou wu (fo ti), rehmannia, lycium and ligustrum. Typical Chinese formulas are Shou Wu Pian and Rehmannia 6.

II.9
NERVOUS SYSTEM DISORDERS

The ancients considered nerve impulses to be a kind of wind or air travelling through the body. Vata, the biological air humor, is the energy that moves through the brain and the nerves, controlling both voluntary and involuntary functions. Hence, Vata derangements always involve some weakness, disturbance or hypersensitivity of the nervous system.

Nervous system disorders are called 'Vatavyadhi', Vata diseases, in Sanskrit. They can also be brought on by imbalances of the other two doshas. High Pitta can burn out the nervous system, causing disruption in nerve impulses. High Kapha can clog it.

These disorders are due to obstruction or wrong flow of prana or nervous energy in the subtle channels. Blockage of flow causes spasms, rigidity, numbness or paralysis. Wrong flow causes tremors and involuntary movements.

In Ayurveda, nervous system disorders are linked with mental disorders; the mind and nerves are directly connected by a system of special channels. Therefore, mental conditions should be examined carefully with any nervous disorder.

Nervous system disorders include such minor problems as insomnia, headache and tremors, major malfunctions like epilepsy or paralysis, and such degenerative nervous diseases as multiple sclerosis and Parkinson's disease, many of which are difficult to treat with Western medicine.

GENERAL TREATMENT OF THE NERVOUS SYSTEM

Nervous system diseases arise either through blockage of nerve impulses or through wasting away of nerve tissue. Flow of nerve energy can be blocked by accumulation of any of the doshas, as well as by Ama, the undigested food mass. Emotional or psychological blockage cause nervous diseases, as well. Wasting away of nerve tissue is caused by malnutrition, poor digestion and hyperactivity or by blockage of nerve energy over a period of time. Lack of emotional nourishment or mental grounding, or excessive meditational practices are other disease-provoking factors.

For blockage conditions nervine and antispasmodic herbs work well: they have the power to clear and open the channels. Calamus is an important herb for opening up the flow of nerve impulses and restoring nerve function. Basil, particularly holy basil (tulsi) is cleansing and clearing to the brain and nerves. Other good herbs include bayberry, guggul, myrrh, turmeric, bay leaves and mint. The same herbs work well as essential oils for aromatherapy.

Gotu kola is important for clearing the nervous system and relieving inflammation. Other good herbs for overheated nerves include skullcap, bhringaraj, passion flower, hops and betony.

For a general nervine tonic, Kapha constitution individuals can take gotu kola and calamus in equal parts along with honey. For Pitta gotu kola is better alone or with a slight amount of calamus (1/4 that of gotu kola) and taken with ghee. For Vata, calamus is preferable, although gotu kola in small amounts can be beneficial (up to equal amounts with calamus), taken with ghee or warm water.

For deficiency or degenerative conditions, such as MS or Parkinson's, tonic herbs and supplementation therapy are needed. Ashwagandha is the best herb, and can be combined with gotu kola or calamus, as above. Other good tonic nervines are haritaki, guggul, and bala, or nervines such as calamus and gotu kola prepared in ghee or as herbal jellies (Brahma Rasayana). For formulas, use the Energy tonic (no. 2) and Brain Tonic (no. 6).

A number of herbs possess special analgesic, or pain-relieving, properties and can be added to formulas to dispel nerve pain. These include the narcotic herbs, marijuana and datura, commonly used in Ayurvedic formulas, and milder herbs such as valerian, camomile, hops, corydalis, cloves, wild ginger, guggul, myrrh and prasarini.

A good general patent formula for protecting the nervous system is the Brain Tonic (no. 6). For Vata types it can be taken with milk and ghee or warm water. For Pittas take it with milk and ghee, aloe gel or cool water. For Kaphas take it with honey.

Spiritual Therapies for The Nervous System

As the nervous system is subtle, the spiritual therapies of Ayurveda are important here. Yoga therapy is a major part of treatment; it is specific to mind, nerve and bone disorders. Sitting asanas, such as the lotus pose or siddhasana help calm internal wind, but should not be forcefully attempted. Pranayama done correctly is also essential. Using breathing exercises, the prana can be directed through the various channels, removing blockages and restoring nutrition.

A very useful Ayurvedic Pranayama therapy is to plug one of the nostrils, as with a piece of cotton, for a period of days or weeks. This may cause some initial discomfort but it is usually quickly gotten over. Generally the flow of the breath will be stronger in the nostril needing to be plugged.

- Plugging the left nostril is good for conditions caused by cold and is used for nervous disorders where rigidity and lack of movement prevail, as in Parkinson's disease.
- Plugging the right nostril is best for conditions caused by heat or hyperactivity, as in insomnia or hallucinations.

Mantra, meditation and visualization are important to help guide nerve impulses back along the proper channels. The mantra, SOM, is good for nourishing the nerves in wasting or long-term, debilitating nervous disorders. The mantra SHAM calms the nerves. OM itself is very effective for clearing and calming the nervous system.

Gems have strong action on the nervous system, strengthening nerve function and relieving pain. Most important are those for Mercury, the planet of the nerves, which are emerald, jade or peridot. Those for Jupiter, ruling hormonal function, are also important. These are yellow sapphire, yellow topaz or citrine. Pearl, for the moon, has a calming and nurturing effect on the mind and emotions. Gold stimulates the nerves and revives function; silver calms the nerves and builds substance.

The colors of these gemstones can be used for color therapy: green (Mercury) for stopping pain, gold (Jupiter) for strengthening the nerves, white (Moon) for calming hypersensitivity.

Treatment of the Nervous System

Lowering high Vata is the focus because Vata is the underlying vitiated dosha behind all nerve function. Special anti-Vata herbs or an anti-Vata diet may be taken temporarily, even by other constitutions. Sleep, rest, relaxation or meditational retreat are helpful.

Special emphasis is on medicated oils given externally, along with massage, as the nerves can be nourished through the skin. Simple sesame oil or almond oil can be used, or a medicated sesame oil such as Mahanarayan. For calming the nerves, oil application to the head is best; like an essential oil such as sandalwood to the forehead. For stimulating the nerves, such essential oils as camphor, musk, myrrh and frankincense are useful when applied to the temples. Nasal application of herbs is also important; for example, take several drops of gotu kola or calamus ghee morning and night.

INSOMNIA

Insomnia is our most typical sign of nervous distress. Frequent insomnia is most commonly a Vata disorder involving nervousness, anxiety, ungroundedness, hypersensitivity, excess thought and worry. Sleep patterns include difficulty in falling asleep, easily disturbed sleep and difficulty in returning to sleep once awakened. Dreams may be frightening, filled with flying, falling, nightmares, encounters with ghosts or other disturbing experiences.

Causes of insomnia include stress, anxiety, excessive think-ing, taking of drugs or stimulants, too much travel, overwork and other Vata increasing factors.

General Treatment for Insomnia

The diet should be anti-Vata, emphasizing heavy or ground-ing foods. These include dairy, whole grains and root vegetables. Coffee, tea and other stimulants, including stimulant herbs like ma huang or ginseng, should be avoided. Warm milk with a little nutmeg can be taken an hour before sleep. Mental activity should be avoided in the evening, listening to loud music, or watching stimulating movies. Sleep hours should be adjusted, so that one retires early (around 11 pm) and rises early (by 6 am). Apply warm sesame oil to the feet, the top of the head or forehead, or to the whole body, followed by a warm shower.

Yoga asanas can be done, but avoid aerobic exercises. A calm-ing meditation before sleep consciously releasing all the worries and tensions of the day can work wonders. Surrendering the mind to the Divine, giving complete faith to the Divine will to take care of the world is a good part of this. The bed and the sleeping room should be a place of peace, comfortable, clean and well kept. Peace-inducing mantras such as RAM or SHAM can be repeated. The mind should be concentrated on the breath or centered in the heart.

Important Ayurvedic herbs for insomnia are jatamamsi, gotu kola, nutmeg, valerian and ashwagandha. Simple jatamamsi by itself is often enough, 1/2 teaspoon of the powder in a little honey. Formulas include Ashwagandha compound, Saraswat powder, the Brain Tonic (no. 2) or the Herbal Sedative (no. 14), taken with ghee.

A good formula is 2 parts ashwagandha, 2 parts jatamamsi, 2 parts nutmeg and 1 part licorice. For chronic insomnia take 3-6 grams of this mixture with warm milk and ghee before bed.

Chinese medicine uses heavy mineral sedatives such as drag-on bone and oyster shell for severe insomnia. Heart-nourishing sedatives, zizyphus seeds and biota seeds, are indicated for milder conditions and safer for long-term usage. Formulas include Bupleurum and Dragon Bone or Zizyphus combination.

Western herbs are valerian, skullcap, betony, hops, passion flower and camomile. For insomnia, tinctures often work well because their main effect is on the brain. Take a tincture of valerian or skullcap, 10-30 drops two hours before sleep and when you go to bed. Skullcap and other cooling nervines are more helpful taken with the warmer ones like nutmeg or valerian because their cold and light nature in excess can aggravate Vata.

PITTA TYPE INSOMNIA

Pitta insomnia involves turbulent emotions like irritability, anger, jealousy, resentment and hatred. It may follow an argument or stress or may be part of a febrile disease or infectious condition. Dreams may be dramatic and sleep disturbing. Sleep is agitated and broken but one is usually able to fall back to sleep. Causes include unresolved emotions, excessive willfulness, over-eating of hot or stimulant foods, and exposure to sun and heat.

The diet should be anti-Pitta, avoiding all spices and stimulants as well as too much sour food or salt. The best Ayurvedic herbs are gotu kola, bhringaraj, jatamamsi, aloe, and shatavari taken before sleep. Formulas include Brahmi compound or Sarasvat powder, as well as most of the formulas for Vata. Bhringaraj or Brahmi oil can be applied to the feet or the top of the head. Sandalwood oil is excellent applied to the forehead.

Western herbs include skullcap, betony, hops and passion flower. Skullcap and passion flower in equal parts is very effective. Valerian may aggravate the condition.

KAPHA TYPE INSOMNIA

Kapha constitutions tend towards excess sleep, so insomnia is seldom a problem for them. But it sometimes temporarily occurs as a congestive disorder, with Kapha blocking the channels of the mind, preventing sleep from occurring. In this case warming nervines like calamus, nutmeg and valerian are indicated. A little calamus, approximately 1/2 teaspoon, is excellent, taken with honey. Sometimes, simple hot spices like ginger and cinnamon or the formula Trikatu are sufficient. But they should be taken throughout the day, not merely before sleep.

HEADACHE/MIGRAINE

Headache can be due to many causes: indigestion, constipation, colds and fluís, hormonal imbalances, pollutants, poor posture or muscle tension. As a nerve pain condition, we will examine it in this section of the book, though it could go in other categories as well. Migraine, a more severe type headache, is often related to congenital factors.

Headaches often relate to hypertension, and the corresponding increased pressure in the head. Therefore, many of the treatments for hypertension are helpful for it.

Types of Headaches

- Headache is another common Vata disorder. Vata headache is characterized by extreme pain, anxiety, depression, constipation, and dry skin. It is aggravated by lack of sleep, irregular diet, excessive activity, and mental stimulation, worry and stress.
- Pitta headache symptoms are burning sensation, red face and red eyes, sensitivity to light, anger, irritability and possible nosebleeds. It is often associated with liver disorders or toxic blood conditions.
- Kapha type is more a dull headache with feelings of heaviness and tiredness. There may be nausea, phlegm, excess salivation or vomiting. It is usually caused by congestion of phlegm in the head and may be associated with pulmonary disorders.

Ayurvedic Healing

Treatment of Headaches

Many headaches are sinus based, such as those associated with the common cold, cough or allergies. These are usually Kapha conditions, but sometimes Vata as well. Generally follow an anti-kapha diet; avoid sugars, oils and dairy products. Decongestant and expectorant herbs are used such as calamus, ginger, bayberry, angelica and wild ginger. Calamus powder can be snuffed or calamus ghee applied to the inner nose. The powder is better for Kapha, the ghee for Vata. Basil, particularly holy basil (tulsi), is excellent as a tea.

Ginger paste can be applied to the lower nose and temples. Helpful essential oils for external application are camphor, wintergreen and eucalyptus. Inhaling the steam of such herbs or their oils is also good. Nasya is excellent, applying medicated sesame oil prepared with herbs like calamus, camphor, ginger or eucalyptus.

Treating the colon is important for many headaches, particularly those caused by indigestion or toxins in the colon. In all nervous disorders and pain conditions, the colon, the home of Vata, is the main site of the problem. Vata types often experience headaches from irregular eating habits, wrong food combinations, insomnia or constipation. They benefit from Triphala as a laxative. Useful herbs include valerian, jatamamsi, calamus and gotu kola. The formula, Sarasvat powder, is good. Adequate sleep is essential, so herbal sedatives are indicated.

Pitta type headaches are generally based upon internal heat from the liver and hyperacidity. The best herbs for this are aloe powder or rhubarb root as a purgative. The liver should also be cleansed. Gotu kola is excellent by itself or with passion flower or as Gotu kola compound. Sandalwood oil should be applied to the head. Sun and heat should be avoided; cool walks in the moonlight and flower fragrances like rose or lotus are excellent.

Kapha does well with formulas such as Trikatu or Clove combination. Camphorated oils can also be applied to the head. Strong exercise is helpful. The herbal Brain Tonic (no. 6) is useful for all these conditions with honey for Kapha and ghee for Pitta and Vata.

310

Migraine headaches are usually due to Pitta and Vata. Causes include lack of sleep, overwork, stress, poor digestion or muscular tension. They can be treated as above, but long-term tonification therapy is usually needed, with Chyavan Prash, Brahma Rasayana or Ashwagandha compound. Premenstrual headaches can be treated as under Dysmenorrhea.

PARKINSON'S DISEASE

Certain Ayurvedic herbs are excellent for Parkinson's disease, most notably Kapikacchu, which is a natural source of L-dopa. Take 1-3 grams of the powder twice a day, or add 1/4 cup of the herb (it is a pleasant tasting bean) to your rice or bean dishes. The herb is not expensive and has no side effects. In fact it also improves Ojas and strengthens our overall vitality.

Other nervine tonics like ashwagandha, shatavari and bala are also good. They do well taken along with nervine sedatives like brahmi (gotu kola) and jatamamsi. Such cooling nervines are helpful, even though Parkinson's as a nervous system disease is connected to Vata, it usually has a Pitta component as well. Pitta pushes Vata to the point that nerve impulses cease to flow properly.

EPILEPSY

Epilepsy is usually a Kapha disease but can be caused by any of the doshas. In Kapha types it is phlegm blocking the channels. In Pitta types it is related to nerve inflammation. For Vata types it is due to hypersensitivity. Much of the treatment is as per constitution, as it is a constitutional problem.

Purgation therapy is helpful and can prevent seizures. The best purgative is castor oil, which is generally the best strong laxative for nervous system disorders. Take it with a little ginger juice and honey. Triphala is also good but should be taken with meals 1 gram of the powder or tablets.

Nervines such as gotu kola compound or Brahma Rasayana are excellent. Calamus with ashwagandha is good for Vata (with ghee) and by itself for Kapha (with honey). Calamus relieves the channel blockage behind most epileptic seizures and is one of the best and simplest herbal treatments of the condition. Chyavan Prash is a useful tonic between attacks. Sesame oil can be applied to the feet for a general calming effect.

EYE DISEASES

The eyes relate to Pitta as an organ of perception. Pitta types are sensitive to light, prefer sunglasses and are more likely to need prescription glasses than other types. Most inflammatory diseases of the eyes, such as conjunctivitis, are Pitta disorders and treated like infectious diseases (see section).

As we age our vision and other sensory functions gradually lose their acuity. Increased Vata causes us to gradually lose these functions. Debilitating diseases, particularly those of the liver, can also damage the vision, as can weakness of the blood.

Gazing at a ghee lamp is a simple but effective practice to improve vision. Put a wick of cotton in a small vessel fixed with ghee. Fix your gaze upon the flame for twenty minutes. Make this into a daily practice. This is helpful for treating photophobia or photophobic headaches. Another good practice is to go out on dark nights and gaze at the stars. This cools and cleanses the eyes as well as sharpening vision.

Ghee itself is the most important food for the eyes, and by taking 1-2 teaspoons twice a day, vision can be improved. Triphala ghee is a special medicine for the eyes. It can be used both in infectious conditions and as a general tonic.

Triphala itself can be used externally as a wash for inflamed eyes. Camomile, chrysanthemum, and rose flowers are also good herbal eyewashes for pain, irritation or inflammation. Put a cool infusion of the herbs into the eye with the help of an eyedropper. Aloe gel or ghee can be applied to the eyelid. A paste of mung bean flour is also very soothing to the eyes. Never put essential oils or spicy herbs into the eyes. A good tonic food for the eyes is Chyavan Prash, since amalaki, its main ingredient, nourishes the eyes.

Many other anti-Pitta formulas are good for improving vision. The common formulas, Sudarshan powder and Mahasudarshan powder, mean literally 'the formula for good vision' and 'the great formula for good vision.' These formulas are mainly bitter herbs as bitter taste helps cool and cleanse the eyes.

Crying or making tears can cleanse the eyes. Onion juice can be applied to the eye for this purpose, but care must be taken as it is a little irritating. Crying also helps cleanse the nerves, the liver and the blood. Crying is a natural therapy, another route for dispelling toxins. Suppressing emotions and not crying can cause a build up of subtle toxins. A good cry often improves our moods and restores our perception. But such crying should come out of love, not out of grief or pity.

Gem therapy is an important treatment for the eyes. The right eye relates to the Sun and the left eye to the Moon. The gemstones for these planets help improve vision. Pearl set in silver is good for dry or inflamed eyes, photophobia, and for Pitta and Vata conditions. Ruby set in gold is good for lack of visual acuity, turbidity, congestion in the eyes, and Kapha and Vata conditions. When these two stones are not available, moonstone and garnet can be used as substitutes. Diamonds (or other Venus stones including quartz crystal) are also good for the eyes and give better perception of colors.

Color therapy is also good. Deep blue has the most soothing effect upon the eyes and counters inflammation. Gold and orange are the best colors for increasing visual acuity.

EAR DISEASES

The ears, governing the ether element, are a Vata organ and benefit from anti-Vata therapies. Regular application of sesame oil to the ears is a good preventative measure for most ear diseases and should be a regular practice, particularly for the elderly.

Intolerance of sound is one of the main indications of high Vata that occurs in many Vata diseases. It also indicates low plasma (low rasa dhatu), which means internal dryness and

313

dehydration, with possible anemia in the case of women. Treat it with tonics like ashwagandha, shatavari and amalaki.

Ear infections are a complication of colds, flus and other congestive Kapha disorders. Treat them like the common cold for Kapha with aromatic spices like sage, thyme or calamus. Severe infections aggravate Pitta and require natural antibiotics like goldenseal and echinacea, or the Ayurvedic katuka.

Another good practice for the ears is to listen to the inner sounds. Close your ears with your fingers and try to hear the sounds not only within your body but also within the mind. The soul has an internal music that we can listen to and bathe the mind and heart with higher vibrations. Be good to your ears and donít subject them to unnecessary harsh sounds. The ears are our gateway to the worlds of space beyond. Learn to listen to the sounds of silence that contain nature's healing powers.

II.10
AYURVEDIC PSYCHOLOGY:
Mental and Emotional Conditions

As a comprehensive system of medicine Ayurveda treats diseases of both body and mind. It also recognizes the link between the two, prescribing meditation to treat physical diseases and diet and herbs for psychological conditions. The very concept of the doshas or biological humors contains a psychological as well as physiological orientation with Vata, Pitta and Kapha having mental and physical profiles. The Ayurvedic treatment of mental disorders also follows a doshic model.

Disease usually involves an underlying psychological or emotional imbalance. All physical diseases, particularly chronic or severe diseases that involve pain or diminished functioning, disturb our psychology. In addition, most physical diseases result from underlying psychological factors. We become unable to give proper care to our bodies when we are preoccupied with psychological or emotional problems. Similarly, psychological diseases can result in physical disorders disrupting patterns of sleep, eating and exercise. A pattern of imbalance on the mental level, with disturbed thoughts and emotions, is usually reflected and reinforced on a physical level.

As a general rule in treatment, psychological factors outweigh physical factors. A patient may have the right diet and herbs, but if their mental state is agitated or if there is a negative attitude about the treatment, it will likely not be effective. So we cannot forget the emotional implications of treatment on any level.

Ayurveda as a holistic system treats every type of mental disorder, from mild stress to severe conditions, including schizophrenia. It has methods for enhancing mental, as well as physical, well-being. For the healing of the mind, Ayurveda employs a whole series of yogic and spiritual therapies including meditation, pranayama, mantra, prayer, visualizations and rituals called 'spiritual therapy' (daiva cikitsa).

This chapter examines the Ayurvedic treatment of common psychological problems. However, we should be careful in trying to treat individuals with severe emotional imbalances who require medical supervision or are under heavy sedation. This chapter also looks into the psychological side effects of yoga and meditation practices. Yoga and meditation can raise our consciousness, if done rightly, but if done wrongly or excessively can disturb the mind and prana.

MANAGEMENT OF EMOTIONS

The main psychological problems that people suffer from are emotional in nature such as painful or disturbing emotions of fear, anger, desire, grief and jealousy. Ayurvedic treatment for the mind is based on the right management of emotions, which includes developing positive emotions and releasing those which are negative.

Expression of emotions is a common treatment in the new psychology today. The idea is that if we express an emotion, particularly one that has been hidden or suppressed, then the emotion can be released and peace of mind will be restored. This is true in some cases. Whatever has been blocked inside us must come out, just as a toxin in the body has to be eliminated for health to be restored. However, expression can aggravate emotions in some people. Much of this can be understood in terms of the doshas.

Kapha people generally do better if they express their emotions because their emotional energy tends to be heavy, blocked and congested. While Kaphas are generally emotional people, they are often too kind or complacent to really deal with negative emotions. For them, expressing their anger or fear can help them open up emotional blockages and promote emotional healing.

Pitta and Vata people usually do better learning to control their emotions. Pittas usually express their emotions anyway, particularly anger, which is often harmful. They must learn to be circumspect about venting their anger, particularly around more sensitive types. The exception is that Pittas have a harder time expressing positive emotions of love and appreciation. This they should cultivate.

Vata types are already caught in excessive emotional fluctuations and expressions. They can get disturbed by an overexpression of emotions, particularly fear and anxiety. They need to develop calm, quiet and evenness of mind, avoiding emotional ups and downs. Yet some Vatas, particularly of a Saturnian bent and an isolated life-style, suffer from lack of emotional expression, particularly a lack of the feeling of love. They need to cultivate emotional warmth and reach out to others.

Repression of emotions should be avoided because the restrained energy eventually works itself out in disturbed subconscious reactions. We should not supress our emotions, which are energies, but should treat them with love and respect. We should learn to manage our emotions, like cultivating plants in a garden, favoring the flowers and pulling out the weeds. Generally, we have many emotional urges that we cannot possibly all follow or fulfill. So we must choose the best emotions to give attention to. Above all, we must learn to control negative emotions that direct us to harm others, like anger and hatred.

Emotional healing occurs when emotions are spontaneously released. Neither expression nor repression can bring this about. Release means that the energy trapped in the emotion is let out and allowed to assume a positive form. This means transforming negative emotions like lust and hatred into positive emotions like devotion and compassion.

The Role of the Astral Body

Behind the physical is a subtle or astral body composed of prana, emotions and thoughts. The astral is the underlying energy pattern of the physical, from which the physical is produced. In our waking life, we experience the astral through the physical. In the dream state, the astral body is free to function on its own and we can experience it directly through conscious dreaming.

317

There is another plane of existence, an astral universe, which we can experience through the astral body. Its experience can be developed through yoga and other occult techniques.

Just as there are channels in the physical body, so there are channels in the astral or emotional body through which prana and thought flow. These are the nadis, or subtle channels, which run from the different chakras, the energy centers of the astral body. Disruption in the flow of these energies causes psychological disease, just as disruption in the channels of the physical body produces physical disease. Our mental energy can stagnate or move in the wrong direction, resulting in various forms of misapprehension and confusion.

It is important to keep these subtle channels pure. This is one of the main purposes of Pranayama, yogic breathing practices. The extra prana taken in opens these channels and circulates through them. Many herbs help clear the channels as well, particularly spicy and bitter herbs of an aromatic nature that contain large amounts of the ether elements. Such are calamus, basil, turmeric, guggul, bayberry, camphor, myrrh, frankincense and cedar. They can also be employed as aromas and incense.

There is a shield between the astral and physical bodies, protecting the physical from the negative effect of astral forces. When this breaks down we can no longer discriminate the physical from the astral, between our actual sensory perceptions and our thoughts, fantasies and emotions. When this link becomes weak, other astral influences (which may be entities from that plane or just emotional influences of the people or environment around us) can take temporary control of our physical body. We may do things we do not really wish to do, such as harming others.

According to Ayurveda, modern psychology is not yet a mature science of the psyche because it does not understand these subtle forces. It treats psychological problems merely as personal issues. Ayurveda regards them as an imbalance of energies on an inner level. Psychological energies are woven into the whole of the collective consciousness, with cosmic ramifications such as astrological influences. Ayurveda focuses more on provid-

318

ing practical tools for correcting imbalances rather than on analyzing the particular configuration of the imbalance in terms of personal experience.

Causes of Mental Disorders

Mental disorders are as diverse and variable as the mind itself. They are caused by emotional stress, trauma, poor upbringing, coming under the influence of disturbed individuals, sexual abuse or perversion, and taking of drugs. They can be brought on by excess thinking or by strain in yogic or meditation practices. Naively opening up to the influences of the astral plane, through various occult methods, can also cause mental imbalances.

As a culture, we are reconnecting with the astral plane. As is perhaps to be expected at the start, it is mainly the lower astral that we are accessing, reflected in the mass media, sexual liberation, and the use of mind-altering drugs. The new interest in channeling, shamanism and the occult is part of this process as well. This can bring new knowledge, and is a necessary stage in the evolution of the human mind, but it can also create mental disorders. Once we have opened up our minds to astral forces or entities, they can gain a power over us, which cannot be simply eradicated by the power of will or by physical methods.

The Place of Sattva (Purity of Mind)

Psychological disorders are caused by a vitiation of sattva—by a disturbance of the inherent clear quality of the mind. This occurs through rajas and tamas, turbulence and darkness in the mind. Rajas involves anger, hatred and fear, nervousness, worry and anxiety. Tamas involves excess sleep, dullness, apathy, inertia and the inability to perceive things as they are.

Modern society is excessively rajasic. We are constantly moving, travelling, taking on new stimulations, and ever on the go. We are always preoccupied with one thing or another, working, playing, or entertaining ourselves. We have little time for peace, silence and meditation, or for heart-to-heart communication.

Sattva, the clear essence of the mind, can only be truly renewed in silence and space. It is worn out by too much mental activity, including excessive intellectual or philosophical thinking. Most of our relaxation today involves entertainment, movies, television or watching sports. These are a kind of passive mental activity that still wears out the mind. We have lost the sattvic mental pursuits of traditional cultures such as prayer, meditation, chanting and selfless service, which nourish the heart. We are lacking in love, faith, openness and peace. With our agitation and distraction comes mental stress or psychological disease.

Psychological unrest is a sign of lack of connection with the soul, which is the source of our joy and creativity. It occurs when we forget our soul's purpose in incarnation, when we are not following a spiritual path that brings us peace. The spiritual implications behind mental unrest are always important.

MENTAL DISORDERS AND THE DOSHAS

The simplest way to understand psychological conditions is through their doshic profile.

Vata (Air) Type

Mental, like nervous, disorders are mainly due to high Vata (high air), which, as the nervous force, also governs the mind. The mind, like Vata dosha, is composed of air and ether. Vata's excess of air causes instability in the mind. It involves increased rajas: a disturbed, agitated, excessively thinking nature, which causes lack of control and internal hypersensitivity. Too much exposure to the mass media, loud music, taking of drugs or stimulants, excessive exercise, overwork and excessive or unnatural sexual activity make Vata hyperactive, creating a predisposition for mental disturbance. Misguided meditation and excessive practice of Pranayama can also aggravate Vata.

High Vata, as excess ether, makes us ungrounded, spaced out and unrealistic in our expectations and beliefs. It weakens our connection with the physical body, disrupting our harmony with the physical world. We live too much in our thoughts, which take the place of reality and disperse our life-force. Fear, anxiety, unrest and rapid shifts of mood occur. Insanity or schizophrenia is an extreme form of this disruption of the mind from physical reality.

Pitta (Fire) Type

Pitta psychological disorders are also due to too much Rajas, but usually directed outwardly, against other people. There is aggression, ambition and anger, an unyielding and sometimes ruthless pushing to achieve our aims. Typical Pitta is the overly critical type who cannot see any other view of things than his own. We blame other people for everything, see enemies everywhere, are always on guard and ready for a fight. We are even at war with ourselves and our past. This causes anger and hostility that at the extreme leads to psychotic behavior.

Kapha (Water) Type

Kapha psychological unrest involves excessive Tamas. There is too much sleeping, sleeping during the day, day dreaming, attachment to the past, and a general dullness and lethargy. The mind may be incapable of abstract, objective or impersonal thinking. There is a lack of drive and motivation along with passivity and dependency. We want to remain a child and to be taken care of. We become preoccupied with what others think about us. We lack a proper self-image and passively reflect our immediate environment. We have many attachments and cannot let go of the past.

Ayurvedic Treatment of Psychological Unrest

Mild mental disorders, what we call 'neurosis', is indicated here. Such mental imbalance does not generally prevent us from functioning but makes our lives unhappy, much like a chronic disease. It is a condition that we can treat on our own at least to some degree.

Treatment of psychological unrest first involves restoring sattva, the natural clear quality of the mind. This involves a sattvic diet, being careful not to aggravate the constitutional dosha in the process. Fruit harmonizes the mind, whole grains strengthen the mind, dairy products nourish the heart, and oils like ghee nourish the nerve tissue.

A sattvic life-style should be followed with due regard to one's constitution. Preferably, this includes arising early in the morning and practicing yoga; asana, pranayama, mantra and meditation. A mere thirty minutes of silent meditation or chanting can be very helpful if done on a regular basis.

Sattvic qualities such as faith, love, compassion, honesty and truthfulness should be cultivated. We should practice self-examination and self-inquiry. Or we can open up to the Divine in whatever form is dear to our heart, and engage in some sort of service work for the benefit of humanity, ceasing to focus on our personal lack of fulfillment.

Application of oils to the head is calming and nourishes the mind. Heavy fatty oils are best for sedation and to aid in sleep—sesame oil for Vata and coconut oil for Pitta. These can be combined with nervine herbs, gotu kola in coconut oil for Pitta (called Brahmi Oil), or ashwagandha in sesame oil for Vata.

Essential oils such as sandalwood are good to promote calm and peace. Basil, myrrh, frankincense, sage or mint clear the channels and promote perception. Essential oils can be applied warm to the forehead (to improve perception), to the top of the head (to give greater intelligence), or to the base of the neck (to calm the unconscious).

Oils can also be applied to the nose, to directly influence the brain. Calamus ghee is best applied this way for clearing purposes (for Kapha and Vata). Gotu kola ghee is also good for calming (for Pitta and Vata). Enemas are important for Vata conditions. Use sesame, a calming oil, or mind-nourishing herbs such as ashwagandha or haritaki. Massage of the abdomen is good for releasing emotions, which are generally held in the region of the navel, the pranic center in the body.

For calming the mind and improving the psychic atmosphere, incense is important, much like essential oils. Sandalwood is the best and most harmonizing incense. Burning of camphor, sage or cedar cleanses the psychic environment. Myrrh and frankincense cleanse the aura and purify the air. Rose calms and nourishes the heart, as does lotus. Jasmine cleanses the emotions and increases love and compassion. Gardenia purifies the heart.

Flower remedies are helpful in this way—not only the fragrances but having the flowers around us for their influence on the heart. Certain plants in the house help improve the psychic as well as the physical atmosphere. These include aloe, basil and hibiscus.

Color therapy is very helpful. White gives peace and purity. Deep blue gives peace and detachment. Gold gives discrimination. Green gives harmony, balance and healing energy. Gems for the mind include pearl or moonstone to calm emotions; emerald which gives balance and equanimity; yellow sapphire or topaz to increase wisdom; and red coral which calms anger.

Ayurvedic herbs for improving sattva (the mind) are gotu kola, calamus, holy basil (tulsi), bhringaraj, shankha pushpi, haritaki, sandalwood, ashwagandha and guggul. They are better prepared in ghee or taken with it. Sarasvat powder is good for all types, as is the Brain Tonic (no. 6). Take these herbs with ghee for Pitta, with milk for Vata, with honey for Kapha.

The best herbs per dosha are ashwagandha for Vata, gotu kola (brahmi) for Pitta and calamus for Kapha. Chinese herbs for calming the mind are zizyphus, biota seeds or schizandra. Western herbs for improving mental function include sage, bayberry, cedar, myrrh, skullcap and camomile. Tinctures of these herbs are preferable as the alcohol helps draw their effects into the brain.

Herbs to nourish the heart and promote positive emotions may also be necessary to calm the mind. These include shatavari, saffron, rose, lotus and licorice, particularly as prepared in milk decoctions. They are good for balancing negative Pitta (fiery) emotions and for calming Vata (airy) sensitivity. Formulas include Shatavari compound.

Other specific nervine and sedative herbs can be used for calming the mind. Such herbs include jatamamsi, valerian, nutmeg, passion flower, hops and asafoetida.

DEPRESSION

Depression is probably the most common mental health complaint and also the most common psychological problem that accompanies the disease process. Much of depression is cultural and has reached almost epidemic proportions today. As we depend upon stimulation through coffee, tea and drugs, or through the mass media and other forms of entertainment, when that stimulation is gone we naturally feel depressed. Our lonely and isolated life-style is another factor. Without our living creatures around us our prana sinks and stagnates. Depression often results from grief.

Many people today are on anti-depressant drugs. While natural therapies do work they should be brought in over time, gradually reducing these medications as it becomes possible.

Depression follows stress, overwork, overexertion and trauma, particularly adrenal fatigue. It is generally a sign of low Ojas and weak immune function. Depression is the most common Kapha psychological disorder. Kaphas suffer from low energy and reduced functioning, slow metabolism and obesity. Psychologically, they are prone to conservative attitudes and attachment. All this leads to depression. Yet Vata and Pitta have their types of depression as well.

Vata people tend to be melancholic and with their sensitive natures are easily disturbed in life. Their low body weight and poor stamina makes them easily feel hurt. Vata causes quickly shifting moods that in the long run can render them unhappy. Vata type depression is associated with feelings of abandonment, lack of love and nurturing in life. It can become severe or even suicidal. Its onset can be sudden and variable. Vata type depression is often the manic-depressive type with periods of depression alternating with periods of high energy, hyperactivity, hypersensitivity or even excessive joy. It is closely connected with anxiety and insomnia. Inability to sleep quickly causes depression in Vatas.

Pitta type depression usually follows some failure in life in which the person was not as successful as he or she expected to be. Pitta's have high expectations and high goals that can be difficult to reach. When they fail to achieve these this results in depression. Pitta depression is often mixed with anger.

General Treatment of Depression

Depression is usually difficult to treat because the depressed person is usually unable or unwilling to initiate positive therapies. The first treatment principle in depression is to initiate change and encourage activity on any level, to arouse the patient's interest and enthusiasm in life. Positive association is an important factor.

The diet should be light and stimulating and there should be an effort to restore a sense of taste and relish in food. Lack of desire to eat itself is a sign of possible depression. Take spices like ginger, cardamom and basil that open the mind and heart. There should be walks in nature and the intake of positive impressions through the sky, rivers and lakes, forests and mountains. Stimulating fragrances like eucalyptus, camphor and frangipani are excellent for aromatherapy. Color therapy should emphasize warm and bright tones like yellow, gold and orange. Pranayama is helpful, taking in plenty of fresh air in the sunshine, opening the lungs and heart. Exercise is good to stimulate circulation, including walking and running.

Calamus is the best basic herb for depression. Take it as a tea, 1/4 teaspoon of the powder per cup of hot water, with a little ginger and honey. Basil, particularly holy basil or tulsi, is also excellent and can be taken as a daily beverage. Mints and sages of all types are helpful. Depression usually involves blocked sinuses or stagnation of energy in the head. Try nasya therapy to open the sinuses through applying herbal oils and powders like calamus to the nostrils. Keep the bowels open with Triphala. The mantra HRIM, which opens the spiritual heart and our higher aspiration, is good for countering depression.

KAPHA TYPE DEPRESSION

Follow an anti-Kapha diet avoiding sweet, heavy, greasy and salty food. Also avoid eating in the early morning or late evening. Nervines and stimulant herbs are indicated like Trikatu, cayenne, cardamom, cloves and calamus. Myrrh and guggul are excellent for improving circulation and opening the channels of the body and mind. Pippali is great, 1/4 teaspoon with honey every few hours to stimulate the mind and body. Avoid sleeping during the day or sleeping after sunrise.

PITTA TYPE DEPRESSION

Follow an anti-Pitta diet avoiding greasy, oily and heavy food. More raw food in the diet is helpful, with a free use of salads, greens and sprouts. Cooling nervines like gotu kola and skullcap are excellent, particularly mixed with mild stimulants like coriander, turmeric or peppermint.

VATA TYPE DEPRESSION

The person should have plenty of social interaction, staying around family and friends, sharing nice meals with warm and nutritive food. Tonic herbs like ashwagandha and shatavari should be taken along with nervines like shankha pushpi, calamus and sage. Oil massage is very helpful, with sesame oil to the head to stimulate sleep. Proper rest is essential. If insomnia exists, target that first. Try to do some creative work and physical activity like yoga postures.

ANXIETY

Anxiety is another common psychological complaint arising from stress, strain and uncertainty in life and relationship.

Anxiety is the main Vata psychological disorder, a feeling of ungroundedness caused by a lack of earth and water in the system. It follows from fear and uncertainty and usually goes along with low Ojas.

Ashwagandha is the herb of choice for anxiety. For Vata types take 1/2 teaspoon of the powder morning and evening in warm milk. For Pitta take ashwagandha with gotu kola in equal parts. For Kapha take ashwagandha, with a little ginger, in honey. Mantras like SHRIM are good for countering anxiety and creating a mood of faith and a sense of Divine support in life.

VATA TYPE ANXIETY

Vata anxiety is a result of excessive nervous activity, too much thinking, worrying or excessive change. Ashwagandha, jatamamsi, Triphala and garlic are helpful herbs. Ashwagandha and jatamamsi in equal parts are excellent, taken with honey.

KAPHA TYPE ANXIETY

Kapha type anxiety usually results from loss of ones possessions and attachments. Shilajit, pippali, myrrh and guggul are excellent. Pranayama is very helpful.

PITTA TYPE ANXIETY

Pitta type anxiety usually occurs from an unwillingness to let go. Pitta types want to control their lives and circumstances and feel anxiety when this control is somehow lost or diminished. The best herbs are gotu kola, jatamamsi and skullcap. Flower fragrances like rose and jasmine can help settle the heart.

ANGER

Anger is the main psychological problem for Pitta or fiery types, who often suffer from irritability and bad temper. Anger usually accumulates in the liver and gives rise to heat and inflammation and other Pitta problems. Yet Vata types can also suffer from anger, generally of an erratic nature. Kapha types suffer least from anger but they can hold a deep-seated anger, accumulated over the years and never expressed.

Anti-Pitta nervines like jatamamsi, gotu kola, passion flower and skullcap are excellent for reducing anger. Shatavari is a good tonic for soothing it. Coconut or Brahmi oil to the head is excellent. Flower fragrances like rose, jasmine and lilac are good. Sandalwood oil or incense often gives quick relief. Cultivate peace and forgiveness with mantras like SHAM or OM SHANTI.

Vata people can suffer from bouts of anger but these are usually temporary in nature. Vata people get most angry when their security is threatened. Vata anger is not vindictive. Though it may exhibit exaggerated emotions, it simply wants a restoration of security. For treating this, an anti-Vata diet and calming herbs are helpful, particularly jatamamsi and ashwagandha.

INSANITY

Insanity occurs when the mental unrest is so severe that an individual is unable to function in physical reality. It is the ultimate result of neurosis or mental disturbance. Yet, some of what is called insanity may be a higher state of consciousness or a consciousness outside of social norms. According to Vedanta, all of us, save the enlightened, are caught in an underlying ignorance and false perception of life. Our whole ego is an illusion. Each culture has its basic social illusion as well, so that what we call sanity is not as fixed as we would like to think.

Often there are physical imbalances involved with insanity. Toxic poisoning, malnutrition, trauma and other factors may cause or aggravate it. While insanity is a clinical condition, the Ayurvedic understanding of it can provide new insight into its origins and new methods on how to resolve it.

Types of Insanity

- Vata type insanity is characterized by excessive singing, laughing, weeping, loss of memory, incoherent talk, erratic gestures and sometimes loss of motor function control. The individuals are usually emaciated, dry and of Vata constitution. Emotionally, fear, anxiety and depression dominate them. They suffer from insomnia and nightmares.

• Pitta type insanity is characterized by anger and violence. There are delusions of grandeur and power with an inflated sense of ego. Such individuals are usually very fiery, proud and contentious, wanting to impose their will on everyone. They have paranoid fantasies and feel they are oppressed by great enemies, the government or the police.

• Kapha type insanity is characterized by dullness, lethargy, sentimentality, attachment to the past or childhood, dependency on the parents (particularly the mother), trying too hard to please people, feeling unloved and not cared for. The individual is usually overweight and often addicted to sugar.

Treatment of Insanity

Treatment is similar to mental unrest but stronger sedative substances should be used. Pancha Karma is very important, as it is a stronger method.

For Vata type, nourishing and sedating herbs are required, especially ashwagandha and its various preparations. Sarpagandha (Rauwolfia serpentina) is an important Ayurvedic herb for mental disorders. From it is derived some of the chemical drugs used to treat insanity today. Other good herbs include valerian, guggul, jatamamsi and calamus. Oil enemas are helpful, as above.

For Pitta type purgation, even with strong purgatives, is often helpful. The more violent the type, the more purgation is indicated. Good herbs for this include rhubarb root, senna and aloe. Gotu kola is the best herb generally; others are bhringaraj, sandalwood and passion flower. Shatavari is good for promoting a sense of love and compassion and is better for weaker Pitta types.

For Kapha, spicy brain-stimulant herbs are indicated. The treatment is mainly expectorant, to clear phlegm from blocking the channels and obstructing mental functioning. Important herbs are calamus, pippali, basil, bayberry, sage, myrrh and guggul, which have good expectorant action. Formulas include Trikatu with ghee or Calamus ghee.

POSSESSION

In most ancient cultures mental disorders were attributed to various kinds of possession by ghosts or evil spirits and some sort of exorcism was prescribed. Ayurveda shares this view but in a more sophisticated way, through the knowledge of yoga. So does Tibetan medicine. This view is not a naive superstition but reflects a scientific knowledge of the occult worlds. Our physical world is intimately linked with subtler worlds and has a constant interplay of energies with them. Forces from these planes can affect us in both positive and negative ways.

Ayurveda distinguishes different forms of possession, according to the entities involved. Possession is most common in individuals who are passive, dependent, vulnerable, open and impressionable. There is often low self-esteem, an extreme sensitivity and a capacity to take on the influences of the environment. The aura is usually weak and the sense of self is not well-defined. Yet people who suffer from trauma, depression, low vitality or insomnia (mainly Vata disorders) become vulnerable to astral influences as well.

Possession can also occur with groups, as in mob actions, and can affect whole countries, like Germany under the Nazis. We must respect these subtle forces, learn to recognize them, and learn to ward off their negative effects. Otherwise we are like children in the dark, and can bring upon ourselves many negative experiences that are not necessary. Here astrology is particularly important, giving us a picture of the astral forces at work in our lives.

General Treatment of Possession

The treatment of possession is similar to that for mental disorders but specific exorcising methods should be used. These include chanting, incense, bells, and calling upon protective deities. Various demon-destroying deities in the Hindu tradition include Durga, Rama and the terrible form of Shiva known as Rudra. Durga is the wrathful form of the Divine Mother. Rama is the Divine Son as the protector, warrior and hero. Rudra is the terrible form of the Divine Father. The Buddhists, particularly the Tibetans, also have their demon destroyers. But any divine power can help in clearing out negative forces in our psyche, whichever form of the Divine is closest to our heart.

Types of Possession

- Possession is more commonly a Vata disorder because Vata types are easily dissociated from physical reality or the physical body. They often have low energy, so more easily come under a stronger force. Vata-type possession is most dominated by fear.
- Pitta type possession usually arises from too much wrath in the nature. One is taken over by an entity that appeals to pride, ambition and power (see Asuric possession).
- Kapha type possession usually comes from excess sentimentality and attachment. Often souls who have died but are unwilling to leave earth, owing to excessive attachment, are able to enter us.

Possession by Gods

By the gods here are the lesser deities of the midastral world, not the truth principles of our higher pure awareness. These lesser gods enjoy a life of play, beauty, and drama in a world of vibration, color and delight. We contact their energy in the aesthetic part of the mind.

They possess human beings for the purpose of play. They do not harm their victims directly; in fact they may provide them with knowledge or inspiration. Many mediums and channels are possessed by gods and find the experience exhilarating.

According to yoga, however, any form of possession is dangerous. Possession by the gods also aggravates Vata, weakening our connection with our own soul. It can cause such Vata disorders as insomnia, arthritis or premature aging.

These lesser gods can be removed by opening up to higher divine forces. We should develop a strong connection with a great teacher or form of the divine and regularly worship it. Generally, we have to take control of our own minds and follow an appropriate life-regimen to remove their influence.

Possession by Ghosts

Many souls are overly attached to the physical world. Death may be sudden so it may be hard for them to pass on. Such entities can continue their stay on the earth plane by becoming connected with the living.

Calamus is a special Ayurvedic herb for clearing the effects of ghosts from the mind. Calamus ghee is good, or calamus enemas. Holy basil also cleanses our psychic environment and connects us with the immanent Divine power (Vishnu). Clearing incense such as camphor is helpful as is the use of bells.

Remove any stagnant air in the house. Attics or basements should be cleared of old possessions and have fresh air brought in. Negative psychic entities usually require some negative air space to live in. Consciously direct the entity away, sending it on to its next life, telling it that its fulfillment is only possible in a new birth.

Possession by Demons (Asuras)

Human life has been described as a war between the Devas and Asuras, the gods of light and the demons of darkness. The Asuras are always trying to enter into and influence human life. They run the underworld, encourage crime, and are behind most wars. Their purpose is to block human evolution, to keep us ignorant of our true spiritual nature; they serve to make us weak in our inner purpose.

This is the most dangerous form of possession. The Asuras cause the more violent forms of insanity, including psychosis.

They can enter into us in a state of excess anger, hatred and fanaticism which causes us to lose self-control.

This is largely a Pitta condition and treatment is similar to Pitta mental problems. Love and forgiveness are important. Purgation is helpful. Gotu kola with ghee is the best herb for this condition. Jatamamsi is also very good.

Mantras for Possession

HUM (pronounced as in our word 'whom') is the best mantra for driving off the Asuras. It is a special fire mantra and sound of Divine wrath that relates to Shiva. It can neutralize all negativity. It is also useful for warding of ghosts. But one must be pure to use it, as it will also attack any negativity that may be inside us.

RAM is the best mantra for giving the protection of the Divine light. It opens up our aura to the guiding intelligence of the Creator and closes it off to the lower influences of the astral plane. It is good in all mental and psychic diseases and is totally safe.

POSSIBLE SIDE-EFFECTS OF CHANNELING

Channeling is a very complex phenomena and, though it may offer us much, does have some possible side-effects. Whenever we allow another entity to work through our minds we are risking both physical and mental health. On a physical level we have to die a little. We have to weaken the hold of our own life-force on our mind in order to let another being work through it. On a psychological level we tend to lose control of our emotional energy.

Channeling in general will aggravate Vata. Those of this constitution should be especially careful with it. Long-term Vata disorders including arthritis, insomnia, epilepsy or paralysis may occur. Jane Roberts, who started the channeling movement with her channeling of Seth, died at a relatively young age of rheumatoid arthritis, a typical Vata disorder. Ayurveda would think that it was caused by her practice. Channeling can have as many health risks as smoking and the taking of drugs.

It may take a number of years for these to manifest. Those who practice channeling may notice certain disorders after a period of time.

An important consideration for channelers is that unconsciousness during channeling is likely to have a damaging effect on the body and mind. If we retain our awareness, this is less likely to occur. Relative to body types, channeling is better for Kapha types. Some weight will keep us grounded. Those who are emaciated, malnourished, with irregular appetite and lack of physical strength, face more danger.

Channelers often become a conduit for various forms of imagination. This is particularly true of Kapha types who have a dreamy, lunar nature. Such channelers are often heavy, if not obese. They generally have less health problems but can still suffer from illusions.

When channeling becomes a problem, it can be treated under mental disorders generally, and specifically under possession. Usually it is a possession by the gods or higher forces but even this can have negative implications. To calm the mind from the side-effects of channeling the best herbs are gotu kola, jatamamsi, calamus and shankha pushpi.

Blue stones such as amethyst or blue sapphire are good for keeping any negative influences away, particularly when set in gold. Hessonite garnet is a good stone for protecting the aura.

MEDITATION DISORDERS

Meditation properly practiced helps cure both physical and mental diseases and promote health and well-being on all levels. Most forms of meditation are safe. Wrongly practiced, however, or done with strain, some can damage the body or mind. True meditation develops peace and the release of tension and anxiety. False meditation is indicated by restlessness, conflict and negative imagination.

In both Ayurvedic and Tibetan medicine, cultures where a great deal of meditation is practiced and often with great effort, a whole series of meditation diseases are recognized. Such disorders are not so common in the West, but with the new and sometimes naive practice of meditation techniques, we are beginning to see them here as well. Of course, western medicine does not have much to offer in their treatment, as its understanding of the process of meditation is limited.

Meditation works to make the mind subtler, which results in the creation of more space or ether in the mind. This, in excess, can make a person feel spaced out and ungrounded. It can cause Vata disorders; so most meditation disorders are of this dosha. Both symptoms and treatment for these problems are similar to that for nervous system diseases.

Some meditation practices involve sensory deprivation. This can produce certain experiences, like colorful visions. Other practices involve sleep deprivation. These will also produce experiences usually of a dream nature. Such practices, however spiritually useful, if not done correctly, can aggravate Vata. One should not confuse a Vata (high air) deranged fantasy or abnormal energy movement with spiritual awareness. Vata disturbances will result in agitation, while true spiritual awareness results in peace.

According to yoga and Ayurveda, meditation practices should be done naturally, through our own aspiration. What we can produce through harsh or forceful methods is likely to have side effects. The mind is capable of any illusion, including a fantasy of enlightenment. We should not put ourselves in positions that may artificially enhance this illusion-building power of the mind.

PRANAYAMA DISORDERS

Pranayama involves efforts at controlling the breath and increasing its energy. Prana as air is connected to Vata. Excessive straining at breath control can aggravate Vata, the air humor. Exhalation or inhalation when unduly suppressed can disturb the flow of energy in the nervous system. It is important, therefore, while performing breathing practices not to use force to hold the breath. The goal is not just to stop breathing, which deprives the body of oxygen. It is to calm the breath in order to increase our vitality, and this requires peace of mind.

In holding our breath we should not forget to breathe. For this reason, many yoga teachers recommend performing retention after exhalation rather than after inhalation. Then we will naturally be compelled to inhale.

In addition, we should not confuse the energy of hyperventilation, which may be brought on by rapid breathing, with spiritual awareness. Energetic forms of Pranayama, such breath of fire (bhastrika), are more likely to cause difficulties. Such stimulating breath control methods can agitate the mind, unless developed carefully.

Pranayama should be increased gradually, extending ones overall practice a few minutes a day. If we suddenly attempt Pranayama practices for long periods of time, difficulties are more likely. Breath control can give us psychic experiences, but if our mind is not pure and our personal will is in operation, these experiences may be unwholesome.

Excessive pranayama causes ungroundedness, anxiety, palpitations, insomnia, involuntary movements, ringing in the ears, dizziness, fainting, vertigo and other conditions of high Vata.

Treatment of Pranayama Disorders

The treatment should begin with a cessation of all breathing exercises. Calming and protecting mantras such as SHAM and RAM should be chanted. An anti-Vata diet should be followed by taking heavy, nutritive and grounding foods, yet avoiding spices. Nothing should be taken that might overstimulate the Prana. One should take adequate rest and relaxation.

Herbs for strengthening the nervous system and calming the mind are indicated such as ashwagandha, gotu kola, jatamamsi, shankha pushpi, haritaki or sandalwood, taken with ghee. Important formulas are Ashwagandha combination or Sarasvat powder with milk or ghee. In severe cases take stronger sedatives like jatamamsi, valerian, nutmeg and sarpagandha. Avoid nervine stimulants like coffee, tea, ephedra and camphor.

Apply oil massage to the feet, head and spine using warm sesame oil or a medicated anti-Vata oil, like Mahanarayan Taila. A warm bath and sleep are prescribed. Mild exercise such as walking in the woods is all right, but strong aerobic exercise should be avoided.

KUNDALINI DISORDERS

Kundalini is the root energy of the astral body. It lays dormant at the base of the spine and a reflection of it maintains our ordinary nervous activities. Pranayama, mantra, or other meditation activities work to awaken it. It can also awaken spontaneously according to past karma. Many modern recreational and hallucinogenic drugs artificially stimulate but do not awaken it in full or in a wholesome manner.

Most Ayurvedic remedies for improving Ojas, such as ghee or ashwagandha, facilitate Kundalini without artificially stimulating it. Good stimulating herbs for it are calamus and shankha pushpi. Makaradhwaj, a mineral remedy, has this effect and should be taken with milk.

One method of spiritual development is to awaken the Kundalini and follow its movement up the spine towards the awakening of cosmic consciousness in the head. Other more direct approaches to spiritual development may circumvent the Kundalini. A few regard it as a power of illusion to be avoided.

Kundalini is not always a beneficent force. It can be aroused artificially or prematurely or be turned on too strongly. This can result in the burning out of the nervous system or various high Vata or high Pitta conditions. It may cause delusions or false imaginings.

Kundalini is not a force to be toyed with and requires the proper guidance in order to use. It is better not to use it at all than to approach it without the right orientation. Before attempting to arouse it, the body and mind should be purified. Its awakening is more appropriately part of Rejuvenation Therapy. Soma was an ancient Vedic herbal preparation that was given along with Rejuvenation Therapy for this purpose. Given to those with doshic imbalances, it would cause disease or even death.

Kundalini disorders generally arise from a forceful or misguided effort to awaken it, though transient Kundalini disorders can happen to anyone on the spiritual path. Such disorders involve pain in the lower back and swelling pain of the genitals. There may be a burning pain along the base of the spine to the solar plexus. Sexual desire may become excessive, or other powerful emotions such as anger may become overwhelming. There will be an inability to sleep, and the need for sleep will be low. Heightened imagination will bring visions of strong colors but with a lack of sensory control. Fantasies may turn negative or destructive. Visions of heaven and hell, feelings of being a great guru, god or bodhisattva may occur. Contact with astral beings may happen and they may encourage such fantasies.

Naturally this is a difficult condition to recognize. The individual may mistake it for a true spiritual experience. Long-term pain, anxiety and mental unrest, however, reveal its true character. Even a great yogi may go through periods of such negative experience.

Treatment of Kundalini Disorders

All meditation techniques should be given up, except for devotional practices. An effortless meditation of peace and calm should be followed or a simple surrender to the Divine. Rest and relaxation are important. Avoid any forceful holding of the breath or breath of fire (bhastrika). Perform gentle lunar pranayama—breathing in through the left and out through the right nostril only—or Shitali.

A combined anti-Vata, anti-Pitta diet is prescribed, avoiding spices, except for turmeric, fennel and coriander. Milk and ghee can be taken but not pure forms of sugar, including honey. All drugs and alcohol should be strictly avoided. Herbal wines generally will not be good.

Calming and nourishing herbs like ashwagandha, shatavari, sandalwood, haritaki, amalaki, gotu kola, jatamamsi and aloe gel are best. Stimulant herbs like calamus, camphor, bayberry and sage should not be used.

Good formulas are Ashwagandha compound, Ashwagandha ghee, Brahmi ghee or Brahma Rasayana, and Shatavari compound.

Oil massage is very helpful, applying warm sesame oil to the pelvic region, genitals and base of the spine. Brahmi oil to the head is particularly good. Essential oils such as sandalwood, rose and lotus should be applied to the top the head, the third eye and navel chakras.

Helpful gems for balancing and regulating Kundalini energy are yellow sapphire, yellow topaz, emerald, jade, pearl and moonstone. Ruby, garnet and cat's eye should not be used as they stimulate Kundalini. The best mantras for calming Kundalini are SHAM and RAM. Using OM a lot can arouse it. The mantra HUM is strongest to arouse it and should not be used.

Above all one should seek the counsel and the company of a true guru. If this is not possible one should pray to the Divine in whatever form most appeals to ones heart.

ADDICTIONS

Addictions are another form of psychological disorder. They occur from too much tamas or inertia in the mind. This is often caused by excess rajas, or mental disturbance, which is compensated for by providing an artificial calm. All addictions tend to increase Vata by creating nervous dependency. The individual becomes mentally destabilized and is not able to look at the condition objectively.

- Kapha individuals with strong physiques can withstand more bad habits such as smoking, drinking and taking of stimulants or drugs. They also have the greatest difficulty in giving up addictions.
- Vata types will be damaged by addictions very easily. They can give them up short-term but tend to return to them, or to shift from one habit to another.
- Pitta types, with their strong self-righteousness, have greater

339

difficulty in giving up addictions unless they are convinced it is their own best choice in the matter. The typical drinker turned fundamentalist religious fanatic is usually of Pitta constitution.

Treatment of Addictions

Ayurvedic treatment of different addictions is similar. The doshic imbalance behind the problem must be addressed. Specific herbs to help reduce the emotional need for the addicting substances are given. These are mainly nervines like calamus, gotu kola, skullcap or camomile. Other herbs are necessary to repair the tissue damage done by the addictive substance: lung tonics for smoking, liver tonics for drinking, and brain or nerve tonics for drugs.

Addictions indicate a wrong-life style, so our whole life-regimen needs to be examined. All addictions are part of a psychological pattern of dependency. This must be addressed. Addictions either involve association, like the drunk at a bar, or isolation, like the drug addict hiding in his bedroom. Right association is important in curing any addictive pattern. Self-honesty is also very important. Generally the addict is unwilling to recognize his or her addiction or blames someone else or society for it.

SMOKING

Addiction to smoking can occur in any of the three doshas but particularly Vata. Vata types like to smoke as a nervous habit to calm anxiety and provide distraction from worry and agitation. Pitta types like the addition of more fire into their systems and the increased feeling of power. Kapha types like the clearing and stimulating effect of tobacco, which activates them and removes lethargy.

The herb calamus helps counter the nervous habit behind addictions. It can be added in small amounts to cigarettes or taken as a powder or ghee; in the latter form it is particularly good to apply several drops to the nose two or three times a day, particularly when the urge to smoke arises.

Gotu kola is excellent for addictions in Pitta and Kapha types. Ashwagandha is good for Vata types. Camomile can be used for calming the nerves in most addictions. Kapha types benefit from herbal cigarettes and can take these as a substitute. Ayurveda recommends smoking of herbs for many Kapha problems.

Treatment for Quitting Smoking

Treatment should follow the predominant dosha, but generally there will be an increase in mucus as a reaction, which necessitates keeping Kapha in check. Kapha types in particular experience congestion after giving up smoking. They do best with more spices and expectorants—calamus, ginger or cloves with honey—or formulas such as Clove compound or Trikatu. Milk decoctions of pippali (pippali) help rebuild the lungs. Elecampane can be taken in the same way. Bayberry, haritaki and bibhitaki are good for any throat congestion.

Smoking causes lung weakness, dry cough and constipation in Vata types. Tonic foods for the lungs like milk, almonds, pine nuts and sesame seeds are good for this. Tonic herbs for the lungs —ashwagandha, shatavari, bala, ginseng, comfrey root and marshmallow—are excellent. These are better taken in milk decoctions with raw sugar and ghee, 1-2 teaspoons of herbs per cup. Formulas include Ashwagandha compound.

Smoking in Pitta types causes infectious diseases of the lungs, liver and blood. Detoxification is required. Good herbs include aloe gel, barberry, shatavari and burdock. Take these with jatamamsi and gotu kola to calm and cool the nerves. Formulas such as Sudarshan churna are excellent.

ALCOHOLISM

Alcohol is a means of adding fire to the body. It overheats and damages the liver and the blood, creating various Pitta disorders.

Alcohol is also a sugar. Addiction to it may be part of a sugar addiction. This occurs more in Kapha and Vata types. Ayurvedic herbal wines can substitute for alcohol and help reduce dependency. Make sure to use good oils in the diet to help cleanse the liver, particularly ghee.

Aloe is the best general herb for balancing liver function. The gel or herbal wine is preferable. Gotu kola is the best herb for clearing out toxins from the brain tissue and reducing disturbed emotions in the liver. Bitters such as katuka, gentian or goldenseal are helpful for cleansing the liver and the blood. Turmeric and barberry together help clear congested emotions from the liver. Good formulas include Brahma Rasayana and Saraswat powder.

Skullcap is a good Western herb for calming addiction and also helps cleanse the liver. Passion flower, betony, hops, jatamamsi and other cooling nervine herbs are helpful in both Pitta and Kapha types. Bitters in general are very good.

A good formula for detox from alcoholism is turmeric, barberry, gotu kola and licorice in equal parts, 1-3 grams of the powder taken with aloe gel after meals. This is mainly for Pitta types. To this formula Vata types can add licorice and take with warm milk, and Kapha types can add dry ginger and take with honey.

The Chinese herb bupleurum has been found to be good for cleansing the liver, as well as reducing emotional factors behind drinking and other addictions. It is available in such formulas as Major Bupleurum for strong body types and Minor Bupleurum for weak types.

DRUG DISORDERS

We live in a culture of drug abuse, both recreational and medicinal. Long-term taking of drugs severely aggravates Vata. Most drug disorders are also Vata disorders. Many drugs are diuretic and have a drying affect, causing constipation, weakening the kidneys and depleting Ojas. However, stimulant drugs, particularly in their short-term use, aggravate Pitta and can burn out the nervous system and damage the eyes.

Drugs damage Sattva, the basic clear nature of the mind. Artificially driving the mind and nerves they create tamas, dullness, inertia, darkness and loss of perception, even though their temporary action appears to be opposite this.

Hallucinogenic drugs function by temporarily increasing Tejas, the mental fire. This results in the experience of color and heightened perception, which may give a sense of the deeper powers of our consciousness. But these drugs function by burning up Ojas, our subtle vital reserve, causing long-term depletion of our primary vitality. Once Ojas is brought below a certain threshold, it is very difficult for it to reconstitute itself. The result is drug burnout, a vegetative state of mind. Hence, the number of times we can take hallucinogenic drugs in a positive way is very limited.

Sleep-inducing medicines, in the long run, tend to cause insomnia, just as laxatives cause constipation. Amphetamines and other stimulants also increase Vata and Pitta. Downers usually increase Kapha (Tamas). Marijuana, particularly when smoked, is much like tobacco addiction and can be treated in a similar way. Also like tobacco it causes lung and liver cancer.

Treatment for Drug Disorders

The diet should be according to the dosha involved, most commonly anti-Vata or anti-Pitta. Take ghee 1-2 teaspoons 2-3 times a day with food, to nourish the nerve tissue. Pitta types should avoid spices except for coriander, fennel, turmeric and saffron. Garlic, onion, asafoetida, nutmeg and other grounding spices are good for Vata. For a Kapha-like lethargy nervine stimulants like calamus, pippali and ginger are excellent.

Gotu kola is the best herb to cleanse hallucinogenic drugs from the liver and brain. Gotu kola ghee or Brahma Rasayana is good for cooling and calming high fire in the mind (too much Tejas).

Ashwagandha is the best herb for rebuilding the nervous system depleted by drug use. Shatavari helps restore emotional sensitivity and balance. Calamus is important for restoring mental

343

acuity, including powers of perception and self-expression. It is especially good for the dullness and depression that follows excessive use of drugs.

Valerian is good to counteract the effects of stimulants and is an effective sedative in drug disorders. Take 3 teaspoons per cup of warm water. Ayurvedic jatamamsi is even better and is also safe for Pitta. Such herbs are best taken with a little ghee.

Guggul and myrrh are important for cleansing and fortifying the deeper tissues. Yogaraj guggul and Mahayogaraj guggul are the best, particularly the latter. Triphala guggul has better cleansing, but weaker tonifying, action.

The Chinese herb, zizyphus seeds, is particularly good for nourishing and tonifying brain tissue damaged through excess use of drugs. Also useful are biota seeds.

II.11
TREATING THE LIFE-FORCE/PRANIC HEALING

B esides the treatment of specific bodily systems and their diseases, it is important to get an overview of the person's vitality or prana as a whole. Ayurveda is not a physically based or symptoms-approach medicine but looks at underlying issues of energy and motivation. It is a life science that requires understanding of life and its forces. Everything that we do in life is a form of reception and transmission of energy, which includes not only eating and breathing, but also sensing, feeling and thinking.

The physical body is a manifestation of prana. Our prana reflects how we think, feel, perceive and breathe, as well our outer patterns of food, rest and exercise. Pranic imbalances lie behind all diseases. The doshas are merely three different statuses or orientations of prana and can all be worked upon through it.

All Ayurvedic treatment methods from diet and herbs to bodywork and meditation are ways of treating prana. Food is a vehicle for prana, which is the deeper energy that we extract from it. Herbs correct the movements of prana and its functions like digestion, elimination or sweating. Touch is the sense through which prana is conveyed. It conveys prana from the therapist to the client. Bodywork loosens pranic blockages in the muscles and bones. Meditation opens the prana or energy of the mind, while mantra energizes it.

The healer's prana should awaken the prana of the patient and direct it towards healing. The rapport between the healer and the patient transmits prana and connects the patient with the will of the therapist. This is the power of counseling. A doctor with an awakened or spiritually energized prana can heal by touch alone. Sometimes the very presence of such a doctor is healing and soothing to the mind and prana of the patient and can work miracles.

345

Many people today suffer from low energy and chronic fatigue. Others suffer from excess or disturbed energy patterns. We should address these energy problems specifically and not just look at particular disease conditions that arise from them.

LOW ENERGY

Behind most disease states—particularly those that are chronic, degenerative or hard to treat—is a state of low energy. Most modern methods of treating disease, such as the use of antibiotics or sedatives, reduce vitality further. Our modern isolated life-style disrupts our connection with nature and with other people and makes us prone to low energy. A person alone can lack the pranic connections to feel really healthy and happy.

There are several sources of energy. First, there is our congenital vitality or inherent Ojas. This depends upon karmic factors and is given at birth, often making it difficult to change. Some people are blessed with strong constitutions. Others are not. Generally Kapha types have the best congenital Ojas and vitality, while Vatas have the least, with Pitta in-between.

Second, there is the energy that we draw in from outside sources. These are primarily twofold as food and breath. Wrong diet decreases our true energy input from food and is a causative factor in most diseases—thus the importance of dietary therapy. Eating freshly cooked organic food removes many cases of low energy. Wrong breathing, including shallow or hurried respiration, is another important factor—thus the importance of pranayama or breath control. Daily pranayama improves energy and counters many diseases, particularly those of the heart, lungs and brain.

Third are factors that produce energy through the mind. These start with sensory perception. When the impressions that we take in are wholesome, like the beauty of nature, the mind receives positive energy and creativity. When these are unwholesome, like artificial stimulation of the senses through

346

images of violence or from an unnatural living environment, the mind develops negative energy and becomes destructive.

Our sensory impressions can either stimulate our higher faculties or dull us and put us to sleep. Meditation, silence and peace of mind increase mental energy. Distraction of mind, excess pursuit of entertainment, gossip, worry and any excess thinking dissipate mental energy.

Deep sleep is also important for renewing the mind. This is our natural form of meditation that regenerates our entire being. When this does not occur, our energy is not able to renew itself and we get unhappy or diseased.

We also receive from other people. Association is a key source of vitality, which is why we naturally congregate together. To have a positive energy in life we should ally our wills with those individuals whom we can emulate and are seeking to do what we think is truly valuable in life.

Love itself is the highest and most nourishing form of prana. Love can keep people alive who would otherwise die. It can raise our prana from its deepest depths. That is why love has such a healing force to it. A person who feels really loved will not be depressed or debilitated. Similarly, a person who can give love becomes a source of life itself.

The most important source of energy is our own soul (Jivatman), which is the ultimate source of Prana and Ojas. If we are not in contact with that internal source of energy, we are entirely dependent upon external sources of energy, which are limited and possess a certain entropy or tendency towards decay. Connecting with our internal source of inspiration, discovering our spiritual aspiration in life, and following our true dharma or right vocation, are ways of attuning ourselves to our soul. For spiritual healing we must awaken in our souls. We must be conscious of ourselves not as mere bodies seeking pleasure or longevity but as spiritual beings, immortal portions of consciousness, seeking enlightenment and Self-realization.

To Increase Energy

Increasing energy requires first of all removing the factors that reduce it. We must change our negative attitudes and emotions, and take a positive view of life and healing. We must remove ourselves from locations or situations that are devitalizing. For example, many people sleep in rooms that have a negative energy or emotional history, or they are tied to relationships that drain them. Without removing these energy drains we cannot expect our energy to grow.

We must establish right diet, right breathing, adequate restful sleep (deep sleep) and moderate use of sexual energy. Important also are right thinking and not dissipating mental energy, which depend upon the proper intake of impressions from the external world. Right association and a spiritual purpose in life are perhaps the key.

If our energy is chronically low we are either dissipating it or not renewing it properly. There is really nothing mysterious about low energy, though it may consist of a combination of subtle factors that cannot be treated simplistically or mechanically. If we donít have energy we must be wasting it in some way that should be obvious to an objective observation of our behavior.

For renewing energy, tonic and supplementation therapy is indicated. Substances to increase Ojas—foods like milk, ghee and almonds, and herbs like ashwagandha and shatavari—are important. Chyavan Prash or Ashwagandha compound or the Energy Tonic (no. 2) are helpful.

For mental energy, mantras are the simplest way to increase it, particularly energizing mantras such as OM, RAM and HUM. Gems for chronic low energy are ruby, garnet, and red coral, which revive and circulate energy, set in gold. Also useful are diamond, zircon, yellow sapphire or yellow topaz which have a tonifying effect.

Treating Blocked Energy

There are two states of low energy, which are often related. The first is energy that is simply low or insufficient. The second is blocked energy, which we cannot use. When energy is blocked it appears low but it is simply not flowing properly. This is more common in young people, whose congenital energy source is not yet exhausted by time. Symptoms of blocked energy involve feelings of suppression, tension, and being pent up, with occasional agitation or even major outbursts. However, blocked energy leads to deficient energy in the long run because if energy is not allowed to flow it eventually dissipates. Complicated cases of combined deficient and blocked energy exist that can be hard to treat.

Blocked energy is treated differently than deficient energy. Activity is required to move the energy, such as purification therapy including Pancha Karma. For the diet, spices to promote the digestive fire are indicated, particularly aromatics like ginger, cardamom, bay leaves or basil, which should be used freely with food. Herbs to move and clear the energy pathways are important like calamus, guggul, myrrh or turmeric. Aromatic oils have important clearing energy, particularly camphor and eucalyptus. Physical exercise and creative mental activity are required. Sweating therapy is great in all of its different forms. Pranayama is excellent, including more active forms.

Often it is necessary to make some move to break stagnation in our life style. This may require change of job, residence or relationship, or otherwise breaking up our pattern of inertia. Some diseases cannot be changed until we change how we live.

EXCESS ENERGY

Generally excess energy is not a problem. But some diseases arise from excess energy, which if not used properly can become toxic. This is mainly too much energy of an inferior quality that comes from eating meat or taking alcohol and stimulants. It can come on a psychic level from being controlling or dominating others. It is often related to a condition of too strong an ego.

Most infectious, congestive and acute diseases are excess conditions because they involve a strong pathogenic factor and acute symptoms. Such excesses can lead to deficiencies because after the excess results in a disease the disease eventually weakens our vitality.

Reducing therapies are indicated for excess energy, including stronger forms of Pancha Karma, like purgation, that eliminate negative energy from the body. Mild sedative herbs are also helpful like jatamamsi and gotu kola. Jatamamsi is excellent for those who feel their energy unstable and about to erupt or cause agitation. Peaceful forms of meditation are helpful along with peaceful mantras like SHRIM or SHAM.

HYPERACTIVITY

Hyperactivity is usually a sign of dissipation. It leads to low energy, and is often a sign that our energy level is in decline. When our energy falls to a certain level it no longer has the power to hold or consolidate itself. This results in hyperactivity, which in turn results in exhaustion.

Some individuals are karmically or congenitally hyperactive. While they may get away with this when young, it causes low vitality or chronic diseases when older. This is often the case with Vata types who often live on nervous energy. Eventually they suffer from an energy collapse, which often follows a period of strong exertion or lack of sleep. Psychologically, hyperactivity is often a form of distraction and indicates that there is something in life we are trying to avoid. We should always remember that inaction is important both for health and longevity. If a muscle is used all the time, for example, it easily gets worn out.

Hyperactivity requires a combination of mildly tonifying and sedating (reducing) therapies. Usually a rich and grounding diet is indicated that is mainly anti-Vata in nature and emphasizing complex carbohydrates and adequate proteins. It should be combined with mild sedative herbs like jatamamsi, ashwagandha or skullcap. Adequate rest, relaxation and meditation are necessary.

In the case of children, hyperactivity often arises from lack of proper attention or emotional regard from the parents. Children need to have their energy contained by an adult or they can easily get hyper. A balanced diet is essential for them as well.

STRENGTHENING THE ENERGY FIELD

Disease involves a disruption in the vital energy field, what is often called the aura. Our energy field reveals any imbalances that we may have. It is the field of our positive vitality, the light emitted by our essential vitality (Ojas). The aura wards off disease and maintains the organic integrity not only of the body but also of the mind.

The condition of the aura can be read through the complexion of the skin, the luster of the eyes, or the pulse. It is revealed by the personís will power, the integrity of their character and the degree of creativity that they possess. By yogic power or the power of concentration, it can be intuited or perceived. Astrology gives us a key to it because it is created by the colors of our planetary rays.

Pranayama, gems, mantra and meditation have the most power to improve the aura. The aura is the total effect of our daily thought and action, so right life-regimen in general improves it.

Dark gems, such as blue sapphire or amethyst, seal off or protect the aura. Warm gems like ruby, garnet or red coral, energize it. Nurturing gems like pearl, diamond or yellow sapphire feed and strengthen it.

Mantras like OM expand the aura, while those like RAM protect it. Those like HUM ward off any negative energy that may disrupt it. Peace and silence of mind both energize and consolidate it.

To renew our aura we need to create our own sacred space. This may be a meditation room, an altar or any other defined area where we do a daily practice or ritual, a sacred activity connecting us to the cosmic Being or inner Self.

Most allopathic practices like use of medical drugs, machines, or staying in hospitals, weaken the aura. Excess stimulation or dissipation of any kind damages it. This includes too much travel, too much exercise, excessive sex, over-use of the senses, and such factors as radiation, environmental pollution or overexposure to mass media influences.

The aura is weakened when we give our minds over to an external influence because the aura on an inner level is a function of the power of our attention. External influences are astral and psychological nature, not merely physical. So improving concentration also strengthens the aura

Part III
AYURVEDIC REMEDIAL MEASURES

VEDIC HYMN TO THE PLANTS

Plants, which as receptacles of light were born three ages before the Gods, I honor your myriad colors and your seven hundred natures.

A hundred, oh Mothers, are your natures and a thousand are your growths. May you of a hundred powers make whole what has been hurt.

Plants, as Mothers and Goddesses, I address you. May I gain energy, light, and sustenance, your soul, you who are a conscious being.

Where the herbs are gathered together like kings in an assembly, there the doctor is called a sage, who destroys evil, and averts disease.

As they fell from Heaven, the plants said, "The living soul we pervade, that man will suffer no harm.

The herbs that are in the kingdom of the Moon, manifold with a hundred eyes, I take this plant as the best of them, for the fulfillment of wishes, as peace to the heart.

Plants that are queens of the Soma, spread over all the Earth, generated by the Lord of Prayer, may your energy combine within this herb.

RIG VEDA X.97

Section I of this book examines the basic principles and therapies of Ayurveda. Section II, the treatment of common diseases, introduces a number of formulas. In Section III more information is given on these formulas, as well as additional Ayurvedic healing modalities of oils, incense, gems, mantras and spiritual measures.

III.1
HERB USAGE

DOSAGE

The sections on diseases in the book list individual herbs for different conditions. These herbs can be taken as single remedies, usually one ounce of the herb per pint of boiling water, taken daily in two or three portions. If the herbs are very pungent or very bitter, like cayenne or goldenseal, lower dosages are better, one-quarter to one-half the amount.

Herbs can be taken as powders, 1-4 grams (four grams is one teaspoon or a little more for most powdered herbs), two or three times daily. Again the lower dosage is for the stronger tasting herbs. The appropriate vehicles (anupanas) like honey for Kapha, ghee for Pitta or warm milk for Vata, should be used.

The same dosages and manner of taking can be used for those who wish to prepare for themselves the formulas listed in the text. For the premade medicines listed in this section the dosages are included.

PRINCIPLES FORMULA DEVELOPMENT

To devise Ayurvedic herbal formulas, we must first comprehend the main principles of formula development. We can build on classical Ayurvedic formulas or combinations (Trikatu, for instance), or use similar ideas to make our own base formulas. We can use Western or Chinese herbs and combinations once we understand their energetics. Devising our own formulas and using raw herbs, rather than premade pills and tablets, we can make stronger preparations and have greater variability in our treatment approach. It also allows us to make a remedy when the appropriate Ayurvedic herbs or premade formulas are not available. However, it is less convenient and requires a certain skill and familiarity with herbs that can take some time to acquire.

There is no great mystery about formula development. There are a few major principles with adaptations according to conditions. Yet certain combinations, theoretically no better than others, are found to work especially well.

A good starting principle is to use two to four herbs that most typify the action one wishes to achieve, like the famous three pungent herbs, the Trikatu formula of Ayurveda, just mentioned. Imagine that we want a formula with primarily bitter taste, which can treat a large variety of Pitta and Kapha conditions. We can make a simple formula with three common bitters like gentian, barberry and goldenseal.

To such a base formula we add supplementary herbs to adjust or modify its effects in various directions. We can add herbs to strengthen its action or balancing agents to prevent its action from being too extreme.

Diuretics would aid in its cleansing properties; uva ursi or pipsissewa, also mainly bitter, would strengthen its antibiotic properties against bladder infections.

We could add alteratives like dandelion or isatis to aid in its blood-cleansing action for dealing with boils or severe infections.

Purgatives to aid in its bile cleansing action could be rhubarb root and aloe powder, also bitter.

To increase its weight-reducing action and to prevent these bitter herbs from weakening the digestive fire, we could add spices like dry ginger. This would be especially good for Kapha types.

As it is a fairly reducing formula, we might want to add some tonifying herbs to balance it out. Licorice, marshmallow or shatavari would do this, giving it some nourishing properties but retaining its anti-Pitta action. Moreover, the demulcent property of these tonics, combined with the bitter, makes a good combination for ulcers and hyperacidity, adding a soothing action to the mucus membranes.

As all disease involves stress, tension and disturbed mental or emotional states, we might want to add a nervine or antispasmodic herb. Gotu kola or bhringaraj would be good; they aid in

355

the basic liver-cleansing action of the three bitters. Such a combination would help deal with alcohol and other substances that make the liver toxic.

Disease is commonly based on a stagnation of energy or blockage of the channels. We might want to add some turmeric for opening up the liver and pancreas and relieving any blockage in their systems.

Putting these principles together for a liver-cleansing formula for a strong Kapha type who has eaten too much meat, sugar and fats, we might use gentian, goldenseal and barberry, along with dry ginger, turmeric and gotu kola, taken with honey.

For a weak Pitta type suffering from chronic hepatitis, we might use the three bitters with shatavari, licorice, turmeric and gotu kola, taken with ghee. We might even take out one of the bitters, like goldenseal, to prevent the formula from being too reducing.

With the appropriate strategy, avoiding any excessive or one-sided action, we have much latitude in combining herbs to treat conditions. Yet, whatever the condition, we must take care to treat the underlying dosha and not just proceed symptomatically. Then we must adjust the formula based upon the experience of the patient. In this process we can learn to make our effective combinations.

Herbs, whether classically formed and commercially made or formulas made by ourselves, do not always have the expected result, even if all factors appear correct. Experience must always be our final teacher. Using these Ayurvedic herbs and formulas, we may find that their effectiveness varies according to time, place and culture, requiring some adaptation and adjustment.

POTENTIZATION OF HERBS

Not only must we have the right diagnosis and right prescription to adequately treat a condition, the herbs must have the right potency. Many old or commercially prepared herbs may lack this.

Potentization of herbs is not just a physical or chemical matter. It requires strengthening the prana or life-force of the herbs, which in turn requires an act of consciousness. It cannot be done by mechanical methods alone. A physically oriented medicine must fail because it cannot serve as a vehicle for the life-force.

In some respects it is misleading to speak of the general properties of an herb. These vary, particularly by degree, according to how the herb is grown, prepared and combined. They are general guidelines, not rigid rules. Miraculous powers can be found in very ordinary herbs when they are specially grown and prepared. All herbs are vehicles of prana or cosmic healing power. As such, they all possess a certain neutrality and can be made into vehicles for that power on different levels.

SPECIALLY POWERFUL HERBS

Some herbs, like ginseng or ashwagandha, are endowed with special power. They tend to retain this power even when other supporting factors are lacking. Generally roots hold their power longer than other plant parts, thenbarks and fruit; leaves and flowers deteriorate first.

SPECIALLY GROWN HERBS

Fresh herbs maintain a special power, having more prana or chi than dry ones. Their juice is particularly strong. Fresh herbs, even singly or in small dosages, can affect the body and mind directly, and have better healing power, than large amounts of old herbs. Homegrown herbs, grown with love and attention, possess a more gentle, yet consistent, healing power.

How an herb is grown is as important a factor in healing as what the herb is. A few well grown or prepared herbs can cure diseases that manyherbs otherwise cannot touch. Some herbalists, therefore, choose to use a few herbs, perhaps very common ones, grown and prepared with care. This is not a lack of sophistication but sophistication of a different nature.

WILD HERBS

Wild herbs possess the strongest prana. Handpick your own with care, love and respect. They transmit the force of Nature herself. Wildcrafted herbs also tend to be stronger than those cultivated.

SPECIAL COMBINATIONS OF HERBS

The right combination of herbs allows the individual herbs to function synergistically, with geometrically increased powers. Each herbal tradition has such combinations. We can discover others ourselves.

SPECIAL EXTRACTION

The active ingredients of herbs are best extracted by the appropriate medium. These include water, alcohol, vinegar, milk, honey and oils. These may be used as vehicles for taking the herbs also.

ADDITION OF POTENTIZING HERBS

Some herbs are able to potentize others in different directions and can be added as an activating principle. These include stimulants such as cayenne, ginger, camphor and mint which serve as guiding herbs.

Vehicles (anupanas), or special media such as honey or ghee, also help to direct the effects of herbs.

HERBAL PREPARATIONS

Herbal wines, oils and jellies not only extend the life of herbs but also can heighten their powers.

TRITURATION

This process involves stirring an herb with a mortar and pestle. Usually a powder or a liquid paste is used. Juices or decoctions, or the herb or other herbs, can be added. This allows a more uniform energy to the herbal preparation as well as greater strength. The properties of the substance the mortar and pestle are made of is important. Stone, copper, silver or gold add their special qualities to the herbs triturated in them.

ALCHEMICAL PREPARATIONS

Spagyric tinctures are very powerful. The combination of herbs with specially incinerated minerals (bhasmas) is commonly used in Ayurveda.

GEMS AND MINERALS

Gems can be used to energize plants, using gem waters or gem tinctures along with the herbs. Gold, silver, copper and iron also can help energize herbs. Prepared or cooked in vessels of these metals, herbs gain additional power. Tinctures of metals transmit their properties to the herbs, without causing any toxicity. Gold aids in reducing Vata and Kapha. Silver reduces Pitta and Vata. Copper reduces Kapha. Iron reduces Vata. Bronze reduces Pitta.

ATTUNEMENT METHODS

Attunement is the growing, preparing or prescribing of herbs according to the right time. Astrology is the main attunement method. Proper power and aspect of the Moon is important, as it rules plants generally. Mercury, which rules healing, and Jupiter, which gives vitality, are also considered.

MENTAL METHODS

Methods of mental empowerment are mantra, meditation and prayer. They may involve the energization of a particular wish or intention. Some use an energy pattern in the mind on a subtle level to empower that in the herb on a gross level. Others concentrate on a certain deity or divine power to work through the herb.

Some may be a part of, or involve, physical actions or rituals. All preparation of herbs should be a ritual, a sacred action in harmony with the rhythm of the cosmos to facilitate the cosmic healing force. Such methods are essential to any form of holistic healing. Otherwise, on a subtle or astral level the herbs, with their sensitivity and neutrality, may pick up negative energies.

MANTRAS FOR POTENTIZING HERBS

Many different mantras can be used for potentizing herbs. Deities may be called on as part of this process, as each mantra is a Divine Name. OM affirms and empowers whatever we direct it towards. It also empowers other mantras. The mantra SOM increases the energy of plants, their Soma.

OTHER FACTORS

Herbs have better effect when applied close to the site of the problem; for instance, the use of enemas for Vata. Also, herbs have to be integrated into an appropriate life-regimen in harmony with an individual's nature. They can only work through the tree of our own soul.

III.2
CLASSICAL AYURVEDIC FORMULAS

The classical Ayurvedic formulas mentioned in the book reflect both common usage in Ayurveda and accessibility of their main ingredients in the West. There are many other formulas of equal quality. The formulas are limited primarily to purely herbal products. Ayurvedic mineral preparations or compounds of minerals and herbs are very common and have better potency but are not yet available here.

The same formula may be offered in several forms: powder, tablet, herbal jelly or herbal wine. Ayurveda offers the largest variety of herbal preparations of any herbal tradition. Some preparations preserve the potency of herbs; others enhance their properties.

Powders have the shortest shelf life, six months to one year, particularly if exposed to sunlight or dampness. Tablets are good up to two years if well coated and kept out of the sunlight. Herbal oils, wines and jellies last up to three years. Medicated ghees may last only six months unless refrigerated.

Powders, tablets, pills and gugguls are taken with appropriate vehicles (anupanas) – warm or cool water, milk, buttermilk, ghee, honey, butter, yogurt, or teas of other herbs. Such appropriate vehicles are listed after each formula. This vehicle can guide the energy of the herbs to a certain location of the body or change its effect altogether. The same herbs can target different doshas depending upon the medium that we take them with.

Formulas are not always specific for lowering one dosha. The dosha a formula treats can be modified not only by the vehicle used to take it but also by the formulas with which it is combined. In this way some formulas can be good for lowering two or even all three doshas.

The properties of a formula are usually determined by the primary herb it is named after, or by its largest constituent. When a particular formula is not available, a decoction of the main herb or chief ingredients is generally sufficient.

Classical formulas come from Ayurvedic source books. However, the ingredients and their proportions vary according to different formulations, modern adjustments, or the standards of the company that manufactures them. Usages generally remain the same. Modern Ayurvedic companies modify classical formulas to make them more useful today and rename them to appeal for sales. I have translated the Ayurvedic names of these formulas when this can be done easily.

POWDERS/TABLETS

Many herbal powders are used in Ayurveda. Herbs are seldom used in the raw form, partly because raw herbs deteriorate quickly in India's tropical climate. Powders are prepared by reducing the herbs to a fine powder and mixing them together. As powders tend to deteriorate quickly, many powders are made into tablets, particularly for export to the West, and given special protective coatings.

Tablets, however, are not made only of powdered herbs. Many use herbal pastes and herbal extracts, which give them a superior quality over simple tableted powders.

Asafoetida 8 Compoun/Hingashtak Churna

Ingredients	Asafoetida, Trikatu, rock salt, cumin, black cumin, ajwan
Doshas	Decreases Vata and Kapha, increases Pitta, for Vata indigestion
Properties	Carminative, stimulant, antispasmodic
Uses	Abdominal distention, gas, colic, indigestion
Dose	1-4 grams or 2-8 tablets, 2-3 times a day
Vehicle	Warm water

Ashwagandha Compound/Ashwagandha Churna

Ingredients	Ashwagandha, vidari kanda
Doshas	Lowers Vata, mildly increases Kapha and Pitta
Properties	Tonic, aphrodisiac, antirheumatic, astringent, analgesic, rejuvenative

Uses	Arthritis, debility, wasting diseases, impotence, nocturnal emissions, leucorrhea, anxiety, insomnia, general tonic for elderly, convalescence
Dose	1-6 grams or 2-12 tablets, 2-3 times a day
Vehicle	Milk or ghee

Avipattikar Churna

Ingredients	Trikatu, Triphala, cyperus, vidanga, cardamom, cinnamon leaf, cloves, trivrit, raw sugar
Doshas	Good for Pitta type digestive disorders
Properties	Laxative, carminative, cholagogue
Uses	Hyperacidity, heartburn, biliousness, vomiting, indigestion, dropsy, rheumatism
Dose	1-4 grams or 2-8 tablets, 2-3 times a day, after meals
Vehicle	Warm water

Bilva Compund Powder/Bilvadi Churna

Ingredients	Bilva, ginger, fennel, cardamom, bombax, woodfordia, and others
Properties	Astringent, alterative
Uses	Diarrhea, dysentery, malabsorption
Dose	1-3 grams or 2-6 tablets, 2-3 times a day
Vehicle	Buttermilk, water

Cardamom Compound/Eladi Churna

Ingredients	Cardamom, cloves, keshara, kolamajja, laja, priyangu, cyperus, sandalwood, pippali
Doshas	Decreases Kapha and Vata
Properties	Carminative, antiemetic, stomachic
Uses	Vomiting, cough, asthma, indigestion, anorexia
Dose	1-4 grams or 2-8 tablets, 2-3 times a day
Vehicle	Honey or raw sugar (some formulations of it already contain rai sins or other forms of sugar)

Chitrak Compound Tablets/Chitrakadi Bati

Ingredients	Chitrak, 5 salts, Trikatu, ajwan, chavya, asafoetida
Doshas	Decreases Vata and Kapha, increases Pitta and Agni
Properties	Stomachic, antacid, carminative
Uses	Indigestion, gas, hyperacidity, colic
Dose	2-4 tablets twice a day after meals
Vehicle	Warm water

Cloves Compound/Lavangadi Churna

Ingredients	Cloves, camphor, cardamom, cinnamon, nagakeshar, nutmeg, vetivert, ginger, cumin, valerian, bamboo manna, jatamamsi, pippali, sandalwood, cubeb, raw sugar
Doshas	Reduces all doshas
Properties	Diaphoretic, expectorant, antitussive, antispasmodic
Uses	Colds, cough, whooping cough, intestinal gas, colic, diarrhea, nausea, vomiting, lack of appetite, lumbago
Dose	1-4 grams or 2-8 tablets, 2-3 times a day
Vehicle	Honey

Dashamula/Ten Roots

This formula is very good for Vata conditions as a tonic and sedative. It is used in enema therapy and in medicated oils. Ingredients vary slightly by formulation.

Dhatupaushtic Churna (Tissue Strengthening Powder)

Ingredients	Shatavari, gokshura, cannabis seed, vamsha rochana, sarsaparilla, cubeb, kapikacchu, black musali, white musali, Trikatu, dioscorea, ashwagandha, nishotha
Doshas	Reduces Vata and Pitta, Increases Kapha
Properties	Tonic, rejuvenative, aphrodisiac
Uses	Debility, convalescence, senility
Dose	2-5 grams or 4-10 tablets, 2-3 times a day
Vehicle	Warm milk

Garlic Compound Tablet/Lashundi Bati

Ingredients	Garlic, cumin, rock salt, sulfur, Trikatu, asafoetida, lemon juice
Doshas	Reduces Kapha and Vata, increases Pitta and Agni
Properties	Stimulant, carminative, laxative
Uses	Loss of appetite, distention, gas, borborygmus, constipation, parasites
Dose	2-4 pills (1-2 grams), 2-3 times a day
Vehicle	Warm water

Gotu Kola Compound Tablet/Brahmi Bati

Ingredients	Gotu kola, shankha pushpi, calamus, black pepper, often with various minerals
Properties	Sedative, antispasmodic, nervine tonic, rejuvenative
Uses	Mental weakness, poor memory, neurasthenia, epilepsy, coma, paralysis
Dose	2 pills (1 gram) twice a day
Vehicle	Honey, ghee

Guduchi Sattva/Tinospora Extract

Ingredients	Water soluble extract (starch) of guduchi
Properties	Bitter tonic, diuretic, alterative, rejuvenative
Uses	Liver disorders, fever, malaria, headache, urinary disorders, convalescence
Dose	1-2 grams twice a day
Vehicle	Ghee or water

Kutajghan Bati

Ingredients	Kutaj, ghan, atish
Properties	Alterative, astringent, amoebicide
Uses	Diarrhea, dysentery, hemorrhoids, hematuria. Specific antibacterial and amoebicidal for dysentery
Dose	2-4 pills (1-2 grams), three times a day
Vehicle	Warm water, buttermilk or yogurt

Lavanbhaskar Churna/Five Salts Compound Powder

Ingredients	5 salts, fennel, pippali, pippali root, black cumin, cinnamon leaf, nagakeshar, talisha, rhubarb root, pomegranate seeds, cinnamon, cardamom
Doshas	Decreases Vata, increases Agni and Pitta
Properties	Stimulant, carminative, laxative
Uses	Loss of appetite, malabsorption, constipation, abdominal pain, tumors
Dose	1-4 grams or 2-8 tablets, 2-3 times a day
Vehicle	Warm water, buttermilk

Licorice Powder/Yashtimadu Churna

Ingredients	Licorice
Properties	Demulcent, tonic, expectorant, laxative
Uses	Cough, sore throat, chronic constipation, debility
Dose	2-4 grams or 4-8 tablets, 2-3 times a day
Vehicle	Honey (as laxative or expectorant), milk (as nutritive tonic)

Mahasudarshan Powder

Ingredients	Bitters (such as chiretta, guduchi, barberry), Trikatu, Triphala, cannabis
Doshas	Mainly anti-Pitta
Properties	Antipyretic, diaphoretic, diuretic
Uses	Fever, intermittent fever, debility after fevers, nausea, enlargement of liver and spleen
Dose	1-4 grams or 2-8 tablets, 2-3 times a day
Vehicle	Water, ghee

Nutmeg CompoundD/Jatiphaladi Churna

Ingredients	Nutmeg, cloves, cardamom, cinnamon leaf, cinnamon, nagakeshar, camphor, bamboo manna, valerian, amalaki, haritaki, Trikatu, chitrak, cumin, vidanga, cannabis, raw sugar
Properties	Sedative, astringent, antispasmodic, hemostatic

Uses	Diarrhea, dysentery, malabsorption, lack of appetite, cough, asthma, migraine headache, dysmenorrhea, menorrhagia
Dose	1-3 grams or 2-6 tablets, 2-3 times a day
Vehicle	With honey

Rasayana Churna/Rejuvenation Powder

Ingredients	Guduchi, gokshura, amalaki
Doshas	Good rejuvenative tonic for Pitta, in particular after febrile diseases
Properties	Bitter tonic, demulcent, alterative, diuretic, antacid
Uses	General debility, sexual debility, venereal diseases, skin rashes, allergies, chronic fevers or infections
Dose	1-4 grams or 2-8 tablets, 2-3 times a day
Vehicle	Raw sugar and ghee, in milk

Sarasvat Powder

Ingredients	Ashwagandha, calamus, shankha pushpi, ajwan, cumin, Trikatu, rock salt, and others
Doshas	Mainly for Vata disorders
Properties	Nervine tonic and stimulant
Uses	Mental weakness, nervous strain, mania, epilepsy, hemiplegia, weakness of voice
Dose	1-4 grams or 2-8 tablets, 2-3 times a day
Vehicle	Honey and ghee, in milk

Sitopaldi Churna (Rock Candy Compound Powder)

Ingredients	Rock candy, bamboo manna, pippali, cardamom, cinnamon
Doshas	Major anti-Kapha formula, also reduces Vata
Properties	Expectorant, antitussive
Uses	Colds, cough, lack of appetite, fever, debility, burning sensation in extremities
Dose	1-4 grams or 2-8 tablets, 2-4 times a day
	Vehicle Honey, ghee

Sandalwood Compound Powder/Chandanadi Churna

Ingredients	Sandalwood, fennel, pippali, pippali root, black pepper, cloves
Properties	Diuretic, alterative, febrifuge, urinary antiseptic
Uses	Urinary tract infections, cough, asthma, fever, venereal diseases
Dose	1-4 grams or 2-8 tablets, 2-3 times a day
Vehicle	Water, milk

Sarsaparilla Compound Powder/Chopchinyadi Churna

Ingredients	Sarsaparilla, fennel, pippali, pippali root, black pepper, cloves, ginger, cinnamon, and others
Properties	Alterative, sedative, antirheumatic
Uses	Venereal diseases, sexual debility, gout, arthritis, epilepsy
Dose	1-4 grams or 2-8 tablets, 2-3 times a day
Vehicle	Milk

Shatavari Compound/Shatavaryadi Churna

Ingredients	Shatavari, gokshura, atibala, and others
Doshas	Good tonic for Pitta and Vata
Properties	Tonic, nutritive, demulcent, diuretic, aphrodisiac
Uses	Debility, convalescence, impotence, infertility
Dose	1-6 grams or 2-12 tablets, 2-3 times a day
Vehicle	Milk, ghee

Sudarshan Churna

Ingredients	Chiretta and various mainly bitter or pungent herbs
Doshas	Mainly anti-Pitta
Properties	Anti-pyretic, alterative, antiperiodic
Uses	Fever (old), intermittent fever, debility, weak digestion, liver disorders, enlargement of liver and spleen
Dose	1-4 grams or 2-8 tablets, 2-3 times a day
Vehicle	Warm water

Talisadi Churna

Ingredients	Talisha, Trikatu, bamboo manna, cardamom, cinnamon, raw sugar
Doshas	Mainly anti-Kapha
Properties	Expectorant, antitussive, stimulant
Uses	Colds, flu's, bronchitis, loss of appetite, indigestion, chronic fever
Dose	1-4 grams or 2-8 tablets, 2-3 times a day
Vehicle	Honey

Tikta/Bitter

A compound of bitter herbs, good for all the general indications of bitter taste and used like Sudarshan churna.

Trikatu Powder

Ingredients	Black pepper, pippali, dry ginger
Doshas	Specific for low Agni and high Ama, weak digestive fire and accumulation of toxins; reduces Kapha and Vata, increases Pitta
Properties	Stimulant, expectorant
Uses	Lack of appetite, indigestion, cough, congestion
Dose	1-3 grams or 2-6 tablets, 2-3 times a day
Vehicle	Honey, warm water

Triphala Churna

Ingredients	Haritaki, amalaki, bibhitaki
Doshas	Good for all three doshas, best and safest laxative
Properties	Laxative, tonic, rejuvenative, astringent
Uses	Chronic constipation, abdominal gas and distention, diabetes, eye diseases, chronic diarrhea
Dose	2-10 grams or 4-10 tablets, before sleep, 1- 2 tablets with meals as a tonic
Vehicle	Ghee, honey, warm water

Trisugandhi Churna (Three Aromatics Powder)

Ingredients	Cinnamon, cinnamon leaf, cardamom
Doshas	Decreases Kapha and Vata, increases Pitta and Agni
Properties	Stimulant, carminative, diaphoretic
Uses	Indigestion, lack of appetite, vomiting, gas, distention. Good like Trikatu for improving the digestion of food and herbs; bay leaf can be used in place of cinnamon leaf
Dose	1-3 grams or 2-6 tablets, 2-3 times a day
Vehicle	Honey or warm water

Gugguls

Gugguls are special pills made with the resin of guggul, Commiphora mukul, a relative of myrrh. They are mainly for treating arthritis, nervous system disorders, skin diseases and obesity, many of the same conditions Western herbalists treat with myrrh. Their advantage over myrrh is that they are purified so that the resin does not damage kidney function. Guggul is purified by boiling it in herbal decoctions like Triphala and then straining out the purified resin. Herbal powders or extracts are added to the purified guggul resin, often with ghee.

Gokshuradi Guggul/Tribulis Compound Guggul

Ingredients	Guggul, gokshura, Trikatu, Triphala, cyperus
Properties	Diuretic, alterative, demulcent
Uses	Difficult urination, urinary tract stones, diabetes, leucorrhea, gonorrhea, arthritis
Dose	2-5 pills, 2-3 times a day
Vehicle	Cyperus tea, pashana bheda tea, vetivert tea

Mayayogaraj Guggul

Ingredients	Guggul, Triphala and the ashes of lead, silver, tin, iron, mica, iron sulfate and mercuric sulfide, along with many different, primarily pungent herbs.

Properties	Antirheumatic, alterative, sedative, astringent
Uses	Arthritis, gout, diabetes, nervous disorders, epilepsy, asthma, tumors. This is the main Ayurvedic formula for severe and degenerative arthritis and for difficult nervous disorders like paralysis, MS and Parkinson's disease
Dose	1-3 pills, 2-3 times a day
Vehicle	Galangal tea, Triphala tea or honey

Triphala Guggul

Ingredients	Guggul, Triphala and pippali
Properties	Alterative, anti-inflammatory, antibiotic, antiseptic
Uses	Boils, carbuncles, abscesses, ulcers, hemorrhoids, nasal polyps, edema, and arthritis. Very cleansing and detoxifying for Vata, particularly in Sama conditions or when Vata has entered the lymph or blood
Dose	2-5 pills, 2-3 times a day
Vehicle	Warm water

Yogaraj Guggul

Ingredients	Guggul, Triphala, ginger, black pepper, chavya, asafoetida, ajwan, galangal, vidanga, atish, calamus, chitrak and others.
Uses	Arthritis, gout, nervous diseases, hemorrhoids, epilepsy, anemia
Dose	2-5 pills, 2-3 times a day
Vehicle	Galangal tea, garlic juice, honey

Herbal Wines

Herbal wines are self-generated herbal fermentations. They are prepared similar to grape wine, in big wooden vats. They are quite different than tinctures, though tinctures can substitute for them to some extent. There are two types, asavas and arishtas. Asavas are made without boiling the herbs used in them; usually fresh herbal juices are used. Arishtas are made with decoctions. Fermentation is brought about by the addition of dhataki flowers.

Medicinal wines not only last longer than powders and pills, but they also make the herbs more digestible. Many contain additional spices for improving their assimilation. Their sour taste makes them particularly good for Vata. Draksha is already being made in this country. Herbal wines are a new field of herb preparation for us. At some point we will learn to produce many varieties of our own.

Aloe Herbal Wine/Kumaryasava

Ingredients	Aloe gel, jaggary and honey, with Trikatu, Triphala and other predominately spicy herbs
Properties	Alterative, tonic, hematinic
Uses	Anemia, poor endocrine function, cough, asthma, constipation, liver disorders, chronic hepatitis
Dose	2-4 ounces with meals

Arjunarishta/Arjuna Herbal Wine

Ingredients	Arjuna, raisins, madhuka flower, dhataki and jaggary
Properties	Heart tonic, cardiac stimulant
Uses	All cardiac and pulmonary disorders, heart weakness
Dose	2-4 ounces with meals

Ashokarishta/Ashoka Herbal Wine

Ingredients	Ashoka, dhataki, jaggary, cumin, Triphala, ginger, sandalwood, and others
Properties	Alterative, astringent, hemostatic
Uses	Menorrhagia, leucorrhea, dysmenorrhea, hematuria
Dose	2-4 ounces with meals

Ashwagandharishta/Ashwagandha Herbal Wine

Ingredients	Ashwagandha, white musali, madder, licorice, turmeric, Trikatu, sandalwood, calamus, dhataki and jaggary

Properties	Nervine tonic, sedative
Uses	Nervous debility, loss of memory, epilepsy, insanity. Another good way to take ashwagandha, particularly for its nervine properties
Dose	2-4 ounces with meals

Balarishta/Bala Herbal Wine

Ingredients	Bala, ashwagandha, lily, cardamom, galangal, cloves, vetivert, gokshura, castor root, dhataki, jaggary
Properties	Tonic, nutritive, antirheumatic, diuretic
Uses	rthritis, paralysis, debility, high Vata
Dose	2-4 ounces with meals

Draksa/Grape Herbal Wine

Ingredients	Mainly raisins and various spices; some varieties made with nuts have better tonification properties
Properties	Stimulant, carminative, diuretic
Uses	Loss of appetite, indigestion, general debility, insomnia, cough, pulmonary diseases. Particularly good for Vata type weak digestion
Dose	2-4 ounces with meals

Kutajarishta/Kutaj Herbal Wine

Ingredients	Kutaj, raisins, madhuka, gmetina, dhataki, jaggary
Properties	Astringent, hemostatic, antiperiodic
Uses	Diarrhea, dysentery, malabsorption, parasites
Dose	2-4 ounces with meals

Saraswatarishta/Saraswat Herbal Wine

Ingredients	Gotu kola, shatavari, vidari kanda, haritaki, vetivert, fresh ginger, fennel, honey, raw sugar, dhataki and other herbs and spices
Properties	Nervine tonic, sedative

Uses	Nervous debility, convulsions, stammering, memory loss, sexual debility

Herbal Jellies

Herbal jellies are prepared with raw sugar such as jaggary or honey. They are herbal confections. The sugar acts as a preservative, improves the taste of the herbs and enhances their tonic properties. Herbal jellies serve as herbal foods and are good for tonification therapy. Not all of them, however, taste good.

Brahma Rasayan/Gotu Kola Herbal Jelly

Ingredients	Haritaki, amalaki, gotu kola, shankha pushpi, vidanga, sandalwood, agaru, calamus, Dashamula, raw sugar, and others
Properties	Alterative, tonic, nervine, rejuvenative
Uses	Mental weakness, loss of memory, general debility, senility, neurasthenia, cough; Good brain and meditation food
Dose	1-2 tsps., 2-3 times a day
Vehicle	Milk

Chyavan Prash

Ingredients	Amalaki, pippali, bamboo manna, cloves, cinnamon, cardamom, cubebs, ghee, raw sugar, and others (many varieties are available, some with silver or gold foil)
Properties	Nutritive tonic, rejuvenative
Uses	General debility, old age debility, anemia, sexual debility, cough, tuberculosis
Dose	1-2 tsps., 2-3 times a day
Vehicle	Milk

This is the most famous and widely used herbal jelly, good for almost any weakness condition or as an energy supplement. Many kinds are available, some with gold, silver or other minerals. It is considered a good tonic for all three doshas. Most Indian markets and restaurants in this country carry it. The same formula can be found as a pill or powder.

The best quality is made with fresh Amalaki. Not all Ayurvedic companies do this today because the fresh fruit is only available seasonally.

Musli Pak

Ingredients	White musali, ghee, sugar, Trikatu, cinnamon, cardamom, chitrak, ashwagandha, cloves, nutmeg and special minerals
Properties	Nutritive tonic, aphrodisiac
Uses	Sexual debility, infertility, emaciation, lack of strength
Dose	1-2 tsps., 2-3 times a day
Vehicle	Milk

Vasavaleha/Vasa Herbal Jelly

Ingredients	Vasa, haritaki, bamboo manna, pippali, chaturjat
Properties	Antispasmodic, expectorant, laxative, alterative
Uses	Asthma, bronchitis, cough, bleeding from the lungs
Dose	1-2 tsps., 2-3 times a day
Vehicle	Milk

Medicated Oils

Medicated oils (tailas) are prepared mainly with sesame oil. They are mainly for external use. Dose is largely as needed for massage; Ayurveda uses larger amounts of oil for massage, requiring a shower afterwards to remove excess oil.

These medicated oils are an Ayurvedic specialty. No other herbal system uses so many different herbs in a heavy oil base. Most others are essential oils in a light alcohol base, or else heavier ointments. Ayurveda uses many tonic herbs prepared in oil for external nourishment as well as special analgesic herbs.

Medicated oils are not just supplements; they are a primary treatment and can be a treatment in themselves. They are very important in oleation (snehana) therapy.

Some modern companies are preparing these oils with more pleasant fragrances and better absorbability. Simple oils can be made by adding herbs to sesame oil and water, boiling the water away and straining the excess herbs.

Bhringaraj Taila/Eclipta Oil

Ingredients	Bhringaraj juice and sesame oil
Properties	Antiseptic, hair tonic, nervine
Uses	Premature graying or balding, alopecia, pruritus of the scalp. Can use as a good hair and scalp conditioner, also for calming the mind

Brahmi Taila/Gotu Kola Oil

Ingredients	Gotu kola and other nervine herbs in coconut oil base
Properties	Nervine, sedative, antipyretic
Uses	Insomnia, mental agitation, headache, eye-ache, premature graying or balding. Generally as brain tonic; some varieties commonly sold in this country

Chandanadi Taila/Sandalwood Compound Oil

Ingredients	Sandalwood, licorice, saussurea, etc. and sesame oil
Properties	Antipyretic, hemostatic, sedative
Uses	Fever, headache, neuralgia, burning sensation, nose bleed, hemoptysis

Chandan Bala Lakshadi Taila

Ingredients	Sandalwood, bala, sumac, deodar, saussurea, manjishta, ashwagandha, etc. and sesame oil
Properties	Antipyretic, antispasmodic, antiseptic, analgesic
Uses	Fever, cough, asthma, headache, skin diseases, arthritis

Mahamasha Taila

Ingredients	Masha, Dashamula, castor root, and sesame oil
Properties	Demulcent, emollient, analgesic
Uses	All kinds of pain, paralysis, earache

Mahanarayan Taila

Ingredients	Shatavari, castor root, brihati, bala, and sesame oil
Properties	Demulcent, emollient, analgesic
Uses	Arthritis, rheumatism, gout and paralysis. Most commonly used oil for arthritis

Narayan Taila

Ingredients	Shatavari, ashwagandha, bilva root, brihati, neem, Dashamula, milk, sesame oil
Properties	Demulcent, emollient, analgesic
Uses	Rheumatic pain, paralysis, fever

Pinda Taila

Ingredients	Manjishta, sariva, sarjarasa, licorice, wax, castor oil
Properties	Anti-inflammatory, analgesic
Uses	Rheumatism, gout

Vishagarbha Taila

Ingredients	Vatsanabha, vitex juice, bhringaraj juice, and sesame oil
Properties	Analgesic, sedative
Uses	Good for any kind of muscle ache, neuralgia, gout, rheumatism, earache, sciatica

Medicated Ghee

Medicated ghees are good as nervine tonics, as ghee nourishes the brain and nerves. Ghee also combines well with bitter herbs enhancing their properties by its Pitta reducing action. Most nervines or bitters gain in strength when prepared in ghee or taken with ghee.

Ghees do not require vehicles (anupanas) to take them with but they are usually followed with milk. Simple ghees can be prepared like medicated oils. Ghee itself is prepared by cooking raw unsalted butter over a low flame until all the milk fats settle to the bottom, then straining off the clear liquid.

Ashwagandha Compound Ghee/Ashwagandha Ghrita

Ingredients	Ashwagandha and ghee
Properties	Tonic, nervine, aphrodisiac
Uses	General debility, nervous debility, insomnia, lack of sexual vitality
Dose	1-2 tsps. twice a day
Vehicle	Milk

Gotu Kola Compound Ghee/Brahmi Ghrita

Ingredients	Gotu kola, calamus, saussurea, shankha pushpi, ghee
Properties	edative, nervine tonic
Uses	Insanity, epilepsy, weakness of voice, as brain tonic
Dose	1-2 tsps., twice a day
Vehicle	Milk

Note: a simpler version of this formula can be made with gotu kola 3 parts and calamus or bayberry 1 part. Cook two ounces of the herbs in one pint of water; simmer slowly down to one cup. Add to one cup of ghee and slowly cook until the water evaporates.

Mahatikta Ghrita

Ingredients	Katuka, vasa, mainly bitter tonics and ghee
Properties	Bitter tonic, alterative
Uses	Inflammatory diseases, boils, carbuncles

III.2 Classical Ayurvedic Formulas

Dose	1-2 tsps. twice a day
Vehicle	Milk

Phala Ghrita

Ingredients	Triphala, saussurea, katuka, calamus, sariva, galangal, bamboo manna, ghee
Properties	Tonic, endocrine stimulant
Uses	Sexual debility and infertility in women
Dose	1-2 tsps. twice a day
Vehicle	Milk

Purana Ghrita/Old Ghee

Ingredients	Ghee at least 1 year old, the older the better, (very old ghee, ten years or more, is said to be able to cure all diseases)
Properties	Tonic, expectorant, emollient, antiseptic
Uses	Pulmonary disorders, general debility, externally for sores, boils, carbuncles, etc.
Dose	1-2 tsps. twice a day
Vehicle	Milk

Shatodhara Ghrita

Ingredients	Ghee that has been triturated with water in a copper vessel
Properties	Demulcent, emollient, anti-inflammatory, antiseptic
Uses	Externally for skin rashes, itch, skin sores, burns

Triphala Ghrita/Triphala Ghee

Ingredients	Triphala, vasa, bhringaraj, ghee
Properties	Tonic and alterative for the eyes
Uses	Conjunctivitis, weakening of vision
Dose	1-2 tsps. twice a day
Vehicle	Milk

Mineral and Animal Preparations

These are all specially prepared and are safe for human usage. Many such formulas exist in Ayurveda.

Godanti Bhasma/Gypsum Ash

Ingredients	Gypsum, aloe juice
Properties	Alterative, antacid, febrifuge
Uses	Fever, cough, flu, headache, malaria
Dose	250-500 mg., 2-3 times a day
Vehicle	Honey

Navayas Loha Guti/Iron Tablets

Ingredients	Iron ash, Trikatu, Triphala, cloves, nutmeg, cardamom
Properties	Blood tonic and alterative, One of the main Ayurvedic iron supplements
Uses	Anemia, amenorrhea, dropsy
Dose	1-3 grams, 2-3 times a day
Vehicle	Water or punarnava tea

Shankha Bhasma/Conch Shell Ash

Ingredients	Mainly conch shell
Properties	Carminative, antacid, analgesic
Uses	Hyperacidity, indigestion, gas and distention
Dose	250 mg. to 1 gm., 2-3 times a day
Vehicle	Water

Shilajit Compound

Ingredients	Shilajit, gurmar, neem, various minerals
Properties	Tonic, diuretic, alterative, aphrodisiac
Uses	Urinary tract disorders, kidney stones, edema, sexual debility, diabetes, venereal diseases
Dose	1-2 pills (500 mg. to 1 gm.) twice a day
Vehicle	Honey

Shringa Bhasma/Deer Horn Ash

Ingredients	Deer horn and aloe juice
Properties	Expectorant, diaphoretic
Uses	Lung diseases, cough, pneumonia, chest pain
Dose	125-500 mg.
Vehicle	tHoney

RASA PREPARATIONS

These are special very powerful Ayurvedic herbal preparations using minerals, primarily purified sulfur and mercury. While important to Ayurvedic practice, they are part of an old spiritual, alchemical tradition now lost in the West (and for the most part, in China). Though we cannot import them, owing to FDA restrictions, we can get them in India. We want to introduce them to acquaint the public with their power.

The toxic metals are purified by various procedures. These include soaking and boiling in various herbal preparations and repeated incinerations (up to one thousand times). The result is usually a white powder, an oxide of the metal or gem, which is 'humanized' or rendered safe for human
consumption. Clinical tests in India prove these products, in the normal dosage, do not leave any toxic residues in the tissues.

Makaradhvaj

This is the most famous Ayurvedic rasa preparation, consisting of purified sulfur and mercury, to which herbs like camphor, nutmeg, cloves, black pepper and other minerals like gold may be added depending upon the formulation. It is a stimulant, alterative, aphrodisiac and a heart tonic. It is unexcelled for reviving energy in low vitality or chronic diseases. It is a great energy tonic for the nervous system. Dosage is ½-1 gram daily for periods of up to one month, usually in the winter.

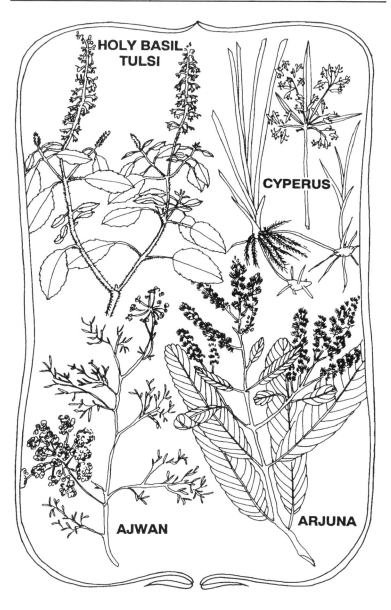

III.3
Modern Ayurvedic Formulas

Ayurvedic practitioners not only use classical formulas, they devise their own formulas. These are usually based on classical models, modified according to experience. Ayurvedic companies have their special proprietary medicines. We ourselves can make Ayurvedic formulas using Ayurvedic principles with herbs we are familiar with. The following are such modern formulas, which I have devised with help from India. They are largely balanced (Tridosha) medicines; but the vehicle we use to take them with, like honey or ghee, can serve to direct their effects to the different doshas.

Additional modern Ayurvedic medicines may be made of only a single herb like bhumyamalaki (phyllanthus), ashwagandha, guggul or shilajit. They may be potentized by preparation along with the fresh juice or decoction of the herb. They may be as potent as formulas but sometimes require higher dosages.

While pre-made and over the counter formulas can be good, usually what we make for ourselves with raw herbs is stronger and has the additional power of bringing us in more direct contact with the herbs and the healing process.

1. Digestive Stimulant/Trikatu plus

INGREDIENTS	Dry ginger, black pepper, pippali, coriander, nutmeg, ajwan (when ajwan is not available cloves can be used); all equal parts
DOSHAS	Decreases Kapha and Vata, increases Pitta, burns up Ama.
PROPERTIES	Stimulant, expectorant, carminative
USES	Lack of appetite, indigestion, nausea, vomiting, colic, intestinal gas, malabsorption, candida, metabolic disorders (overweight or underweight), cough, cold, congestion and poor circulation. Can be used wherever Trikatu is indicated and is safer and more balanced for long-term usage.

DOSE	1-4 grams three times a day, before meals to increase appetite, after to promote digestion.
VEHICLE	Warm water generally. Honey for Kapha, warm water for Pitta and Vata. Pitta can take more safely with raw sugar, ghee or aloe gel. For Vata, warm milk is also good.
PRECAUTIONS	Inflammatory conditions of the g.i. tract. (in such cases it is safer to use it with milk or aloe gel). Use with care on Pitta types.
DIET	Can be combined with all foods to improve absorption, generally a light, warm diet of whole grains and steamed vegetables is preferred. Can be taken during fasting to burn up toxins, as long as there is a tongue coating. Goes well with anti-Ama (detoxifying) or anti-Kapha diets and is usually good for Vata. Taken with milk or dairy, it aids in the absorption. Balances the negative effects of ice cream and other cold and damp foods, like raw vegetable or fruit juices.

2. Energy Tonic/Ashwagandha Plus Compound

INGREDIENTS	Ashwagandha 4, shatavari 2, pueraria (kudzu) 2, pippali (pippali) 1
DOSHAS	Decreases Vata, does not overly increase Pitta or Kapha.
PROPERTIES	Tonic, rejuvenative, aphrodisiac, expectorant, antirheumatic, analgesic
USES	Lack of energy, low vitality, sexual debility, infertility, nervous debility, insomnia, nerve degeneration, emaciation, arthritis, diabetes, weak immune function, chronic bronchitis. Can be used wherever Ashwagandha or its preparations are indicated. More balanced and safer for long-term usage or usage as a general tonic for all three doshas than Ashwagandha by itself.
DOSE	2-5 grams three times a day with meals.
VEHICLE	Warm milk or warm water with ghee (clarified butter). Milk is preferable as a vehicle for its nutritive properties, ghee for its nervine properties. Vata and Pitta can take with milk and ghee, Kapha with honey

PRECAUTIONS	Do not take during colds, flu, fevers and other acute conditions, though it is useful in chronic conditions.
DIET	Good with such invigorating and aphrodisiac foods as dairy products and nuts including almonds, sesame seeds, lotus seeds, chick peas, onions or garlic, or a general rich and nutritive diet. It is particularly good with anti-Vata diet and can be added to any tonification therapy.

3. Lung Tonic

INGREDIENTS	Elecampane root 2, bala or Solomon's seal 2, holy basil (tulsi) 2, bayberry 1, vasa or mullein 1, cinnamon 1
DOSHAS	Decreases Kapha and Vata, increases Pitta.
PROPERTIES	Expectorant, stimulant, diaphoretic, decongestant
USES	Cough, colds, flu, congestion, asthma, bronchitis, weak lungs, shortness of breath, indigestion
DOSE	2-4 grams every two hours for acute conditions; 1-4 grams twice a day as a lung tonic.
VEHICLE	Warm water or honey for its dispersing and expectorant action. Honey for Kapha, raw sugar for Pitta, either for Vata, as a tonic with milk.
PRECAUTIONS	Severe lung infections, high fever without chills
DIET	Should be taken with fasting or a light diet, like rice or steamed vegetables. Heavy foods, meat, dairy or oils should be avoided until the cough, phlegm, cold or flu has been eliminated. As a long-term lung tonic, it goes well with anti-Kapha or anti-Vata diets.

4. Woman's Tonic/Shatavari plus

INGREDIENTS	Shatavari 3, comfrey root 2, cyperus 1, red raspberry 1, saffron ¼
DOSHAS	Decreases Vata and Pitta, does not overly increase Kapha.
PROPERTIES	Emmenagogue, tonic, alterative, laxative: Can be used whenever Shatavari is indicated in treating female reproductive, blood or liver disorders.

USES	Menstrual disorders (PMS, amenorrhea, dysmenorrhea), menopause, female debility, infertility, anemia, swollen breasts, breast or uterine tumors, chronic hepatitis, cirrhosis
DOSE	1-4 grams three times a day before meals.
VEHICLE	Milk (with ghee) as a tonic, warm water or fresh ginger tea to promote menstruation. Honey for Kapha, milk for Vata and Pitta. Taking with aloe gel will increase it effects.
PRECAUTIONS	During pregnancy.
DIET	Should be taken with a nourishing diet to strengthen its tonic action, including milk, ghee (clarified butter), basmati rice, almonds, sesame seeds.

5. Colon Tonic/Triphala Plus

INGREDIENTS	Haritaki 2, amalaki 1, bibhitaki 1, ginger 1
DOSHAS	Good for all three doshas.
PROPERTIES	Laxative, astringent, tonic, rejuvenative
USES	Chronic constipation, colitis, diverticulitis, hemorrhoids, arthritis, nervous debility. Can be used whenever Triphala is indicated. Stronger in action and requires lower dosage (Triphala by itself traditionally requires 3-15 grams for a normal dosage).
DOSE	1-2 grams three times a day, before meals or on an empty stomach; 3-6 grams before sleep as a purgative.
VEHICLE	Water generally. For Kapha with honey or warm water, for Vata warm water or warm milk, for Pitta, with cool water.
PRECAUTIONS	Acute diarrhea, dysentery, uterine bleeding
DIET	Good diet includes oils, ghee (clarified butter), bran or other bulk items to lubricate and strengthen the colon, but can be taken with any good diet relative to the appropriate dosha.

6. Brain Tonic/Gotu Kola Plus

INGREDIENTS	Gotu kola 4, ashwagandha 2, calamus 1, haritaki 1, sandalwood 1, licorice 1

DOSHAS	For Kapha with honey, for Vata with warm water and for Pitta with cool water. Vata and Pitta can also take with milk and ghee.
PROPERTIES	Nervine, antispasmodic, diuretic
USES	Insomnia, headaches, nervousness, irritability, anxiety, mental weakness, poor memory, poor concentration, hypertension, drug detoxification, to counter addictions. Can be used whenever Gotu Kola is indicated. Balanced for all three doshas and a good tonic for the mind.
DOSE	1-3 grams three times a day after meals.
VEHICLE	With cool water to cool the mind, with ghee (clarified butter) or warm milk as a tonic.
PRECAUTIONS	None
DIET	No special dietary recommendations, except to avoid overly tasty, spicy or heavy, processed or junk food which interferes with the proper functioning of the brain. Coffee and other stimulant beverages should also be avoided.

7. Herbal Febrifuge/Blood Purifier

INGREDIENTS	Sandalwood 2, vetivert 2, lemon grass 1, katuka (or barberry) 2, dry ginger 1
DOSHAS	Decreases Pitta and Kapha, increases Vata
PROPERTIES	Antipyretic, alterative, refrigerant
USES	Fever, swollen glands, sore throat, boils, skin rashes, acne, sunstroke, burns, flu, bronchitis, headaches
DOSE	1-4 grams three times a day for general blood cleansing; four tablets (2 grams), three times a day for three days for fever
VEHICLE	Ghee for old fevers, warm water for new. Honey for Kapha, cool water for Pitta, Vata with milk and raw sugar.
PRECAUTIONS	Do not use in cold conditions, or in the absence of fever, infection or inflammation.
DIET	Should be taken with fasting, light diet and rest, along with adequate fluid intake. Sandalwood oil or rose water can be applied to the head. Generally an anti-Pitta diet should be followed with food such as mung water, Kicharee, rice, mung or barley gruel.

8. Liver Tonic

INGREDIENTS	Bhumyamalaki (phyllanthus) 2, katuka 2, turmeric 1, barberry 1, gotu kola 1, Coriander 1
DOSHAS	An excellent anti-Pitta formula, cuts to the root of many Pitta disorders by decongesting the bile. Helpful for many Kapha conditions also; increases Vata.
PROPERTIES	Hepatic, alterative, bitter tonic
USES	Hepatitis, jaundice, gall stones, cirrhosis, genital herpes, venereal diseases
DOSE	1-3 grams three times a day (double dosage during fever)
VEHICLE	Generally with cool water. Specifically, with honey for Kapha, aloe gel or ghee (for tonification property) for Pitta, with milk and ghee or raw sugar for Vata.
PRECAUTIONS	Pallor, chills, nervous debility, high Vata conditions.
DIET	Good with anti-Pitta, anti-Kapha or anti-Ama diet. Emphasis should be on raw vegetables and whole grains, with avoidance of meat, yogurt, oily or greasy food and hot spices.

9. Herbal Absorbtion

INGREDIENTS	Nutmeg, cardamom, cyperus, pippali (pippali), haritaki, camomile, licorice; all equal parts
DOSHAS	Decreases Vata and Kapha, increases Pitta.
PROPERTIES	Stimulant, carminative, astringent
USES	Lack of appetite, indigestion, gas and abdominal distention, colic, nervous indigestion, candida, chronic diarrhea or loose stool, malabsorption
DOSE	1-3 grams three times a day before meals.
VEHICLE	Water, buttermilk, draksha. Buttermilk is the main vehicle for all doshas.
PRECAUTIONS	Do not take where there is constipation or severe inflammation of the digestive tract.
DIET	Hard-to-digest food should be avoided in the beginning, including milk, cheese, oily or greasy food. A simple diet of buttermilk, Kicharee, rice, mung or barley gruel should be taken and gradually built upon, according to the constitution.

388

10. Kidney Tonic

INGREDIENTS	Gokshura 2, pashana bheda 2, corn silk 1, lemon grass 1, coriander 1, fennel 1
DOSHAS	Decreases Kapha and Pitta, does not overly increase Vata.
PROPERTIES	Diuretic, lithotriptic, tonic
USES	Difficult, painful or burning urination, urinary tract infections, sciatica, lower back pain, kidney stones
DOSE	1-3 grams three times a day.
VEHICLE	For Kapha with honey, for Pitta or infectious conditions with cool water or aloe gel, for Vata and as a tonic with milk (and ghee).
PRECAUTIONS	Dehydration, lack of body fluids, high Vata conditions
DIET	Works well with diuretic foods like barley, corn, carrots, celery and anti-Kapha diet, but can be used with any of the diets as per constitution. With stones or infections it should usually be taken with large amounts of water and cooling juices like cranberry or pomegranate.

11. Heart Tonic/ Arjuna Plus

INGREDIENTS	Arjuna 4, ashwagandha 2, guggul 2, sandalwood 1, cardamom 1
PROPERTIES	Cardiac, tonic, alterative, hemostatic
USES	Heart weakness, palpitations, arteriosclerosis, hypertension, coronary heart diseases, angina, after heart attacks, post surgery, cardiac edema: Can be used wherever arjuna is indicated, balanced for all three doshas.
DOSE	1-3 three times a day.
VEHICLE	Water generally. For Kapha with honey, for Pitta with cool water or ghee, for Vata with warm water or ghee. With milk for tonic action.
PRECAUTIONS	None noted
DIET	As per constitution.

NOTE: Another effective heart tonic can be made with arjuna 2, guggul 1, gotu kola 1 and elecampane 1.

12. Antacid Formula

INGREDIENTS	Amalaki 1, shatavari 1, licorice 1, dry ginger 1/2
DOSHAS	Decreases Pitta and Vata, mildly increases Kapha.
PROPERTIES	Antacid, demulcent, analgesic
USES	Indigestion, hyperacidity, heartburn, ulcers, gastritis
DOSE	1-3 grams three times a day, after meals.
VEHICLE	With water or milk generally. With milk or ghee for Pitta and Vata, honey for Kapha.
PRECAUTIONS	Deficient acidity
DIET	Avoid food that is spicy, oily, fried or hot, as well as wine, pickles and sour juices. Irregular eating and food that is light or dry should also be eliminated. Mild demulcent food like whole grains or dairy is often good. Generally diet should be anti-Pitta.

13. Antirheumatic Formula/Guggul Plus

INGREDIENTS	Guggul 4, shallaki 2, cyperus 1, galangal 1
DOSHAS	Decreases Vata and Kapha, does not overly increase Pitta.
PROPERTIES	Antirheumatic, alterative, analgesic
USES	Arthritis, gout, rheumatoid arthritis, bone or ligament injuries, useful in sports medicine: Good wherever guggul is indicated. Decreases Vata and Kapha, does not overly increase Pitta.
DOSE	1-3 grams morning and evening.
VEHICLE	Warm water generally. With honey for Kapha and Vata, ghee for Pitta.
PRECAUTIONS	None noted
DIET	As arthritis is an Ama condition, avoid Ama-forming foods and follow detoxifying diet according to the constitution

14. Herbal Sedative

INGREDIENTS	Gotu kola 2, valerian 1, shankha pushpi 1, ashwagandha 1, nutmeg 1
DOSHAS	Generally balancing but specific for lowering Vata
PROPERTIES	Sedative, nervine, antispasmodic
USES	Insomnia, anxiety, hypertension, nervousness, tremors, palpitations

390

DOSE	2-5 grams in the evening or as needed.
VEHICLE	Warm milk or ghee for increasing calming action on all three doshas.
PRECAUTIONS	Do not use when you need to stay awake
DIET	Heavy, grounding food is useful, mainly anti-Vata diet including dairy, root vegetables, whole grains, nuts and oils

15. Weight Reduction Formula

INGREDIENTS	Haritaki 2, amalaki 2, bibhitaki 2, vidanga 2, dry ginger 1, katuka 1, gotu kola 1
PROPERTIES	Laxative, alterative
DOSHAS	Specific for Kapha but balances all three doshas
USE	Obesity, overeating, hypertension, chronic constipation, sugar addictions
DOSE	1-3 grams before meals.
VEHICLE	Best taken with honey or warm water by all types.
PRECAUTIONS	Emaciation, chronic low weight or sudden weight loss
DIET	Detoxifying, anti-Ama or anti-Kapha diet is indicated, avoiding sweets and heavy, greasy, oily or fatty foods.

NOTE: A slightly modified western version of this formula can be made by combining ginger, prickly ash and bayberry with Triphala, or by taking them along with it.

16. Chyavan Combination

Chyavan Prash is the most famous Ayurvedic herbal tonic food. The jelly, however, is not always convenient to take. This formula can be taken whenever Chyavan Prash is indicated.

INGREDIENTS	Amalaki, gokshura, bhumyamalaki, guduchi, ashwagandha, shatavari, kapikacchu, cyperus, cinnamon leaf and nagakeshar
DOSE	1-3 grams or two to three tablets twice a day morning and evening.
VEHICLE	Warm milk

17. Sexual Vitality Formula

INGREDIENTS	Gokshura, Asteracantha longifolia, kapikacchu, ashwagandha, shatavari; all equal parts
PROPERTIES	Tonic, stimulant, aphrodisiac, rejuvenative
DOSHAS	Decreases Vata and increases Kapha, does not overly increase Pitta
USES	Sexual debility, impotence, swollen prostate, low vitality, poor immune function, lower back pain
DOSE	1-3 grams morning and evening.
VEHICLE	Warm milk (and ghee) - these are also considered aphrodisiacs
PRECAUTIONS	Do not take where there is poor digestion or congestion.
COMBINATIONS	For Kapha take with Digestive Stimulant.
DIET	Take with rich diet of milk nuts, oils and tonifying, nurturing food

III.4
OIL THERAPY, AROMA THERAPY, AND INCENSE

Various fatty oils, whether vegetable-based like sesame or animal-based like ghee, are used in herbal systems throughout the world, but they have their greatest diversity and importance in Ayurveda. Oil therapy is specific for Vata (air or wind) disorders. As these constitute the majority of diseases, oil therapy is helpful in most forms of treatment. It is specifically indicated in diseases of the nervous system, bones and the deeper tissues. Oil therapy useful for the other doshas as well, with cooling oils like coconut being good for Pitta and hot pungent oils like mustard good for Kapha.

Ayurvedic oils are mainly for external usage but some can be taken internally. With their nutritive properties they combine well with tonic herbs like licorice or ashwagandha. Simple oils can be homemade or special preparations can be purchased. External usage in Ayurveda includes application of oils to the nasal passage, the ears, mouth and other orifices and in medicated enemas, as well as massage. Ayurvedic massage uses an abundance of oil. As part of Pancha Karma an extensive oleation therapy is always prescribed.

Essential Oils

Besides fatty oils, essential oils are used in Ayurveda and often combined with them. These are mainly subtle aromatic oils from fragrant or pungent plants like mint or jasmine. They are active in small amounts and, when combined with heavier oils, activate them and give them greater powers of penetration. They work well in alcohol. They should never be taken internally in their pure form, however, nor applied directly to any mucus membranes because their action can be highly irritating with many side effects. Essential oils can be placed on various sites on the skin, like the points of the seven chakras (especially the third eye).

393

OIL THERAPY ACCORDING TO THE DOSHAS

OILS FOR VATA

For Vata types the best general oil is sesame. It is warm, heavy, lubricating, nourishing to the skin, bones and nerves and calms the mind. It is said to be the only oil that has the power to penetrate all seven layers of the skin and to nourish all the organs and tissues. Almond or olive oil are also good but cannot substitute for sesame in severe conditions.

Many tonic herbs are good prepared in sesame oil, such as ashwagandha, shatavari and bala. The nutritive, softening, demulcent action of the oils and tonic herbs works synergistically. This combination is necessary for lowering high Vata. Special Ayurvedic oils for Vata include Mahanarayan and Narayan. Most Ayurvedic oils are good for Vata.

Essential Oils for Vata

Best for Vata are warm, stimulating essential oils like camphor, wintergreen, cinnamon, musk, galangal or cyperus, combined with calming, nutritive and grounding oils like sandalwood, rose or jasmine. Both do better added to the heavy oils and tonics mentioned above, like used in a sesame oil base. In an alcohol base they may be too light to alleviate Vata, which can be irritated by fragrances that are too strong or "perfumy."

OILS FOR PITTA

For Pitta types the best general oil for external usage is coconut oil. It is cooling and calming and relieves thirst and burning sensations. Sunflower oil is also helpful and can be used for inflammatory skin conditions. Sometimes sesame oil is used as a base for anti-Pitta oils with the addition of cooling herbs that neutralize its warming energy. Some Pitta types who cannot tolerate sesame oil (it causes itching) do well with olive oil.

Ghee (clarified butter) is usually the best oil for Pitta, but mainly for internal usage. However, it can be used externally, particularly if aged in a copper or silver vessel. Cooling and calming tonic herbs should be added to these oils including shatavari, gotu kola, and bhringaraj. Formulas include Brahmi oil and Bhringaraj oil.

Essential Oils for Pitta

Pitta types enjoy fragrant flowers as most flowers have cooling and calming properties. Good flowery oils for Pitta include gardenia, jasmine, rose,
honeysuckle, violet, iris and lotus. The best essential oil for Pitta is sandalwood, especially when applied regularly to the third eye. Other good cooling oils are lemon grass, lavender, mint and vetivert.

OILS FOR KAPHA

For Kapha types the best general oil is mustard oil. It is warm, light and stimulating and dispels phlegm. Another good drying oil for Kapha is flaxseed (linseed) oil. Sesame is sometimes used because of its warming nature.
Sunflower can also be good and is lighter in properties.

Essential Oils for Kapha

Kapha does best with essential oils that are warm, light, stimulating and expectorant. Good oils include sage, cedar, pine, myrrh, camphor, musk, patchouli and cinnamon. Kapha can tolerate and should use strong, sharp and stimulating fragrances, though may prefer those that are sweet. Plasters of these herbs, like ginger paste, or the oils in rubbing alcohol can be applied when Kapha cannot tolerate any heavy oils.

INCENSE

Incense is not only for religious purposes but also for healing, particularly for the mind and the nerves. It is also a good preventative to ward off disease and promote longevity. All incenses generally balance the mind, equalize the doshas and increase sattva, mental clarity.

Incense should be used on a daily basis. It purifies the air and the physical environment, the aura and astral environment, increasing prana. It helps counter negative emotions, negative attitudes and confused thoughts, and drives out negative influences and negative entities. Drawing down the energies of the gods (beneficent cosmic powers), incense increases faith, devotion, peace and perception. The properties and application of different types of incense are similar to those of their essential oils.

Vata types benefit from incense to calm the mind and strengthen the nerves, to relieve restlessness, anxiety and fear, and to counter hypersensitivity. For Vata good incenses are those that are warming and energizing yet grounding, stabilizing and give peace and strength.

Pitta benefits from incense to calm the emotions and cool the mind, to relieve agitation, aggression and anger. Most flower fragrances are good for Pitta.

Kapha benefits from incense to stimulate the mind, promote perception and counter dullness. Essential oils of flowers, which increase Kapha and promote Kapha emotions like love, faith and compassion, are better for Pitta and Vata. Incense from tree resins like pine or myrrh are good for Kapha as they have expectorant and cleansing properties.

Incense for the Doshas

Vata	Sandalwood, myrrh, frankincense, rose, almond, musk, basil, camphor, heena
Pitta	Sandalwood, rose, saffron, lotus, jasmine, gardenia, geranium, plumeria, champak
Kapha	Myrrh, frankincense, cedar, sage, basil, camphor, musk, heena

III.5
SPIRITUAL REMEDIAL MEASURES
Gem Therapy and Mantra

1. GEM THERAPY
AYURVEDA AND ASTROLOGY

Ayurveda uses various spiritual therapies to treat both body and mind. These are aligned with astrology but can be applied on their own. In this section we present gems and mantras, which are the main spiritual methods used. Color therapy follows the same logic as gem therapy. Gem therapy is a stronger form of color therapy.

Ayurveda and astrology were originally part of a single spiritual science. While Ayurveda primarily diagnoses and treats the physical body, astrology primarily diagnoses and treats the subtle body or mind. Using both together we can achieve a more integral treatment. Ayurveda gives us a specific view on present physical imbalances, while astrology shows us the long-term trends of the life and vitality.

The Vedic use of gems is grounded in a many thousand year old medical and astrological system. It is integrated with the use of colors and mantras as part of the system of yoga originated by enlightened sages. Ayurvedic doctors have carefully noted the internal effects of gem oxides. Hence, the Vedic system presents the oldest, most continually used and most validated system of gem therapy. Its insights should be carefully considered in any new gem therapy today. The following are introductory ideas. Medical astrology is a complex subject in itself and requires its own study.

ASTROLOGY AND GEM THERAPY

In Vedic astrology gems are correlated to the planets and used specifically to balance their influences. In this way gems are used astrologically to treat physical, mental and spiritual disorders. Gem therapy is the main astrological therapy and is usually prescribed according to astrological indications. It is best to have a professional Vedic astrologer look at ones birth chart before putting on a gem, particularly the more powerful and expensive primary gemstones.

While gems do have an influence on the physical body, their main action is on the level of prana and mind. For this reason gemstones cannot be related rigidly to the doshas. We cannot simply put on a gem to counter the doshas the way that we can take a food or an herb. Some gems, as subtle remedies, help balance all three doshas by harmonizing the prana or the mind.

We can also direct or balance the doshic action of gems according to the metal we set them in which serves as their vehicle. The same gem taken with gold, a warming metal, can have a different doshic effect than if taken with silver, a cooling metal. Different gems can be used to reduce the same dosha as well. For example, a ruby, red coral or yellow sapphire can all reduce Vata. In such instances it is best to use a gem that is more in harmony with ones birth chart.

Gems prescribed according to Vedic astrology can be taken internally for similar effects in Ayurveda. However, for internal usage they are specially treated by complex processes to render them safe and non-toxic to the body. Such gem preparations are still used in Ayurvedic medicines today. They are not available for sale in the United States, but we can use gem tinctures that do not actually involve taking the mineral itself.

Gems are worn externally as rings, bracelets or as pendants hanging down to the throat or heart. According to the Vedic system the fingers of the hand and the elements correspond:

Finger	Elements	Planets
Little finger	Earth	Mercury
Ring finger	Fire and water	Sun and Moon
Middle finger	Air	Saturn
Index finger	Ether	Jupiter

By wearing the gems relating to these respective elements or planets on the appropriate fingers, we can strengthen their influences. Venus stones can be worn on Saturn and Mercury Fingers.

398

Stones for Mars can be worn on the ring finger. Make sure to set the gems to actually touch the skin. This is necessary to transmit their energies fully.

Gem tinctures, like herb tinctures, are prepared by soaking the gem in a 50-100% alcohol solution. Hard gems like diamond or sapphire can be soaked for one month (from full moon to full moon). Soft gems, like pearl and coral, are soaked for shorter periods of time or in weaker solutions. Chanting of planetary mantras aids in giving power to the tincture.

GEMS, COLORS AND THE PLANETS

Planet	Gem	Substitutes Color	
SUN	Ruby	Garnet, Sunstone	Light Red
MOON	Pearl	Moonstone	White
MARS Red	Coral	Carnelian	Dark Red
MERCURY	Emerald	Peridot, Green Zircon	Green
JUPITER	Yellow Sapphire	Yellow Topaz, Citrine	Yellow
VENUS	Diamond	White Sapphire, Quartz Crystal	Variegated
SATURN	Blue Sapphire	Amethyst	Dark Blue
RAHU	Hessonite Garnet		Infrared
KETU	Cat's Eye, Chrysoberyl		Ultraviolet

This is the classical Vedic correspondence between the major precious gemstones and the planets. Since most of these stones are very expensive various substitutes can be used. Red coral is not expensive so substitution for it is not necessary. For those who cannot afford these gems one can use mantras or meditation to balance planetary energies.

USE OF GEMS IN ASTROLOGY AND AYURVEDA

The more expensive gemstones, worn as rings, should be two or more carats. The less expensive or substitutes are better in four or more. Even larger stones can be used, particularly for pendants or necklaces (in which case a good substitute stone would be better than a small size primary stone). Gemstones have stronger effects if they touch the skin. Hence rings made according to the Vedic system are open below, set to come into direct contact with the skin. Below I list the main properties of the primary gemstones. Their substitutes have similar but weaker qualitie

RUBY

Energies	Hot
Elements	Fire, air and ether
Doshas	Increases Pitta and decreases Kapha and Vata

Ruby is used in astrology for strengthening the heart, improving digestion, promoting circulation, reviving fire and increasing energy. Ruby strengthens the will, promotes independence, gives insight and enhances power; it was the gem of kings. It is usually set in gold and worn on the ring finger of the right hand.

Ruby ash (Manikya bhasma) is regarded as a stimulant, nervine and heart tonic for weakness of the heart and nerves, and for general debility.

PEARL

Energy	Slightly cold
Elements	Water, earth and ether
Doshas	Increases Kapha and decreases Pitta and Vata

Pearl is good for promoting body fluids and the blood, nourishing the body tissues and the nerves. It strengthens the female reproductive system, improves fertility, and calms the emotions. It is usually set in silver and worn on the ring finger of the left hand. Pearl ash (Moti bhasma) is said to be tonic, alterative, sedative, nervine and antacid. It is used for hyperacidity, ulcers, epistaxis, hemoptysis, liver and kidney ailments, nervous excitability, and hysteria and as a good general tonic for women and infants.

RED CORAL

Energy	Slightly warm
Elements	Earth, water and fire
Doshas	Decreases Vata, increases Kapha, harmonizes Pitta

Red coral strengthens the blood and reproductive system, improves energy and calms emotion. Red coral is an aphrodisiac, particularly for the male, builds flesh and muscle, gives courage and improves work capacity. It is usually set in silver and worn on the ring or index finger. Red coral ash (Praval bhasma) is alterative, antacid and tonic. It is used for cough, asthma, swollen glands, hyperacidity, impotence, bleeding from the lungs, anemia and sexual debility. It is also good for the bones.

EMERALD

Energy	Slightly cool
Elements	Water, air, ether
Doshas	Harmonizes Vata, decreases Pitta, increases Kapha

Emerald calms mental agitation, regulates the nervous system, helps stop nerve pain and improves speech and intelligence. Emerald promotes healing, energizes the breath, strengthens the lungs and increases flexibility and adaptability of mind. It is a harmonizing stone, good for cancer and other degenerative diseases. For Vata and Kapha it is set in gold, for Pitta silver. It is worn on the middle or little finger.

Emerald ash (Panna bhasma) is nervine, alterative and tonic. It is used for nervous debility, neurasthenia, and general debility and as a heart tonic. It is good for asthma, ulcers, skin diseases, fevers and infections and as a tonic for children.

YELLOW SAPPHIRE

Energy	Slightly warm
Elements	Ether, fire, water
Doshas	Balances doshas, lowers Vata, can increase Pitta

Ayurvedic Healing

Yellow sapphire gives energy and vitality and is the best general stone for promoting health. It regulates the hormonal system and increases Ojas. Yellow sapphire is good for diabetes and all wasting diseases and for convalescence. It is usually set in gold and worn on the index finger.

Yellow sapphire ash is tonic, alterative and nervine. It improves digestion, strengthens the heart and brings about an increase of intelligence.

DIAMOND

Energy	Slightly cooling
Elements	Ether, water
Doshas	Decreases Vata and Pitta but increases Kapha

Diamond strengthens the kidneys and reproductive system and enhances Ojas. Diamond gives beauty, power and charm and enhances our creative abilities. It protects our life in extreme diseases. It is usually set in white gold and worn on the middle or little finger.

Diamond ash (Hira bhasma) is tonic, nutritive and aphrodisiac. It gives strength and firmness to the body, protects the life, and increases sexual power and Ojas. Zircon ash (Vaikrant bhasma) can be used as a substitute.

BLUE SAPPHIRE

Energy	Cold
Elements	Ether, air
Doshas	Decreases Pitta and Kapha, increases Vata

Blue sapphire clears infections and wards off negative energies. It is antitumor and antifat and good for reducing therapy. Blue sapphire strengthens the bones, increases longevity and helps calm the nerves and emotions. It promotes calm, peace and detachments. For Vata and Kapha it is set in gold, for Pitta, silver. It is worn on the middle finger.

Blue sapphire ash is used as an alterative, nervine and antiseptic. It is good for arthritis, rheumatism, fevers, infections, nerve pain and paralysis.

HESSONITE GARNET

Energy	Slightly warm
Elements	Fire, water, ether
Doshas	Balances doshas, lowers Vata, can increase Pitta

Like the yellow sapphire, golden hessonite is a good balancing stone. It calms the nerves, quiets the mind, and relieves depression. This stone is recommended for almost everyone as it counters the negative influence of Maya (illusion). The north lunar node is thought to indicate the influence of Maya, which is predominant in the materialistic age in which we live. Hessonite garnet is usually set in gold and worn on the middle finger. No ash of it is commonly made.

CAT'S EYE

Energy	Hot
Elements	Fire, air, ether
Doshas	Decreases Kapha and Vata, increases Pitta

Cat's eye is hot in energy and composed of the elements of fire, air and ether. It stimulates Tejas, mental fire, and is good for promoting psychic and spiritual perception. Cat's eye is a good nervine stimulant and is helpful for mental disorders. It is the gemstone of seers and astrologers. It also is not usually found as an ash.

Quartz Crystal

The commonly used quartz crystal is also used in the Vedic system. Clear quartz is considered a Venus stone, cloudy or milky is a Moon stone. Clear quartz has an action similar to diamond but much weaker. It is regarded as a very impressionable stone that magnifies whatever influence, good or bad, is around it. Hence, it should be purified and energized properly through mantra and meditation. Rock crystal ash (Sphatika bhasma) is alterative, hemostatic and tonic and used to treat bleeding disorders, anemia, chronic fever, jaundice, asthma, constipation and debility.

GEMS AND HERBS

Gems, when appropriate astrologically, can be used to enhance the effects of various herbs.

- Hot, spicy herbs – Ruby tincture or by wearing a ruby or its substitutes.
- Tonic and rejuvenative herbs – Yellow sapphire or yellow topaz tincture or by wearing these stones or their substitutes.
- Herbs to clear heat, cleanse the blood, detoxify the liver and reduce tumors – Blue sapphire tincture or by wearing the stone or its substitutes.
- Nervine and harmonizing herbs – Emerald tincture or by wearing an emerald or its substitutes.
- Stimulant and aphrodisiac herbs – Red coral tincture or by wearing of red coral.
- Emmenagogue herbs or tonics to the reproductive system – Diamond tincture or by wearing of diamond or its substitutes.
- Demulcent and nutritive tonic herbs – Pearl tincture or by wearing of pearl and its substitute.

2. MANTRA THERAPY

Mantra is the means of energizing healing methods on a subtle or spiritual level. Through mantra we place an energy of Divine sound into healing. We also energize healing methods on a mental or spiritual level with the energy of consciousness. Such mantras can be used to energize herbs, to direct prana or to simply encourage healing at a deeper level.

Generally a mantra should be done on a regular basis for several months for its desired effect to take place, which is to alter the nature of the mind and prana, particularly the subconscious mind and its impulses and instincts which are behind most of our problems in life. One hundred thousand repetitions are recommended for full energization.

Main Bija Mantras: Seed Syllables for Healing

These are powerful mantras for general healing, energy and transformation purposes. They direct the Shakti or the higher power of consciousness.

OM — The most important mantra. Serves to energize or empower all things and all processes. Therefore all mantras begin and end with OM. It clears the mind, opens the channels and increases Ojas. In ancient books OM is the sound of the Sun and carries the energy of Prana.

SHRIM (shreem) — The best mantra for promoting general health, beauty, creativity and prosperity. It has lunar and Venusian properties and can strengthen the feminine nature.

RAM (a-sound as in father) — The best mantra for drawing down the protective light and grace of the Divine. It gives strength, calm, rest and peace and is particularly good for high Vata and mental disorders.

HUM (u-sound as in put) — The best mantra for warding off negative influences attacking us, whether disease-causing pathogens, negative emotions or even black magic. It is also the best mantra for awakening Agni and promoting the digestive fire.

AIM (aym) — The best mantra for the mind, for improving concentration, thinking, for rational powers and for improving speech. It is helpful in mental and nervous disorders. It has a Mercury energy and corresponds to the Goddess of Wisdom, Saraswati.

KRIM (cream) — Gives the capacity for work and action and gives power and efficacy to what we do. It is good for chanting while making preparations as it allows them to work better.

KLIM (kleem) — Gives strength, sexual vitality and control of the emotional nature.

SHAM (a-sound as in shut) — The mantra for Saturn used generally for promoting peace, calm, detachment and contentment. It is good for mental and nervous disorders.

HRIM (hreem) — is a mantra of cleansing and purification. It gives energy, joy and ecstasy but only after atonement. It aids any detoxification process.

Mantras for the Elements

Mantra	Element	Sense	Tissue	Chakra
LAM	Earth	Smell, Nose	Muscles	Root Chakra
VAM	Water	Taste, Tongue	Fat tissue	Sex Chakra
RAM	Fire	Sight, Eyes	Blood	Navel Chakra
YAM	Air	Touch, Skin	Plasma	Heart Chakra
HAM	Ether	Sound, Ears	Prana	Throat Chakra

The five elements and their corresponding senses, tissues and chakras can be strengthened by their respective mantras. In each case the 'a-sound is short, like the e-vowel sound in the.

Part IV
APPENDICES

1. Sanskrit Terms

Alochak Pitta	form of fire governing vision
Ama	toxins, the undigested food mass
Ambhuvaha Srotas	channels carrying water
Annavaha Srotas	channels carrying food
Apana	downward moving air
Arishta	herbal wine made with decoctions
Artavavaha Srotas	channels carrying menstrual fluid
Asanas	yoga postures
Asava	herbal wine made with juice of herbs
Asthi	bone
Atman	true Self
Avalambaka Kapha	form of water giving support
Avaleha	herbal jelly
Ayurveda	Vedic science of life or longevity
Bhakti	devotion
Bhasma	specially incinerated mineral preparation
Bhrajaka Pitta	form of fire governing complexion
Bodhaka Kapha	form of water governing taste
Brahma	reality; the absolute
Brahmacharya	control of sexuality; celibacy
Brimhana	tonification or building therapy
Buddha	the enlightened one; an incarnation of Vishnu
Chikitsa	Ayurvedic treatment
Churna	herbal powder
Dhanvantari	traditional deity of Ayurveda
Dharana	attention
Dhyana	meditation
Ghee	clarified butter
Ghrita	clarified butter
Guggul	pills made with guggul (Commiphora mukul)
Guna	prime quality of nature (Prakriti)
Jnana	Vedic or Hindu astrology
Kapha	biological water-humor
Karma	action
Kledaka Kapha	form of water governing digestion
Kratu	inner will
Kundalini	energy of the subtle body

Langhana	or lightening therapy
Majja	marrow and nerve tissue
Majjavaha Srotas	channels supplying marrow and nerve tissue
Mamsa	muscle
Mamsavaha Srotas	channels supplying muscle
Manas	mind
Manovaha Srotas	channels carrying thought
Mantra	healing sounds, sacred words
Medas	fat tissue
Medovaha Srotas	channels supplying fat tissue
Mutra	urine
Mutravaha Srotas	channels carrying urine
Nasya	nasal application of herbs and oils
Nirama	conditions without Ama
Niyama	yogic observances
Ojas	prime energy of the body
Patch Pitta	form of fire governing digestion
Pancha Karma	the five purification practices of Ayurveda
Pariksha	examination, diagnosis
Pitta	biological fire-humor
Prana	life-force; inward-moving air
Pranavaha Srotas	channels carrying the life-force
Pranayama	breath control, yogic breathing practices
Prakriti	primal Nature; biological constitution
Prash	herbal jelly
Pratyahara	yogic control of the senses
Puja	devotional worship or flower offering
Purisha	feces
Purishavaha Srotas	channels carrying feces
Purusha	pure Spirit
Ranjaka Pitta	form of fire coloring the blood
Rajas	quality of energy, turbulence and distraction
Rakta	blood
Rakta Moksha	blood purification
Raktavaha Srotas	channels carrying the blood
Rasa	plasma; special Ayurvedic mineral reparations
Rasayana	rejuvenative
Rasavaha Srotas	channels carrying plasma
Rig Veda	most ancient scripture of India
Sadhaka Pitta	form of fire governing intelligence
Sama Kapha	Ama condition of Kapha
Sama Pitta	Ama condition of Pitta
Sama Vata	Ama condition of Vata
Samadhi	yogic absorption

Samana	equalizing air, governs digestion
Sattva	quality of clarity and harmony, the mind in its natural state
Shamana	palliation therapy
Shodhana	purification therapy
Shukra	reproductive tissue
Shukravaha Srotas	channels supplying the reproductive tissue
Sleshaka Kapha	form of water lubricating the joints
Snehana	oil application
Srotas	channel system of the body
Stanyavaha Srotas	channels carrying the breast milk
Sveda	sweat
Svedana	therapeutic sweating, steam therapy
Svedavaha Srotas	channels carrying sweat
Taila	medicated oil, mainly with sesame oil
Tapas	asceticism; spiritual work
Tarpaka Kapha	form of water governing emotion
Udana	upward moving air
Upanishads	ancient spiritual teachings of India
Vamana	emesis; therapeutic vomiting
Vata	biological air-humor
Vedas	ancient scriptures of India
Vedanta	final or summary portion of the Vedas
Vikriti	disease nature
Virechana	purgation
Vyana	diffusive or outward moving air
Yama	yogic attitudes
Yoga	practice of spiritual reintegration

2. GLOSSARY OF HERBS

Western Herbs and Commonly Known Ayurvedic Herbs

English	Latin	Sanskrit or Hindi
Agrimony	Agrimonia eupatori	
Alfalfa	Medicago sativa	Lasunghas
Almond	Amygdalus communis	Vatatma
Aloe	Aloe spp.	Kumari
Alum root	Heuchera americana	
American ginseng	Panax quinquifolium	
Angelica	Angelica spp.	Choraka
Apricot seeds	Prunus armenica	Jardalu
Arnica	Arnica montana	
Barberry	Berberis spp.	Daruharidra
Basil	Ocinum spp.	Tulsi
Bay leaves	Laurus nobilis	
Bayberry	Myrica spp.	Katiphala
Betony	Stachys betonica	
Black cohosh	Cimicifuga racemosa	
Black pepper	Piper nigrum	Marich
Burdock	Arctium lappa	
Calamus	Acorus calamus	Vacha
Calendula	Calendula officinalis	Zergul
Camomile	Anthemum nobilis	Babuna
Camphor	Cinnamomum camphora	Karpura
Cardamom	Eletarria cardamomum	Ela
Cascara sagrada	Rhamnus purshianus	
Castor oil	Ricinis communis	Eranda
Catechu	Acacia catechu	Khadir
Catnip	Nepeta cataria	Zufa
Cattail	Typha spp.	Eraka
Cayenne pepper	Capsicum frutescens	Katuvira
Cedar	Cedrus spp.	Devadaru
Chaparral	Larrea divaracata	
Chickweed	Stellaria media	
Chicory	Cichorium intybus	Kasani
Chrysanthemum	Chrysanthemum indicum	Sevanti
Cilantro	Coriandrum sativum (leaf)	Dhanyaka
Cinnamon	Cinnamomum zeylonica	Tvak
Cleavers	Galium spp.	
Cloves	Syzgium aromaticum	Lavanga
Cocklebur	Xanthium strumarium	Arista
Coltsfoot	Tussilago farfara	Fanjuim
Comfrey	Symphytum officinale	

Coptis	Coptis spp.	Mishamitita
Coriander	Coriandrum sativum (seed)	Dhanyaka
Corn silk	Zea mays	Yavanala
Cubebs	Piper cubeba	Kankola
Cumin	Cumin cyminum	Jiraka
Damiana	Turnera aphrodisiaca	
Dandelion	Taraxacum vulgare	Dughdapheni
Dates	Phoenix dactylifera	Kharjur
Datura	Datura alba	Kanaka-dattura
Dill	Anthemum vulgaris	Mishreya
Echinacea	Echinacea angustifolia	
Elecampane	Inula spp.	Pushkaramula
Elder flowers	Sambucus glauca	
Ephedra	Ephedra spp.	Somalata
Evening Primrose	Oenethra biennis	
Eucalyptus	Eucalyptus globulis	Tailaparni
Fennel	Foeniculum vulgare	Shatapushpa
Fenugreek	Trigonella foenumgraecum	Methi
Flaxseed	Linum usitatissimum	Uma
Fo ti	Polygonum multiflorum	
Frankincense	Boswellia carteri	Dhup
Galangal	Alpinia officinarum	Rasna
Gardenia	Gardenia floribunda	Nadihingu
Garlic	Allium sativum	Lashuna
Gentian	Gentiana spp.	Trayamana
Ginger	Zingiberis officinalis	Ardra (fresh), Shunthi (dry)
Ginseng	Panax ginseng	Lakshmana
Goldenseal	Hydrastis canadensis	
Gotu kola	Centella asiatica	Brahmi
Gravel root	Eupatorium purpuerum	
Grindelia	Grindelia robusta	
Hawthorn berries	Crataegus oxycantha	Ban-sangli
Henna	Lawsonia spp.	Mendhi
Hibiscus	Hibiscus rosa-sinensis	Japa
Horehound	Marrubium vulgare	Farasiyun
Horsetail	Equisetum spp.	
Hyssop	Hyssopus officinalis	Zupha
Iris	Iris spp.	Padma-pushkara
Irish moss	Chondrus crispus	
Jasmine	Jasminum grandiflorum	Jati
Juniper berries	Juniperus spp.	Hapusha

Kelp	Fucus visiculosis	
Lavender	Lavendula spp.	Dharu
Lemon	Citrus limonum	Limpaka
Lemon balm	Melissa officinalis	
Lemon grass	Cymbopogon citratus	Rohisha
Licorice	Glycyzrrhiza spp.	Yashtimadhu
Lime	Citrus acida	Nimbuka
Liquidamber	Liquidamber spp.	
Lobelia	Lobelia inflata	Dhavala
Lotus	Nelumbo nucifera	Padma
Male fern	Dryopteris felix-mas	
Marigold	Tagetes erecta	Jhandu
Marshmallow	Althea officinalis	Gulkairo
Mint	Mentha arvensis	Phudina
Motherwort	Leonurus cardiaca	Guma
Mugwort	Artemesia vulgaris	Nagadamani
Mustard	Brassica alba	Svetasarisha
Myrrh	Commiphora myrrha	Bola
Nettle	Urtica urens	Bichu
Nutmeg	Myristica fragrans	Jatiphala
Oak bark	Quercus spp.	Majuphul
Orange peel	Citrus aurantium	Svadu-naringa
Oregano	Origanum vulgare	Sathra
Osha	Ligusticum porteri	
Parsley	Petroselium spp.	
Passion flower	Passiflora incarnata	Mukkopira
Pau d'arco	Tabebuia avellenada	
Peach seeds	Prunus persica	Pichu
Pennyroyal	Mentha pulegium	
Peppermint	Mentha piperata	Gamathi phudina
Pine	Pinus spp.	Shriveshtaka
Pink root	Spigelia marilandica	
Pipsissewa	Chimaphilla umbellata	
Plantain	Plantago spp.	Lahuriya
Plumeria	Plumeria alba	
Potentilla	Potentilla spp.	Spangjha
Prickly ash	Zanthoxylum spp.	Tumburu
Pomegranate	Punica granatum	Dadima
Pumpkin seeds	Curcubito pepo	Kurlaru
Purslane	Portulaca oleracea	Loni
Psyllium	Plantago psyllium	Snigdha-jira
Red clover	Trifolium pratense	Trepatra
Red raspberry	Rubus spp.	Gauriphal
Rhubarb root	Rheum spp.	Amlavetasa

412

Rose	Rosa spp.	Shatapatra
Rosemary	Rosemarinus officinalis	Rusmari
Rue	Ruta graveolens	Sadapaha
Safflower	Carthamus tinctorius	Kusumba
Saffron	Crocus sativa	Kumkum
Sage	Salvia spp.	Shati
Sandalwood	Santalum alba	Chandana
Santonica	Artemesia santonica	Gadadhar
Sarsaparilla	Smilax spp.	Chopchini
Sassafras	Sassafras officinale	
Saw palmetto	Serenoa repens	
Self-heal	Prunella vulgaris	
Senna	Cassia acutifolia	Nripadruma
Sesame	Sesamum indicum	Til
Siberian ginseng	Eleuthrococcus senticosus	
Skullcap	Scutellaria spp.	
Slippery elm	Ulmus fulva	
Spearmint	Mentha spictata	Pahadi phudina
Spikenard	Aralia racemosus	
Squaw vine	Mitchella repens	
Solomon's seal	Polygonatum officinalis	Mahameda
Southernwood	Artemesia abrotanum	
Strawberry leaf	Fragaria spp.	
Sumac	Rhus glabra	Karkata shringi
Tansy	Tanacatum vulgare	
Thyme	Thymus vulgarus	Ipar
Turmeric	Curcuma longa	Haridra
Usnea	Usnea barbata	
Uva ursi	Arctostaphylos uva-ursi	
Valerian	Valeriana spp.	Tagara
Vetivert	Andropogon muricatus	Ushira
Violet	Viola spp.	Banafshah
Wild cherry bark	Prunus virginiana	
Wild ginger	Asarum spp.	Upana
Wintergreen	Gaultheria procumbens	Gandapura
Witch hazel	Hamamelis virgiana	
Wormseed	Chenopodium anthelminticum	Chandanbatva
Wormwood	Artemesia absinthium	Indhana
Yarrow	Achillea millefolium	Rojmari
Yellow dock	Rumex crispus	Amlavetasa
Yerba santa	Eriodityon glutinosum	
Yohimbe	Caryanthe yohimbe	
Yucca	Yucca spp.	

ADDITIONAL SPECIAL AYURVEDIC HERBS

First is the common name and then the Latin and Sanskrit.
When the Sanskrit is the common name it is not repeated.

Common Name	Latin	Sanskrit
Aconite	Aconitum napellus	Visa
Ajwan	Apium graveolens	Ajamoda
Amalaki	Emblica officinalis	
Arjuna	Terminalia arjuna	
Asafoetida	Ferula asafoetida	Hingu
Ashok	Saraca indica	
Ashwagandha	Withania somnifera	
Bakuchi	Psoralea corylifolia	
Bala	Sida cordifolia	
Betel nuts	Areca catechu	Kramuka
Bhallataka	Semecarpus anacardium	
Bhringaraj	Eclipta alba	
Bhumyamalaki	Phyllanthus niruri	
Bibhitaki	Terminalia belerica	
Black musali	Curculigo orchiodes	Kala musali
Chiretta	Swertia chiratata	Kirata tikta
Chitrak	Plumbago zeylonica	
Cuscuta	Cuscuta reflexa	Amaravalli
Cyperus	Cyperus rotundus	Musta
Dhataki	Woodfordia floribunda	
Garcinia camboga		
Gokshura	Tribulis terrestris	
Guduchi	Tinospora cordifolia	also Amrit
Guggul	Commiphora mukul	
Gurmar	Gymena sylvestre	Meshashringi
Haritaki	Terminalia chebula	
Holy Basil	Ocimum sanctum	Tulsi
Indian sarsaparilla	Hemedesmis indica	Anantamul
Isatis	Isatis spp.	Nila
Jatamamsi	Nardostachys jatamamsi	
Kapikacchu	Mucuna pruriens	
Katuka	Picrorrhiza kurroa	
Kutaj	Holarrhena antidysenterica	
Lodhra	Symplocus racemosus	
Pippali	Piper longum	Pippali
Manjishta (Indian madder)	Rubia cordifolium	
Neem	Azadiracta indica	Nimbu
Nirgundi	Vitex negundo	
Nishot	Ipomoea turpethum	
Pashana bheda	Bergenia spp.	

Prasarini	Paedaria foetida	
Punarnava	Boerrhavia diffusa	
Sarpagandha	Rawolfia serpentina	
Saussurea	Saussurea lappa	Kushta
Shankhapushpi	Crotalaria verrucosa	
Shallaki		
Shatavari	Asparagus racemosus	
Shilajit	Asphaltum	
Vamsha rochana	Bambusa arundinacea	
Vidanga	Embelia ribes	
White musali	Asparagus adscendens	Shveta musali
Zedoaria	Curcuma zedoaria	Kachura

SPECIAL CHINESE HERBS

First is the common name, then the Latin and Chinese. When the common name is the Chinese, it is not repeated.

Common Name	Latin	Chinese
Astragalus	Astragalus mongolicus	Huang qi
Biota seeds	Biota orientalis	Bai zi ren
Bupleurum	Bupleurum falcatum	Chai hu
Cimicifuga	Cimicifuga racemosa	Sheng ma
Citrus peel	Citrus reticulata	Chen pi
Corydalis	Corydalis	Yuan hu suo
Dang shen	Codonopsis pilosula	
Desmodian	Desmodian styracifolium	Jin qian cao
Dioscorea	Dioscorea opposita	Shan yao
Du huo	Angelica dahurica	
Eucommia	Eucommia ulmoidis	Du Zhong
Forsythia	Forsythia suspensa	Lian qiao
Fritillary	Fritillaria cirrhosa	Chuan bei mu
Gentiana macrophylla		Qin jiao
He shou wu (fo ti)	Polygonum multiflorum	
Hoelen	Poria cocos	Fu ling
Honeysuckle	Lonicera	Jin yin hua
Ligusticum	Ligusticum wallichi	Chuan xion
Ligustrum	Ligustrum lucidum	Nu zhen zi
Loranthus	Loranthus parasiticus	Sang ji sheng
Lycium	Lycium chinense	Go ji zi
Lygodium	Lygodium japonicum	Hai jin sha
Magnolia bark	Magnolia officinalis	Hou pu
Magnolia flower	Magnolia liliflora	Xin yi hua
Ma Huang	Ephedra sinica	

415

Oldenlandia	Oldenlandia diffusa	Bai hua she she ao
Ophiopogon	Ophiopogon japonicus	Mai men dong
Phellodendron	Phellodendron amurense	Huang bai
Perilla leaf	Perilla frutescens	Zi su ye
Pinellia	Pinellia ternata	Ban xia
Pseudoginseng	Panax pseudoginseng	San qi
Pueraria (kudzu)	Pueraria lobata	Ge gen
Qiang huo	Notopterygium incisum	
Red Peony	Paeonia obovata	Chi shao yao
Rehmannia	Rehmannia glutinosa	Di huang
Salvia	Salvia miltorrhiza	Dan shen
Schizandra	Schizandra chinensis	Wu wei zi
Scute	Scutellaria baicalensis	Huang qin
Spargania	Sparganium simplex	San leng
Tang kuei	Angelica sinensis	Dang gui
Trichosanthes root	Trichosanthes kirlowii	Tian hua fe
White atractylodes	Atractylodes alba	Bai zhu
White peony	Paeonia lactiflora	Bai shao yao
Zizyphus	Zizyphus spinosa	Suan cao ren

CHINESE HERBAL FORMULAS

Anemarrhena, Phellodendron and Rehmannia	Zhi bai di huang wan
Bupleurum and Tang kuei	Xiao yao san
Cannabis seed comb.	Ma zi ren wan
Capillaris comb.	Yin chen hao tang
Cinnamon branch decoction	Gui zhi tang
Citrus and Craetagus	Bao he wan
Coptis and Rhubarb	San huang xie xin tang
Coptis and Scute	Huang lien jie du tang
Dianthus comb.	Ba zheng san
Four Gentlemen	Si jun zi tang
Four Materials	Si wu tang
Gentian comb.	Long dan xie gan tang
Gypsum comb.	Bai hu tang
Honeysuckle and Forsythia	Yin qiao san
Magnolia and Ginger	Ping wei san
Ma huang decoction	Ma huang tang
Minor Bupleurum	Xiao chai hu tang
Minor Pinellia and Hoelen	Xiao ban xia jia fu ling tang
Minor Rhubarb	Xiao cheng qi tang
Major Blue Dragon	Da qing long tang
Major Bupleurum	Da chai hu tang

Major Rhubarb
Ophiopogon comb.
Persica and Rhubarb
Polyporus combination
Pueraria, Coptis and Scute
Rehmannia 6
Rehmannia 8
Shou wu pian
Tang kuei and Gelatin
Tang kuei and Peony
Ten Major Tonification formula
Woman's Precious Pill

Da cheng qi tang
Mai men dong tang
Tao he cheng qi tang
Zhu ling tang
Ge gen huang qin huang lian tang
Liu wei di huang wan
Jing gui shen qi wan

Jiao ai tang
Dang gui shao yao san
Shi quan da bu tang
Ba zhen tang

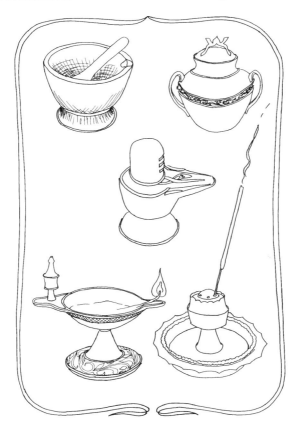

3. Bibilography

Bensky, Dan, Andrew Gamble. *Chinese Herbal Medicine Materia Medica*. Seattle WA: Eastland Press, 1986.

Frawley, David. *Astrology of the Seers*. Twin Lakes, Wisconsin: Lotus Press, 2000.

Frawley. Dr. David. *Ayurveda and the Mind*. Twin Lakes, Wisconsin: Lotus Press, 1997.

Frawley. Dr. David. *Yoga and Ayurveda*. Twin Lakes, Wisconsin: Lotus Press, 1999.

Frawley, Dr. David and Dr. Vasant Lad. *The Yoga of Herbs*. Twin Lakes, Wisconsin: Lotus Press, 1986.

Joshi, Dr. Sunil. *Ayurveda and Pancha Karma*. Twin Lakes, Wisconsin: Lotus Press 1997.

Lad, Dr. Vasant. *Ayurveda, The Science of Self-healing*. Twin Lakes, Wisconsin: Lotus Press, 1984.

Lad, Dr. Vasant. *The Complete Book of Ayurvedic Home Remedies*. New York City: Harmony Books, 1998.

Morningstar, Amadea. *The Ayurvedic Cookbook*. Twin Lakes, Wisconsin: Lotus Press, 1992.

Morningstar, Amadea. *Ayurvedic Cooking for Westerners*. Twin Lakes, Wisconsin: Lotus Press, 1996.

Nadkarni. *Indian Materia Medica*. Bombay, India: Popular Prakashan, 1976.

Smith, Atreya. *Ayurvedic Healing for Women*. Twin Lakes, Wisconsin: Lotus Press, 2007.

Smith, Atreya. *Practical Ayurveda*. York Beach, Maine: Samuel Weiser, 1997.

Tierra, Michael. *Planetary Herbology*. Twin Lakes, Wisconsin: Lotus Press, 1988.

Tierra, Michael. *The Way of Herbs*. New York, NY: Washington Square Press, 1983.

Yeung, Him-che, *Handbook of Chinese Herbs and Formulas* (two volumes). Los Angeles, CA: Institute of Chinese Medicine, 1985.

Sanskrit Texts Used

Charaka. *Charaka Samhita*
Krishna. *Bhagavad Gita*
Patanjali. *Yoga Sutras*
Rig Veda Samhita
Sushruta. *Sushruta Samhita*
Upanishads
Vagbhatta. *Ashtanga Hridaya*

4. Resources

Quintessence Aromatherapy
Attn: Ann Berwick
P. O. Box 4996
Boulder, CO 80306
Ph: 303-258-3791

Ayurveda Centers and Programs
Australian Institute of
Ayurvedic Medicine
19 Bowey Avenue
Enfield S.A. 5085
Australia
Ph: 08-349-7303

Australian School of Ayurveda
Dr. Krishna Kumar, MD, FIIM
27 Blight Street
Ridleyton, South Australia 5008
Ph. 08-346-0631

Ayur-Veda AB
Box 78, 285 22 Markaryd
Esplanaden 2
Sweden
0433-104 90 (Phone)
0433-104 92 (Fax)
E-mail: info@ayur-veda.se

Ayurveda for Radiant Health &
Beauty
16 Espira Court
Santa Fe, NM 87505
Ph: 505-466-7662

Ayurvedic HealingArts Center
16508 Pine Knoll Road
Grass Valley, CA 95945
Ph: 916-274-9000

Ayurvedic Healings
Dr's Light & Bryan Miller
P. O. Box 35214
Sarasota, FL 34242
Ph: 941-346-3581

Ayurvedic Holistic Center
82A Bayville Ave.
Bayville, NY 11709

The Ayurvedic Institute and
Wellness Center
11311 Menaul, NE
Albuquerque, NM 87112
Ph: 505-291-9698
Fax: 505-294-7572

Ayurvedic LivingWorkshops
P. O. Box 188
Exeter, Devon EX4 5AB
England

California College of Ayurveda
1117A East Main Street
Grass Valley, CA 95945
Ph: 530-274-9100
Website: ayurvedacollege.com
E-mail: info@ayurvedacollege.com

Clinical training in Ayurveda
Center for Mind, Body Medicine
P. O. Box 1048
La Jolla, CA 92038
Ph: 619-794-2425

The Chopra Center for Well Being
7590 Fay Avenue
Suite 403
LaJolla, CA 92037
Ph: 619-551-7788
Fax: 619-551-7811

John Douillard
Life Spa, Rejuvenation through
Ayur-Veda
3065 Center Green Dr.
Boulder, CO 80301
Ph: 303-442-1164
Fax: 303-442-1240

East West College of Herbalism
Ayurvedic Program
Represents courses of Dr. David
Frawley and Dr. Michael Tierra in UK
Hartswood, Marsh Green, Hartsfield
E. Sussex TN7 4ET, United Kingdom
Ph: 01342-822312
Fax: 01342-826346
E-mail: ewcolherb@aol.com

Himalayan Institute
RR1, Box 400
Honesdale, PA 18431
Ph: 800-822-4547
E-mail: earthess@aol.com
Website: ayurvedichealing.com

Institute for Wholistic Education
3425 Patzke In. Racine,WI 53405
Ph: 262-619-1798
Beginner and Advanced
Correspondence Courses in Ayurveda.
Website: www.wholisticinstitute.org

Integrated Health Systems
3855 Via Nova Marie, #302D
Carmel, CA 93923
Ph: 408-476-5130

International Academy of Ayurved
NandNandan, Atreya Rugnalaya
M.Y. Lele Chowk
Erandawana, Pune
411 004, India
Ph/Fax: 91-212-378532/524427
E-mail: avilele@hotmail.com

International Ayurvedic Institute
111 Elm Street/Suite 103-105
Worcester, MA 01609
Ph: 508-755-3744
Fax: 508-770-0618
E-mail: ayurveda@hotmail.com
International Federation of Ayurveda

Dr. Krishna Kumar
27 Blight Street
Ridleyton S.A. 5008
Australia
Ph: 08-346-0631

Kaya Kalpa International
Dr. Raam Panday
111 Woodster Rd.
Satto, NY 10012

Life Impressions Institute
Attn: Donald VanHowten, Director
613 Kathryn Street
Santa Fe, NM 87501
Ph: 505-988-2627

Light Institute of Ayurveda
Dr's Bryan & Light Miller
P. O. Box 35284
Sarasota, FL 34242
E-mail: earthess@aol.com
Website: ayurvedichealings.com

Lotus Ayurvedic Center
4145 Clares St.
Suite D
Capitola, CA 95010
Ph: 408-479-1667

Lotus Press
P. O. Box 325/Dept. AH
Twin Lakes, WI 53181 USA
Ph: 262-889-8561
Fax: 262-889-8591
E-mail: lotuspress@lotuspress.com
Website: www.lotuspress.com
Publisher of books on Ayurveda,
Reiki, aromatherapy, energetic heal-
ing, herbalism, alternative health
and U.S. editions of Sri Aurobindo's
writings.

420

Maharishi Ayurved at the Raj
1734 Jasmine Avenue
Fairfield, IA 52556
Ph: 800-248-9050
Fax: 515-472-2496

Maharishi Health Center
Hale Clinic
7 Park Crescent
London, W14 3H3, England

Natural Therapeutics Center
Surya Daya
Gisingham, Nr. Iye
Suffolk, England
New England Institute of
Ayurvedic Medicine
111 N. Elm Street, Suites 103-105
Worcester, MA 01609
Ph: 508-755-3744
Fax: 508-770-0618
E-mail: ayurveda@hotmail.com

Rocky Mountain Ayurveda Health
Retreat
P. O. Box 5192
Pagosa Springs, CO 81147
Ph: 800-247-9654; 970-264-9224

Atreya Smith, Director
European Institute of Vedic Studies
Ceven Point N° 230
4 bis rue Taisson
30100 Ales, France
Fax: 33-466-60-53-72
E-mail: atreya@compuserve.com
Website: www.atreya.com

Vinayak Ayurveda Center
2509 Virginia NE, Suite D
Albuquerque, NM 87110
Ph: 505-296-6522
Fax: 505-298-2932
Website: www.ayur.com

Wise Earth School of Ayurveda
Attn: Bri. Maya Tiwari
90 Davis Creek Road
Candler, NC 28715
Ph: 828-258-9999
Fax: 828-667-0844
Teachers and Practitioners Training
Programs Only.

AYURVEDIC COSMETIC COMPANIES:
Auroma International
P. O. Box 1008, Dept. AH
Silver Lake, WI 53170
Ph: 262-889-8569
Fax: 262-889 8591
E-mail: auroma@lotuspress.com
Website: www.auroma.net
Importer and master distributor of
Auroshikha Incense, Chandrika
Ayurvedic Soap and Herbal Vedic
Ayurvedic products.

Bindi Facial Skin Care
A Division of Pratima Inc.
109-17 72nd Road
Lower Level
Forest Hills, New York 11375
Ph: 718-268-7348

Devi Inc. (for Shivani product line)
Attn: Anjali Mahaldar
P. O. Box 377
Lancaster, MA 01523
Ph: 800-237-8221
Fax: 508-368-0455

Internatural
PO Box 489 CTM
Twin Lakes, WI 53181 USA
800-643-4221 (toll free order line)
262-889-8581 (office phone)
262-889-8591 (fax)
E-mail: internatural@lotuspress.com
Website: www.internatural.com

421

Retail mail order and internet reseller of Ayurvedic products, essential oils, herbs, spices, supplements, herbal remedies, incense, books, and other supplies.

Lotus Brands, Inc.
P. O. Box 325/Dept. AH
Twin Lakes, WI 53181 USA
Ph: 262-889-8561
Fax: 262-889-8591
E-mail: lotusbrands@lotuspress.com
Website: www.lotusbrands.com
Manufacturer and distributor of natural personal care and herbal products, massage oils, essential oils, incense, aromatherapy items, dietary supplements and herbs.

Lotus Light Enterprises
P. O. Box 1008/Dept. AH
Silver Lake, WI 53170 USA
800-548 3824 (toll free order line)
262-889 8501 (office phone)
262-889 8591 (fax)
E-mail: lotuslight@lotuspress.com
Website: www.lotuslight.com
Wholesale distributor of essential oils, herbs, spices, supplements, herbal remedies, incense, books and other supplies. Must supply resale certificate number or practitioner license to obtain catalog of more than 10,000 items.

Siddhi Ayurvedic Beauty Products
C/O Vinayak Ayurveda Center
2509 Virginia NE, Suite D
Albuquerque, NM 87110
Ph: 505-296-6522
Fax: 505-298-2932

Swami Sada Shiva Tirtha
Ayurvedic Holistic Center
82A Bayville Avenue
Bayville, NY 11709
Ph/Fax: 516-628-8200

TEJ Beauty Enterprises, Inc.
(an AyurvedicBeauty Salon)
162 West 56th St. Rm 201
New York, NY 10019
(owner: Pratima Raichur, founder of Bindi)
Ph: 212-581-8136

Ayurvedic Herbal Suppliers:
Auroma International
P. O. Box 1008
Dept. AH
Silver Lake, WI 53170
Ph: 262-889-8569
Fax: 262-889 8591
E-mail: auroma@lotuspress.com
Website: www.auroma.net
Importer and master distributor of Auroshikha Incense, Chandrika Ayurvedic Soap and Herbal Vedic Ayurvedic products.

Ayur Herbal Corporation
P. O. Box 6390
Santa Fe, NM 87502
Ph: 262-889-8569
Manufacturer of Herbal Vedic Ayurvedic products.

Ayush Herbs, Inc.
10025 N.E. 4th Street
Bellevue, WA 98004
Ph: 800-925-1371

Banyan Trading Company
Traditional Ayurvedic Herbs - Wholesale
P. O. Box 13002
Albuquerque, NM 87192
Ph: 505-244-1880; 800-953-6424
Fax: 505-244-1878

Bazaar of India Imports, Inc.
1810 University Avenue
Berkeley, CA 94703
Ph: 800-261-7662; 510-548-4110

Dhanvantri Aushadhalaya
Herbs of Wisdom and Love, Ayurvedic
Herbs and Classical Formulas.
P. O. Box 1654
San Anselmo, CA 94979
Ph: 415-289-7976
Email: ayurveda@dhanvantri.com

Dr. Singha's Mustard Bath and More
Attn: Anna Searles
Natural Therapeutic Centre
2500 Side Cove
Austin, TX 78704
Ph: 800-856-2862

Bio Veda
215 North Route 303
Congers, NY 10920-1726
Ph: 800-292-6002

Earth Essentials Florida
Dr's Bryan and Light Miller
4067 Shell Road
Sarasota, FL 34242
Ph: 941-316-0920

Frontier Herbs
P. O. Box 229
Norway, IA 52318
Ph: 800-669-3275

HerbalVedic Products
P. O. Box 6390
Santa Fe, NM 87502

Internatural
PO Box 489 CTM
Twin Lakes, WI 53181 USA
800-643-4221 (toll free order line)
262-889-8581 (office phone)
262-889-8591 (fax)
E-mail: internatural@lotuspress.com
Website: www.internatural.com
Retail mail order and internet reseller
of Ayurvedic products, essential oils,

herbs, spices, supplements,
herbal remedies, incense, books
and other supplies.

Lotus Brands, Inc.
P. O. Box 325/Dept. AH
Twin Lakes, WI 53181
Ph: 262-889-8561
Fax: 262-889-8591
E-mail: lotusbrands@lotuspress.com
Website: www.lotuspress.com

Lotus Herbs
1505 42nd Ave./Suite 19
Capitola, CA 95010
Ph: 408-479-1667

Lotus Light Enterprises
P. O. Box 1008/Dept. AH
Silver Lake, WI 53170 USA
800-548-3824 (toll free order line)
262-889-8501 (office phone)
262-889-8591 (fax)
E-mail: lotuslight@lotuspress.com
Website: www.lotuslight.com
Wholesale distributor of Ayurvedic
products, essential oils, herbs, spices,
supplements, herbal remedies,
incense, books and other supplies.
Must supply resale certificate number
or practitioner license to obtain
catalog of more than 10,000 items.

Maharishi Ayurveda Products
International, Inc.
417 Bolton Road
P. O. Box 541
Lancaster, MA 01523
Info: 800-843-8332 Ext. 903
Order: 800-255-8332 Ext. 903

Planetary Formulations
P. O. Box 533
Soquel, CA 95073
Formulas by Dr. Michael Tierra

Quantum Publication, Inc.
P. O. Box 1088
Sudbury, MA 01776
Ph: 800-858-1808

Seeds of Change
P. O. Box 15700
Santa Fe, NM 87506-5700
Catalog of rare Western and
Indian seeds.

Vinayak Panchakarma Chikitsalaya
Y.M.C.A Complex, Situbuldi
Nagpur (Maharastra State)
India 440 012
Ph: 011-91-712-538983
Fax: 011-91-712-552409

Retail/Wholesale
Yoga of Life Center
2726 Tramway N.E.
Albuquerque, NM 87122
Ph: 505-275-6141

The Center For Release
and Integration
450 Hillside Drive
Mill Valley, CA 94941

Dr. Jay Scherer's Academy of
Natural Healing
1443 St. Francis Drive
Santa Fe, NM 87505

The Rolf Institute
205 Canyon Blvd.
Boulder, CO 80302

The Upledger Institute
1211 Prosperity Farms Rd.
Palm Beach Gardens, FL 33410

Correspondence Courses:
American Institute of Vedic Studies
Dr. David Frawley, Director
P. O. Box 8357

Santa Fe, NM 87504-8357
Ph: 505-983-9385
Fax: 505-982-5807
E-mail: vedicinst@aol.com
Website: consciousnet.com/vedic
Correspondence courses in Ayurveda
and Vedic Astrology

Light Institute of Ayurvedic Teaching
Dr's Bryan & Light Miller
P. O. Box 35284
Sarasota, FL 34242
Ph: 941-346-3518
Fax: 941-346-0800
E-mail: earthess@aol.com
Website: www.ayurvedichealing.com

Ayurvedic Pratitioner Training,
Correspondence Course, Books
Lessons and Lectures in Ayurveda by
Dr. Robert Svoboda
P. O. Box 23445
Albuquerque, NM 87192-1445
Ph: 505-291-9698

Institute for Wholistic Education
3425 Patzke In. Racine,WI 53405
Ph: 262-619-1798
Beginner and Advanced
Correspondence Courses in Ayurveda.
Website: www.wholisticinstitute.com

To train in Ayurvedic Facial Massage
and Beauty practices:
Melanie Sachs
"Invoking Beauty with Ayurveda"
Seminars
P. O. Box 13753
San Luis Obispo, CA 93406

Beauty and Quality Ayurvedic
Supplements:
Auroma International
P. O. Box 1008/Dept. AH
Silver Lake, WI 53170

Ph: 262-889-8569
Fax: 262- 889 8591
E-mail: auroma@lotuspress.com
Website: www.auroma.net
Importer and master distributor of
Auroshikha Incense, Chandrika
Ayurvedic Soap and Herbal Vedic
Ayurvedic products.

Ayur Herbal Corporation
P. O. Box 6390 AH
Santa Fe, NM 87502
Ph: 262-889-8569
Fax: 262-889 8591
Manufacturer of Herbal Vedic
Ayurvedic products.

Internatural
PO Box 489 CTM
Twin Lakes, WI 53181 USA
800-643-4221 (toll free order line)
262-889-8581 (office phone)
262-889-8591 (fax)
E-mail: internatural@lotuspress.com
Website: www.internatural.com
Retail mail order and internet reseller
of Ayurvedic products, essential oils,
herbs, spices, supplements, herbal-
remedies, incense, books and other
supplies.

Lotus Brands, Inc.
P. O. Box 325/Dept. AH
Twin Lakes, WI 53181
Ph: 262-889-8561
Fax: 262-889-8591
E-mail: lotusbrands@lotuspress.com
Website: www.lotuspress.com
Manufacturer and distributor of
natural personal care and herbal
products, massage oils, essential oils,
incense and aromatherapy items.

Lotus Light Enterprises
P. O. Box 1008/Dept. AH
Silver Lake, WI 53170 USA
800-548-3824 (toll free order line)

262-889-8501 (office phone)
262-889-8591 (fax)
E-mail: lotuslight@lotuspress.com
Website: www.lotuslight.com
Wholesale distributor of Ayurvedic
products, essential oils, herbs, spices,
supplements, herbal remedies,
incense, books and other supplies.
Must supply resale certificate number or practitioner license to obtain
catalog of more than 10,000 items.

Maharishi Ayur-Veda Products
International, Inc.
417 Bolton Road
P. O. Box 54
Lancaster, MA 01523
Ph: 800-ALL-VEDA
Fax: 508-368-7475

New Moon Extracts
P. O. Box 1947
Brattleborough, Vermont
05302-1947
Ph: 800-543-7279

Spectrum NaturalOmega 3 Oil
The Oil Company
133 Copeland Street
Petaluma, CA 94952

Universal Light, Inc.
P. O. Box 261/Dept. AH
Wilmot, WI 53192
Ph: 262-889 8571
Fax: 262-889 8591
E-mail: universallight@lotuspress.com
Importer and Master Distributor for
Vicco Herbal Toothpaste

COLOR, SOUND, AND GEMS:
PAZ
615 Carlisle S.E.
Albuquerque, NM 87106
Telephone: 505-268-6943
E-mail: ehecatl@wans.net

425

For open-backed gemstone settings
Color Therapy Eyewear
C/O Terri Perrigone-Messer
P. O. Box 3114
Diamond Springs, CA 95619

Lumatron (light device)
C/O Ernie Baker
3739 Ashford-Dunwoody Rd.
Atlanta, GA 30139
Ph: 404-458-6509

Genesis (sound device)
Good Medicine
Attn: Tina Shinn
831 Grandview Ave.
Columbus, Ohio 43215
Ph: 614-488-5244

Essential Oil Supplies
Aromatherapy Supply
Unit W3
The Knoll Business Center
Old Shoreham Road
Hove, Sussex BN3 7GS
England

Aroma Vera
3384 South Robertson Pl.
Los Angeles, CA 90034
Ph: 800-669-9514

Auroma International
P. O. Box 1008/Dept. AH
Silver Lake, WI 53170
Ph: 262-889-8569
Fax: 262- 889 8591
E-mail: auroma@lotuspress.com
Website: www.auroma.net
Importer and master distributor of
Auroshikha Incense, Chandrika
Ayurvedic Soap and Herbal Vedic
Ayurvedic products.

Earth Essentials Florida, Inc.
P. O. Box 35214
Sarasota, FL 34242

Ph: 800-370-3220
Fax: 941-346-0800
E-mail: earthess@aol.com
Rare Essential Oils

Fenmail Tisserand Oils
P. O. Box 48
Spalding, LINCS PE11 ADS
England

Internatural
PO Box 489 CTM
Twin Lakes, WI 53181 USA
800-643-4221 (toll free order line)
262-889-8581 (office phone)
262-889-8591 (fax)
E-mail: internatural@lotuspress.com
Website: www.internatural.com
Retail mail order and internet reseller
of Ayurvedic products, essential oils,
herbs, spices, supplements, herbal
remedies, incense, books and
other supplies.

Lotus Brands, Inc.
P. O. Box 325/Dept. AH
Twin Lakes, WI 53181
Ph: 262-889-8561
Fax: 262-889-8591
E-mail: lotusbrands@lotuspress.com
Website: www.lotuspress.com
Manufacturer and distributor of
natural personal care and herbal
products, massage oils, essential oils,
incense and aromatherapy items.

Lotus Light Enterprises
P. O. Box 1008/Dept. AH
Silver Lake, WI 53170 USA
800-548 3824 (toll free order line)
262-889 8501 (office phone)
262-889 8591 (fax)
E-mail: lotuslight@lotuspress.com
Website: www.lotuslight.com
Wholesale distributor of Ayurvedic
products, essential oils, herbs, spices,

supplements, herbal remedies, incense, books and other supplies. Must supply resale certificate number or practitioner license to obtain catalog of more than 10,000 items.

Private Universe
P. O. Box 3122
Winter Park, FL 32790
Ph: 407-644-7203

Oshadi Ayus -Quality Life Products
15, Monarch Bay Plaza, Suite 346
Monarch Beach, CA 92629
Ph: 800-947-1008
Fax: 714-240-1104

Primavera
D 8961 Sulzberg, Germany
08376-808-0
(American Office)
110 Landing Court Unit B
Novato, CA 94945
Toll Free: 888-588-9830
Telephone: 415-209-6688
FAX: 415-209-6677

Original Swiss Aromatics
P. O. Box 606
San Rafael, CA 94915
Ph: 415-459-3998

Smitasha
26961 Ayamonte Dr.
Mission Viejo, CA 92692
Ph: 949-982-8777; 714-785-6891

Exercise Programs and Information:
Diamond Way Ayurveda
P. O. Box 13753
San Luis Obispo, CA 93406
Ph/FAX: 805-543-9291
Toll Free: 877-964-1395
E-mail: diamond.way.ayurveda@thegrid.net
(for Sotai, Tibetan Rejuvenation
Exercises)

Natural Ingredients:
Aloe Farms
P. O. Box 125
Los Fresnos, TX 78566
Ph: 800-262-6771
For aloe vera juice, gel, powder and capsules.

Arya Laya Skin Care Center
Rolling Hills Estates, CA 90274
For carrot oil.

Aubrey Organics
4419 North Manhattan Avenue
Tampa, FL 33614
For rosa mosquita oil and a large variety of natural cosmetics and shampoos.

Body Shop
45 Horsehill Road
Cedar Knolls, NJ 07927-2014
Ph: 800-541-2535
Aloe vera, nut and seed oils, cosmetics, make-up, brushes, loofahs, and much more.

Culpepper Ltd.
21 Bruton Street
London W1X 7DA, England
Variety of natural seed, nut, and kernal oils, essential oils, herbs, books, and cosmetics.

Desert Whale Jojoba Co.
P. O. Box 41594
Tucson, AZ 85717
Ph: 602-882-4195
For jojoba products and many other natural oils, including rice bran, pecan, macadamia nut and apricot kernal.

Everybody Ltd.
1738 Pearl Street
Boulder, CO 80302
Ph: 800-748-5675

Large variety of oils, oil blends, and cosmetics.

Flora Inc.
P. O. Box 950
805 East Badger Road
Lynden, WA 98264
Ph: 800-446-2110
For flax seed oil, herbal supplements for skin, hair, nails and cosmetics.

Green Earth Farm
P. O. Box 672
65 1/2 North 8th Street
Saguache, CO 81149
For calendula oil, creme, and herbal bath.

The Heritage Store, Inc.
P. O. Box 444
Virginia Beach, VA 23458
Ph: 804-428-0100
Castor oil, organic ghee, cocoa butter,massage oils, flowerwaters, essential oils, cosmetics, and natural home remedies.

Internatural
PO Box 489 CTM
Twin Lakes, WI 53181 USA
800-643-4221 (toll free order line)
262-889-8581 (office phone)
262-889-8591 (fax)
E-mail: internatural@lotuspress.com
Website: www.internatural.com
Retail mail order and internet reseller of Ayurvedic products, essential oils, herbs, spices, supplements,herbal remedies, incense, books and other supplies.

Janca's Jojoba Oil andSeed Company
456 E. Juanita #7
Mesa, AZ 85204

Ph: 602-497-9494
Jojoba oil, butter, wax and seeds. Also a large variety of naturally pressed unusual oils, such as camellia, kukui nut, and grapeseed. Also have clay, aloe products, essential oils, and their own line of cosmetics.

Lotus Brands, Inc.
P. O. Box 325
Dept. AH
Twin Lakes, WI 53181
Ph: 262-889-8561
Fax: 262-889-8591
E-mail: lotusbrands@lotuspress.com
Website: www.lotuspress.com
Manufacturer and distributor of natural personal care and herbal products, massage oils, essential oils, incense and aromatherapy items.

Lotus Light Enterprises
P. O. Box 1008/
Dept. AH
Silver Lake, WI 53170 USA
800-548 3824 (toll free order line)
262-889 8501 (office ph.)
262-889 8591 (fax)
E-mail: lotuslight@lotuspress.com
Website: www.lotuslight.com
Wholesale distributor of Ayurvedic products, essential oils, herbs, spices, supplements, herbal remedies, incense, books and other supplies. Must supply resale certificate number or practitioner license to obtain catalog of more than 10,000 items.

Weleda, Inc.
841 South Main Street
Spring Valley, NY 10977
For calendula oil and a large variety of natural cosmetics.

Organic Milk/Certified Raw Milk Suppliers:
Pancha Karma Kitchen Equipment
Earth Fare
Attn: Roger Derrough
66 Westgate Parkway
Asheville, NC 28806
Ph: 704-253-7656
Carries hand grinders and suribachi clay pots and bowls.

Sesam Muhle Natural Products
RR1
Durham, Ontario
Canada, NOG 1RO
Ph: 519-369-6326
Carries a line of hand grinders and flakers for grains and legumes, made in Germany.

Taj Mahal Imports
1594 Woodcliff Drive, N.E.
Atlanta, GA 30329
Ph: 404-321-5940
Carries a full line of Indian kitchen equipment.

Pancha Karma Supplies:
Vicki Stern
P. O. Box 1814
Laguna Beach, CA 92651
Ph: 949-494-8858
For steam boxes.

To Receive Pancha Karma:

Ayurvedic Healings
Dr's Bryan & Light Miller
P. O. Box 35284
Sarasota, FL 34242
Ph: 941-346-3518
Fax: 941-346-0800
E-mail: earthess@aol.com
Website: www.ayurvedichealing.com

Pancha Karma, Kaya Kalpa, Jarpana, Shirodhara
Diamond Way Ayurveda
P.O. Box 13753
San Luis Obispo, CA 93406
Ph/FAX: 805-543-9291
Toll Free: 877-964-1395
E-mail: diamond.way.ayurveda@thegrid.net

Dr. Lobsang Rapgay
2206 Benecia Ave.
Westwood, CA 90064
Ph: 310-282-9918

SPA MEDICINE:

RejuveNation
Attn: Dr. Dennis Thompson
3260 47th St.
#205A
Boulder, CO 80301
Ph: 303-417-0941
E-mail: drtdrt@concentric.net

Transformational Seminars:

Vedic Astrology
American Council of Vedic Astrology (ACVA)
P. O. Box 2149
Sedona, AZ 86339
Ph: 800-900-6595; 520-282-6595
Fax: 520-282-6097
Website: vedicastrology.org
E-mail: acva@sedona.net
Conferences, tutorial and training programs

American Institute of Vedic Studies
Dr. David Frawley, Director
P. O. Box 8357
Santa Fe, NM 87504-8357
Ph: 505-983-9385
Fax: 505-982-5807

E-mail: vedicinst@aol.com
Website: consciousnet.com/vedic
Correspondence courses in Ayurveda
 and Vedic Astrology

Jeffrey Armstrong
4820 N. 35th St.
Phoenix, AZ 85018
Ph: 602-468-9448
Ayurvedic Astrologer, Author,
Lecturer, Teacher

VIDEOS:

Wishing Well Video
P. O. Box 1008
Dept. AH
Silver Lake, WI 53170
Ph: 262-889-8501
Wholesale & retail

5. Index

431

HERBAL INDEX

437

441

Turmeric creams 188, 276
Turmeric ghee 218, 222

Uva ursi 231-233, 235, 261
Valerian 169, 182, 183, 216, 243,
    246, 247, 250, 254, 304, 308-310,
    324, 329, 336, 344
Vamsa rochana 203
Vasa 200, 203, 205, 206
Vasa herbal jelly 375
Vasanta Kusumakara 237
Vetivert (khus) 221, 270, 395
Vidanga 192
Vidanga compound 192, 193
Vidari 281
Vishagarbha oil 377

Weight reduction formula 391
White musali 256, 286
White oak bark 219
White peony 247, 250,254
Wild cherry 201
Wild ginger 208, 249, 280, 283
Wintergreen 203, 207, 279, 310, 394
Woman's Precious Pill 168, 223, 253,
259
Woman's tonic 385
Wormseed 192
Wormwood 187, 192

Xanthium 207
Yarrow 199, 219, 224, 251
Yellow dock 155, 223
Yerba santa 201
Yin Qiao San 199
Yogaraj guggul 280, 344, 370
Yohimbe 260
Yucca 281
Yunnan Bai Yao 219

Zedoaria 286
Zizyphus 214, 254, 308, 323, 344

6. About the Author

Dr. David Frawley

Dr. David Frawley (Pandit Vamadeva Shastri) is one of the few Westerners recognized in India as a Vedic teacher (Vedacharya). His many fields of expertise include Ayurvedic medicine, Vedic Astrology, Yoga, Vedanta and the Vedas themselves. He is the author of over twenty books on these subjects, including half a dozen books on Ayurveda. He has also written many articles for different newspapers, magazines and journals, and has taught and lectured throughout the world, including all over India.

Dr. Frawley is regarded as one of the 25 most influential Yoga teachers in America today according to the *Yoga Journal*. *The Indian Express*, one of India's largest English language newspapers, recently wrote: "a formidable scholar of Vedanta and easily the best known Western teacher of the Vedic wisdom." *India Today*, the *Time Magazine* of India, has called him, "Certainly America's most singular practicing Hindu." He also works closely with Dr. Deepak Chopra on various projects.

Currently Dr. Frawley is the director of the American Institute of Vedic Studies and the president of the American Council of Vedic Astrology (ACVA). He is on the editorial board for the magazine *Yoga International*. The American Institute of Vedic Studies features his extensive correspondence courses on Ayurveda and on Vedic Astrology.

7. American Institute of Vedic Studies

The American Institute of Vedic Studies is an educational center devoted to the greater system of Vedic and Yogic knowledge. It teaches related aspects of Vedic Science including Ayurveda, Vedic astrology, Yoga, Tantra, and Vedanta with special reference to their background in the Vedas. Identifying the Vedas with the broader system of Hindu Dharma, the Institute is engaged in educational projects in the greater field of Hindu studies. Long term Institute research projects include:

- Ayurvedic Psychology and Yoga: the mental and spiritual aspect of Ayurveda relative to Raja Yoga and Vedanta.

- Medical Astrology: relative to both health and disease for body and mind.

- Translations and interpretations of the *Vedas*, particularly the *Rig Veda*, and an explication of the original Vedic Yoga.

- Vedic History: the history of India and of the world from a Vedic perspective and also as reflecting latest archaeological
  work in India.

- Vedic Europe: explaining the connections between the Vedic
  and ancient European cultures and religions.

- Projection of Vedic and Hindu knowledge in a modern context for the coming millennium.

For information on the Institute and its programs please contact:

American Institute of Vedic Studies
PO Box 8357, Santa Fe NM 87504-8357
Ph: 505-983-9385, Fax: 505-982-5807
Dr. David Frawley (Pandit Vamadeva Shastri), Director
Web: www.vedanet.com, Email: vedanet@aol.com

American Institute of Vedic Studies
AYURVEDIC HEALING CORRESPONDENCE COURSE

This comprehensive practical program of over six hundred pages, based upon the book *Ayurvedic Healing* by David Frawley, covers all the main aspects of Ayurvedic theory, diagnosis and practice, with special emphasis on herbal medicine and on dietary therapy. It goes in detail into Yoga philosophy and Ayurvedic psychology, showing an integral approach of mind-body medicine that includes aromatherapy, gem therapy, mantra and meditation. There is almost no aspect of life that it does not address for healing and transformation. It contains all the material covered in two-year Ayurvedic programs for foreign students in India. It is not merely introductory but goes into great detail and depth into its subject.

The course is designed for Health Care Professionals as well as serious students to provide the foundation for becoming an Ayurvedic practitioner. It has been taken by Doctors, Chiropractors, Nurses, Acupuncturists, Herbalists, Massage Therapists, Yoga Therapists, and Psychologists. However, there is no required medical background for those wishing to take the course and many non-professionals have completed it successfully.

Since 1988 over two thousand people have taken the course, which is the most comprehensive correspondence course on this subject offered in the West. It is the basis of Ayurvedic programs taught in the United States, UK, Europe, Australia and India through the California College of Ayurveda, International Institute of Ayurveda, East West School of Herbalism (UK), Australian College of Ayurveda and others.

American Institute Of Vedic Studies
ASTROLOGY OF THE SEERS CORRESPONDENCE COURSE

Vedic astrology, also called Jyotish, is the traditional astrology of India and part of the greater system of yogic knowledge, with its profound wisdom and cosmic understanding. This comprehensive homestudy course of over six hundred pages, based upon the book *Astrology of the Seers* by David Frawley, explains Vedic astrology in clear and modern terms, providing practical insights on how to use and adapt the system. For those who have difficulty approaching the Vedic system, the course provides many keys for unlocking its language and its methodology for the Western student. The extensive course explains Vedic astrology in modern terms and relative to Western astrology, affording easy access to this often arcane system.

The goal of the course is to provide the foundation for the student to become a professional Vedic astrologer. The orientation of the course is twofold:

- To teach the language, approach and way of thinking of Vedic astrology from planets, signs and houses to Nakshatras, Dashas, Ashtakavarga and Muhurta.

- To set forth the Astrology of Healing of the Vedic system or Ayurvedic Astrology, including the use of herbs, gems, deities, mantra and meditation.

The course can be taken as part of a longer tutorial program of training in Vedic astrology through the American Council of Vedic Astrology (A.C.V.A.), the largest Vedic astrology organization outside of India, and counts for two hundred credit hours of the total six hundred hour program.

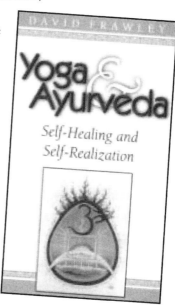

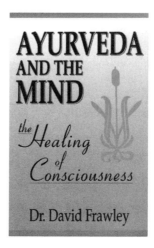

The Yoga of Herbs
An Ayurvedic Guide to Herbal Medicine
Second Revised and Enlarged Edition

by Dr. Vasant Lad & Dr. David Frawley

For the first time, here is a detailed explanation and classification of herbs, using the ancient system of Ayurveda. More than 270 herbs are listed, with 108 herbs explained in detail. Included are many of the most commonly used western herbs with a profound Ayurvedic perspective. Important Chinese and special Ayurvedic herbs are introduced. Beautiful diagrams and charts, as well as detailed glossaries, appendices and index are included.

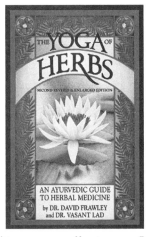

"Dr. Frawley and Dr. Lad have made a truly powerful contribution to alternative, natural health care by their creation of this important book. This book...will serve not only to make Ayurvedic medicine of greater practical value to Westerners but, in fact, ultimately advance the whole system of Western herbalism forward into greater effectiveness. I think anyone interested in herbs should closely study this book whether their interests lie in Western herbology, traditional Chinese herbology or in Ayurvedic medicine."

— Michael Tierra, Author, *The Way of Herbs*

Trade Paper   ISBN 978-0-9415-2424-7   288 pp   pb $15.95

Available at bookstores and natural food stores nationwide or order your copy directly by sending $15.95 plus $2.50 shipping/handling ($.75 s/h for each additional copy ordered at the same time) to:

Lotus Press, PO Box 325, Twin Lakes, WI 53181 USA
toll free order line: 800 824 6396   office phone: 262 889 8561
office fax: 262 889 2461   email: lotuspress@lotuspress.com
web site: www.lotuspress.com

Lotus Press is the publisher of a wide range of books and software in the field of alternative health, including Ayurveda, Chinese medicine, herbology, aromatherapy, Reiki and energetic healing modalities. Request our free book catalog.

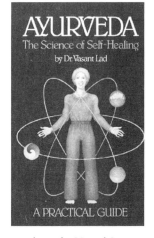

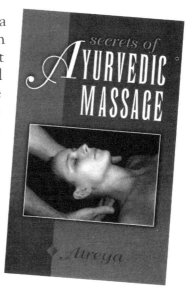

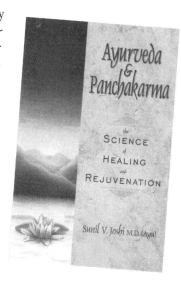

Astrology of the Seers
A Guide to Vedic/Hindu Astrology

by Dr. David Frawley

Vedic Astrology, also called *Jyotish*, is the traditional astrology of India and its profound spiritual culture. It possesses a precise predictive value as well as a deep interpretation of the movement of life, unfolding the secrets of karma and destiny. *Astrology of the Seers*, first published in 1990, is regarded as one of the classic modern books on Vedic astrology, covering all the main aspects of its philosophy, background and practice. The present edition has been thoroughly revised and updated.

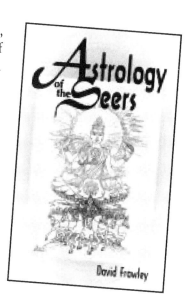

Trade Paper   ISBN 978-0-9409-8588-9   304 pp $17.95

Available at bookstores and natural food stores nationwide or order your 5copy directly by sending $17.95 plus $2.50 shipping/handling ($.75 s/h for each additional copy ordered at the same time) to:

Lotus Press, P O Box 325, Twin Lakes, WI 53181 USA
toll free order line: 800 824 6396   office phone: 262 889 8561
office fax: 262 889 2461   email: lotuspress@lotuspress.com
web site: www.lotuspress.com

Lotus Press is the publisher of a wide range of books and software in the field of alternative health, including Ayurveda, Chinese medicine, herbology, aromatherapy, Reiki and energetic healing modalities. Request our free book catalog.

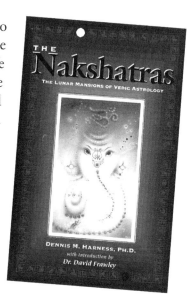

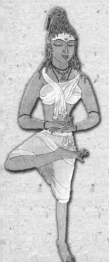

Yoga
and the Sacred Fire
Self-Realization and Planetary Transformation

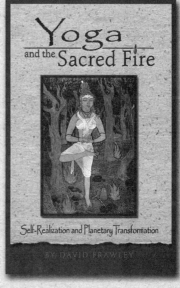

Yoga
and the Sacred Fire

Self-Realization and Planetary Transformation

BY DAVID FRAWLEY

"David Frawley continues to bring the ancient wisdom of Vedic knowledge to contemporary readers with impeccable clarity. *Yoga and the Sacred Fire* will accelerate your journey to enlightenment."
—Dr. Deepak Chopra, Author, *How to Know God*

Yoga and the Sacred Fire
by Dr. David Frawley
Item # 990 521   312 pp pb $19.95
ISBN #978-0-9409-8575-9

Yoga and the Sacred Fire explores the evolution of life and consciousness according to the cosmology and psychology of Fire, viewing Fire not only as a material but also as a spiritual principle. It shows how Yoga's deeper fire wisdom can help us move forward to an enlightened planetary age, where humanity and nature can again be one in a higher awareness.

Dr. David Frawley (Pandit Vamadeva Shastri) is one of the most honored teachers of Vedic spirituality in both India and the West. He brings the full range of his experience and expertise into this present quest for the reader to share.

Herbs and other natural health products and information are often available at natural food stores or metaphysical bookstores. If you cannot find what you need locally, you can contact one of the following sources of supply.

Sources of Supply:

The following companies have an extensive selection of useful products and a long track-record of fulfillment. They have natural body care, aromatherapy, flower essences, crystals and tumbled stones, homeopathy, herbal products, vitamins and supplements, videos, books, audio tapes, candles, incense and bulk herbs, teas, massage tools and products and numerous alternative health items across a wide range of categories.

WHOLESALE:

Wholesale suppliers sell to stores and practitioners, not to individual consumers buying for their own personal use. Individual consumers should contact the RETAIL supplier listed below. Wholesale accounts should contact with business name, resale number or practitioner license in order to obtain a wholesale catalog and set up an account.

Lotus Light Enterprises, Inc.

PO Box 1008 LCH
Silver Lake, WI 53170 USA
262 889 8501 (phone)
262 889 8591 (fax)
800 548 3824 (toll free order line)

RETAIL:

Retail suppliers provide products by mail order direct to consumers for their personal use. Stores or practitioners should contact the wholesale supplier listed above.

Internatural

PO Box 489 LCH
Twin Lakes, WI 53181 USA
800 643 4221 (toll free order line)
262 889 8581 office phone
EMAIL: internatural@internatural.com
WEB SITE: www.internatural.com

Web site includes an extensive annotated catalog of more than 14,000 items that can be ordered "on line" for your convenience 24 hours a day, 7 days a week.